Antioxidants and the Skin

Antioxidants and the Skin

Second Edition

Roger L. McMullen
Principal Scientist, Ashland Specialty Ingredients
Bridgewater, New Jersey, USA
and
Adjunct Professor, Microtoxicity and Biochemistry
School of Natural Sciences, Fairleigh Dickinson University
Teaneck, New Jersey, USA

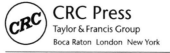

CRC Press is an imprint of the
Taylor & Francis Group, an **informa** business

CRC Press
Taylor & Francis Group
6000 Broken Sound Parkway NW, Suite 300
Boca Raton, FL 33487-2742

© 2019 by Taylor & Francis Group, LLC
CRC Press is an imprint of Taylor & Francis Group, an Informa business

No claim to original U.S. Government works

Printed in Canada on acid-free paper

International Standard Book Number-13: 978-1-1386-3356-8 (Hardback)

This book contains information obtained from authentic and highly regarded sources. Reasonable efforts have been made to publish reliable data and information, but the author and publisher cannot assume responsibility for the validity of all materials or the consequences of their use. The authors and publishers have attempted to trace the copyright holders of all material reproduced in this publication and apologize to copyright holders if permission to publish in this form has not been obtained. If any copyright material has not been acknowledged please write and let us know so we may rectify in any future reprint.

Except as permitted under U.S. Copyright Law, no part of this book may be reprinted, reproduced, transmitted, or utilized in any form by any electronic, mechanical, or other means, now known or hereafter invented, including photocopying, microfilming, and recording, or in any information storage or retrieval system, without written permission from the publishers.

For permission to photocopy or use material electronically from this work, please access www.copyright.com (http://www.copyright.com/) or contact the Copyright Clearance Center, Inc. (CCC), 222 Rosewood Drive, Danvers, MA 01923, 978-750-8400. CCC is a not-for-profit organization that provides licenses and registration for a variety of users. For organizations that have been granted a photocopy license by the CCC, a separate system of payment has been arranged.

Trademark Notice: Product or corporate names may be trademarks or registered trademarks, and are used only for identification and explanation without intent to infringe.

Library of Congress Cataloging-in-Publication Data

Names: McMullen, Roger L., author.
Title: Antioxidants and the skin / by Roger L. McMullen.
Description: Second edition. | Boca Raton, FL : CRC Press/Taylor & Francis Group, [2019] | Includes bibliographical references and index.
Identifiers: LCCN 2018009542 | ISBN 9781138633568 (hardback : alk. paper) | ISBN 9781315207254 (ebook)
Subjects: | MESH: Skin Physiological Phenomena--drug effects | Antioxidants--therapeutic use
Classification: LCC RL96 | NLM WR 102 | DDC 616.5--dc23
LC record available at https://lccn.loc.gov/2018009542

Visit the Taylor & Francis Web site at
http://www.taylorandfrancis.com

and the CRC Press Web site at
http://www.crcpress.com

*To Sílvia Mendiola Buj,
the free radical that entered my life
and made peace with all of the antioxidants.*

Contents

Preface		x
Acknowledgments		xi
1	**Structure and function of skin**	**1**
	Epidermis	1
	Dermal-epidermal junction	5
	Dermis	6
	Cutaneous appendages	7
	Skin immune system	15
	Concluding remarks	18
	References	19
2	**Free radicals in biology**	**21**
	Terminology	21
	Reactive oxygen and nitrogen species	21
	Free radical reactions	25
	Endogenous sources of free radicals	26
	Concluding remarks	28
	References	28
3	**The skin's endogenous antioxidant network**	**30**
	Enzymatic antioxidants	30
	Small-molecule antioxidants	38
	Melanins	44
	Other notable endogenous antioxidants	46
	Antioxidant levels and distribution in skin	46
	Concluding remarks	46
	References	47
4	**Effects of solar radiation, air pollution, and artificial blue light on the skin**	**48**
	Interaction of light with skin	48
	Chromophores in skin	49
	Effects of UV light on skin	54
	Immediate manifestations of UV-induced damage in skin	56
	Photoaging of skin	57
	UV-induced signaling cascades	58
	Photoimmunosuppression	59
	Photocarcinogenesis	61
	Effects of visible and infrared light on skin	63
	Effect of air pollution on the skin	63
	Blue light and its effect on the skin	67
	Concluding remarks	67
	References	68
5	**Lipid peroxidation and its measurement**	**71**
	Lipid peroxidation	71
	Lipid peroxidation measurement techniques for in vitro lipid model systems and biological samples	77
	In vitro lipid peroxidation assays for measuring fat/oil stability	84
	Concluding remarks	88
	References	88
6	**Antioxidant assays**	**92**
	2,2-Diphenyl-1-picrylhydrazyl radical assay	92
	2,2′-Azino-*bis*(3-ethylbenzothiazoline-6-sulfonic acid) assay	93
	Radical trapping parameter assay	95
	Ferric reducing ability of plasma assay	97
	Oxygen radical absorbance capacity assay	98

	Deoxyribose assay	99
	Evaluation of potential skin care antioxidants	100
	Concluding remarks	100
	References	101
7	Electron spin resonance of skin	103
	Electron spin resonance theory	103
	Spin trapping	106
	Detection of free radicals in skin by electron spin resonance	107
	The use of electron spin resonance to measure exogenous antioxidant efficacy in skin	107
	Electron spin resonance imaging of skin	109
	Concluding remarks	110
	References	110
8	Treatment of skin with antioxidants	112
	Vitamin E	112
	Vitamin C	114
	Vitamin A	116
	Selenium	117
	Ubiquinone derivatives	117
	Thiol-based antioxidants	118
	Saccharide-containing antioxidants	119
	Polyphenols	120
	Botanical extracts	129
	Fullerenes and their use in cosmetics	130
	Effects of dietary intake of antioxidants on skin health	131
	Topical application of antioxidants	134
	Formulation challenges	134
	Antioxidant combinations	135
	Use of antioxidants in sunscreen formulations	137
	Antioxidant rating systems	139
	Concluding remarks	139
	References	139
9	Antioxidant properties and application information	145
	N-Acetyl cysteine	145
	Apigenin	146
	Arbutin	147
	L-Ascorbic acid	148
	tert-Butylhydroquinone	149
	2-*tert*-Butyl-4-hydroxyanisole and 3-*tert*-butyl-4-hydroxyanisole	150
	Butylated hydroxytoluene	151
	Caffeic acid	152
	Beta-carotene	153
	Curcumin	154
	Ellagic acid	155
	(−)-Epicatechin	156
	(−)-Epicatechin gallate	157
	(−)-Epigallocatechin	157
	(−)-Epigallocatechin gallate	157
	Equol	158
	Ferulic acid	159
	Genistein	160
	Glutathione	161
	Kojic acid	162
	Alpha-lipoic acid	163
	Lycopene	164
	Nordihydroguaiaretic acid	165

Pogostone	166
Propyl gallate	167
Quercetin	168
Resorcinol	169
Resveratrol	169
Rosmarinic acid	171
Silibinin	172
Theaflavin	173
Thearubigins	174
Thioglycolic acid	174
Tocopherols	175
Tocotrienols	176
Trolox	177
Ubiquinone-10	178
References	179
Appendix 1: Glossary of terms	181
Appendix 2: Biologically important molecules and mechanisms	184
Appendix 3: Cellular signaling in skin	192
Appendix 4: Thermodynamic and kinetic factors that contribute to antioxidant behavior	197
Index	202

Preface

Exposure to solar radiation, other environmental insults, and inflammation all produce reactive oxygen species and free radicals in skin. This imbalance of the redox state is the root cause of many pathological diseases, including skin cancer. That is why, for more than three decades now, researchers have diligently continued to explore the use of antioxidants to mitigate the damage caused by reactive oxygen and free radical species. It is now a well-known fact that treatment of skin with antioxidants is a clinically efficacious way to combat the perils of free radical-induced skin damage. Early research exploited the benefits of common antioxidants, such as vitamins E and C, to prevent photoaging, photoimmunosuppression, and photocarcinogenesis of skin. Accordingly, most skin preparations launched in the marketplace during that period contained these and other small molecule antioxidants, such as butylated hydroxytoluene or butylated hydroxyanisole. More recently, research on the protective benefits of botanical extracts containing powerful phytoantioxidants shed light on the advantages of this class of compounds in combating free radical damage in skin. As a result, phytoantioxidants are now much more prevalent in today's modern skin care preparations. One need only look at the extensive list of botanicals on skin cream ingredient labels currently on store shelves to see that this is true.

The amount of scientific information available about antioxidants can be, to put it mildly, overwhelming. Book chapters appear here and there and new articles are published regularly in an ever-increasing number of journals. So, it is easy to find one's self adrift in a large pool of information, not knowing how to stay afloat or in which direction to swim. *Antioxidants and the Skin* attempts to bring all of this information together in one logically organized and easy-to-digest text. It reaches out to investigators of all disciplines to provide a comprehensive treatise on the subject. The book is suitable for a wide range of readers—whether it be someone just starting their journey in the realm of antioxidants or a more seasoned antioxidant veteran who has need of a valuable reference tool. Moreover, this text features fundamental aspects of skin biochemistry, an introduction to reactive oxygen and free radical species and how they damage biological systems, a thorough overview of the skin's endogenous antioxidant network, and sources of free radical damage including solar irradiation, air pollution, and artificial light.

In addition, a chapter is included that presents concepts of lipid peroxidation and how it affects both the skin (its lipids) and formulations. It provides key information about lipid peroxidation in vivo, in vitro, and in formulation (colloidal) systems. This book also includes an overview of the essential technique for measuring free radicals, electron spin resonance, as well as discussion of the efficacy of antioxidant treatments. Another chapter cites key antioxidants used in formulations, along with their physical/chemical properties; it also references analytical and efficacy studies that substantiate their performance and effectiveness.

It is my hope that many researchers, formulators, clinicians, dermatologists, and academic instructors will find the contents of this book beneficial in their investigations with antioxidants and the skin.

Roger L. McMullen

Acknowledgments

The task of bringing this text from concept/ideation to final manuscript required a great deal of effort and persistence. As with any task of this magnitude, it could not have been accomplished without the help and support of many individuals, including family, friends, and colleagues. First and foremost, I received substantial encouragement from Janusz Jachowicz to embark on this journey with the first edition of this book. His foresight and guidance helped make this concept a reality. The late Johann Wiechers was also very supportive and inspirational when I initially started work on the manuscript. He is and always will be missed by many of his fellow scientists in the personal care industry.

Many colleagues reviewed various chapters in the book and offered critical advice and useful suggestions. I owe a great debt of gratitude to them for the generous offering of their time and expertise. They are: Tony Rawlings, Gopi Menon, Phil Wertz, Joseph Albanese, and Maurício da Silva Baptista. I would also like to extend my gratefulness to my dear friend and colleague, Bret Clark, who reviewed several chapters and often inquired about the progress of the manuscript and encouraged me to follow through with this project. Tim Gillece, Guojin Lu, and Mihaela Gorcea, three good friends and laboratory associates, read sections of the text, were instrumental in offering suggestions, and often engaged in constructive discussions about the chemistry of antioxidants.

Over the course of the book preparation, family backing was a key motivating force behind the scenes. Much appreciation is due to my mother, Carol Jean McMullen, my sister, Kimberly Price, and my grandmother, Maria Giannetti Schultheis, for their moral support and encouragement. Also, to the late Roger L. McMullen, my father, and the late Richard L. Schultheis, my grandfather—two exemplary figures throughout my entire life. Both were with us when I started this journey and sadly were not when this text came to fruition. In addition, many weekends when I needed a break from writing, I enjoyed the company of my cherished nieces and nephews—Seth McLaughlin, Joshua McLaughlin, Alyssa McLaughlin, A.J. Price, Ashley Price, and Justin Price—as well as my brother-in-law Alex Price.

I would be remiss not to mention my dear friend, confidante, spouse, and true love, Sílvia Mendiola Buj, who not only encouraged me to follow through with this endeavor, but also fostered a stimulating environment, which helped me through the most challenging times of composition. I especially thank her for the great deal of help in preparing the second edition of this text. *Moltes gràcies carinyo meu!*

Vull donar les gràcies a la meva família de Barcelona, ja que vaig passar molt temps a casa del Manel Mendiola Querol i la Pepita Buj Poveda fent el manuscrit d'aquest llibre, en un lloc molt acollidor, com són les golfes! També, vull agraïr al Ramón Alías Madrona i a la Maria Àngels Mendiola Buj pel seu suport, ja que em van portar a la biblioteca de l'Universitat de Barcelona en diverses ocasions. A la vegada, estic molt agraït al meus nebots, el Lluís Alías Mendiola, l'Àngels Alías Mendiola, i especialment l'Eva Alías Mendiola, pel seu interès en el tema d'aquest llibre i per les nombroses discussions que hem pogut gaudir junts.

I spent many evenings and weekends working on this monograph at a New York City café known as Tisserie. Much gratitude goes to its baristas who provided an extremely conducive environment for a struggling writer in the midst of a chaotic city. Sadly, the café no longer exists; however, I will always cherish the time spent there.

Finally, a great debt of gratitude is due to the editorial staff at CRC Press. Without the insight and vision of Robert Peden, Senior Editor at CRC Press, the successful implementation of the second edition of this text would not have been possible. I am also very grateful to Kyle Meyer and Angela Graven for their tireless efforts of transforming an unedited manuscript to a cohesive treatise that will be enjoyed by many researchers interested in antioxidants and their use in skin care.

Structure and function of skin

Skin is key to our biology, our sensory experiences, our information gathering, and our relationships with others.

—Nina G. Jablonski
Skin: A Natural History

As the largest organ of the body, the skin provides a protective barrier for the body against the external world and also prevents transepidermal water loss (TEWL), permitting an aqueous organism to live in a rather arid environment. In addition, there are many other functions provided by skin that are often overlooked. For example, the skin maintains body temperature through two mechanisms: one in which the body is cooled by the action of sweating, via sweat glands; the other by the vasoconstriction or vasodilation of the blood vessels in the dermis, which either decreases or increases the flow of blood to the dermis from other internal organs. If the internal organs are overheated, vasodilation occurs in the dermis, allowing increased blood flow, which in turn releases heat to the environment. Through the combined process of sweating, sebum production, and desquamation, a thin film is present on the surface skin, protecting it from bacterial infections and invasion by foreign substances, as well as hydrating and lubricating the surface. Another essential function of skin is sensation, which is provided by a complex network of nerves located in the dermis and at the base of the epidermis.

Morphologically, the skin is composed of two principal components, the epidermis and dermis, which contain various cell types and structural proteins. The hypodermis—also known as the subcutaneous layer—is often categorized as a third component, located below the dermis. Primarily it is composed of adipose tissue. The epidermis is a squamous epithelium that contains several appendages: pilosebaceous unit, nail, and sweat gland. The dermis provides the skin with mechanical strength and elasticity, which is brought about by collagen and elastin. A diagram of skin is provided in Figure 1.1, where the structural components of the dermis and epidermis are shown as well as the various appendages of skin and its vascular network.

In the remainder of this chapter, we review the intricate structural components of the epidermis and dermis as well as the dermal-epidermal junction—the structure that connects the two skin layers. In addition, we discuss the morphology of various appendages of skin, such as the pilosebaceous unit (including both the hair follicle and sebaceous gland), nail unit, eccrine glands, and apocrine glands. Since skin plays such an integral role in immune function, we will survey some fundamental elements of the immune system as it involves skin. Many of the topics touched upon in this chapter are important for our later discussions on free radical mechanisms and antioxidants in skin.

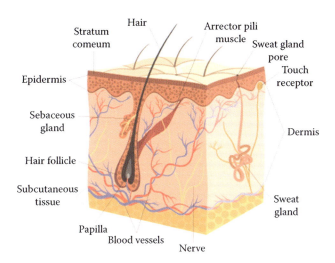

Figure 1.1 Structure of human skin.

EPIDERMIS

This layer of the skin primarily consists of keratinocyte cells, which undergo a process of events leading to terminal differentiation. The keratinocyte begins its journey as a metabolically active cell at the base of the epidermis and eventually makes it way to the outermost layer of skin, where it becomes void of its normal cellular organelles, becomes filled with keratin intermediate filaments (KIFs) and matrix proteins, and contains an unusually tough, protein-rich plasma membrane—known as the cell envelope—which is highly cross-linked. Through this process, the keratinocyte drastically changes shape during its voyage from the bottom to the top of the epidermis. Meanwhile, new organelles are synthesized in preparation for the construction of the ultimate barrier, the stratum corneum. All of the metabolic organelles are eventually degraded by a form of apoptosis. Ultimately, a dehydrated morphological component is formed—the stratum corneum—which prevents H_2O loss to the environment and the entry of foreign pathogens into the viable dermis. While keratinocytes make up the majority of epidermal cells, there are also Langerhans cells, melanocytes, and Merkel cells (Table 1.1). There are several layers of strata within the epidermis, which are categorized based on the level of differentiation of the keratinocyte cells. In the paragraphs that follow, a description of each layer is provided as well as events associated with keratinocyte differentiation in each particular stratum. Figure 1.2 provides a schematic of the epidermis, which illustrates the different cell types present as well as the histological changes associated with the keratinocyte differentiation. As shown in the figure, the lowermost layer of the epidermis (stratum basale)

Table 1.1 Epidermal cell types.

Cell type	Function
Keratinocyte	Differentiation
Melanocyte	Synthesis of melanin
Langerhans cell	Immune system
Merkel cell	Sensation

and the dermis are separated by the dermal-epidermal junction—also known as the basal lamina or the basement membrane zone.

As implied by their name, keratinocytes synthesize KIFs, which ultimately determine the shape of the cell as it makes its way up the epidermis. At the most fundamental level of KIF structure, two molecules (chains) of alpha-keratin wrap around each other to form a coiled-coil. Two coiled-coils then associate together to form a protofilament. Two protofilaments pair to form one protofibril. Four protofibrils constitute one intermediate filament. There are about thirty different known members of the keratin family—twenty of epithelial origin and ten from hair. Keratins are classified as Type I-acidic (K10-K20) or Type II-basic (K1-K9). Coiled-coils are formed by the pairing of two alpha-keratins, one from each class.

Strata of the epidermis

As indicated earlier, one of the primary functions of the epidermis is to provide a medium for the differentiation of keratinocyte cells. Similar to the process that occurs in other epithelial tissues, the keratinocyte begins its journey at the lowest layer of the epidermis (stratum basale) in the shape of a columnar cell, which changes form to a cuboidal-shaped cell and eventually traverses to the outer layers of the skin where the cell assumes a squamous configuration. In addition to the strata outlined below there also exists a lucent layer, called the stratum lucidum, which is present in very thick skin, such as that found on the palms and soles of the feet. This stratum is located between the stratum granulosum and stratum corneum.

Stratum basale

The stratum basale (or stratum germinativum) is the lowest layer in the epidermis and consists of a single layer of cells, which are predominantly keratinocytes. In this part of the epidermis, the keratinocytes are undifferentiated and contain all of the usual organelles that are present in viable cells, such as mitochondrion, Golgi apparatus, ribosome, endoplasmic reticulum, lysosome, and nucleus. The stratum basale is germinative and contains several populations of keratinocytes: stem cells, transient amplifying cells, and postmitotic cells. Stem cells divide rather infrequently and give rise to daughter cells known as transient amplifying cells. In turn, transient amplifying cells divide much more frequently than stem cells, producing postmitotic cells—the cells that actually undergo differentiation.

Keratinocyte cells are joined together by junctions known as desmosomes and are anchored to the underlying dermal-epidermal junction by hemidesmosomes. Desmosomes and hemidesmosomes are rather intricate structures composed of several macromolecules. The cytoskeleton of the keratinocytes consists of keratinocyte intermediate filaments, which provide structural support for the cell by traversing the cytosol. They are long,

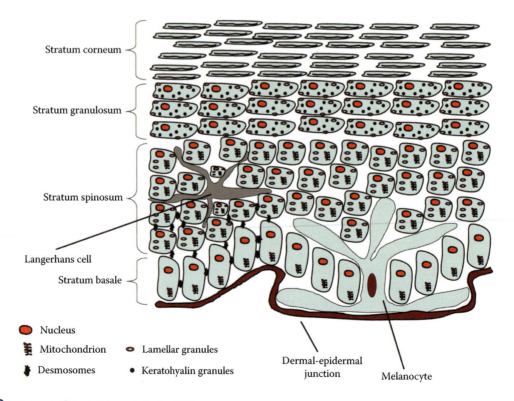

Figure 1.2 Diagram of the epidermal strata of skin.

cylindrical proteins that are arranged concentrically around the nucleus and protrude to the limits of the cell—the plasma membrane—where they anchor to desmosomes and hemidesmosomes. Intermediate filaments anchored to hemidesmosomes are usually referred to as tonofilaments.

In the stratum basale, keratinocytes express K5 (58 kDa) and K14 (50 kDa), which form fine bundles and provide the cell with structural stability and flexibility. At the germinative layer, the cytoskeletal components must confer enough flexibility so that cell replication and division can take place.

Integrins are a family of receptor proteins that are found on keratinocytes in this layer. They participate in the attachment of cells to other cells and cells to extracellular matrix, that is, cell-to-cell and cell-to-extracellular matrix. They contain two subunits, alpha and beta. There are various forms of the alpha and beta subunits, which form many different types of integrins. Nevertheless, integrins play an important part in the stability/adhesion of the multicellular agglomerate of the epidermis.

In addition to keratinocytes, there are also melanocytes interspersed in this layer of the epidermis and to a lesser extent Merkel cells. Melanocytes produce the chromophore melanin, responsible for skin pigmentation, which form aggregates in cellular organelles called melanosomes. In turn, melanosomes are transferred from melanocytes to basal layer keratinocytes in order to protect its cellular components, specifically the chromosomes (DNA) in the nucleus. The Merkel cell, on the other hand, associates with dendritic endings of neurons forming a Merkel disc. The resulting complex (Merkel disc) is a mechanoreceptor; hence, it serves as a sensory receptor for light touch.

Stratum spinosum

In the spinous layer, there is a gradient of shapes adopted by the keratinocyte. At the lower level of the stratum spinosum, the cells have a structure more closely resembling that observed in the stratum basale; however, progressively closer to the stratum granulosum the cells become flatter. The stratum spinosum is extremely rich in desmosomes, providing multiple linkages between the keratinocytes. When the skin is prepared for histological studies, the cells shrink and the connections made by the desmosomes are readily visible, revealing the spinous appearance of this tissue, thus its name.

At this stage of differentiation, typically in cells located at higher levels of the stratum spinosum, we find the appearance of lamellar granules—secretory organelles that carry lipids and enzymes, which will be utilized for the formation of the stratum corneum. The organelles are about 0.2–0.3 μm in diameter, and contain phospholipids, sterols, glycoproteins, glycolipids, acid hydrolases (lipases, proteases, glycosidases, and acid phosphatase), and glucosylceramide.[1]

Residual K5 and K14 from the stratum basale still remain in the keratinocytes, although newly synthesized K1 and K10 appear in the stratum spinosum—forming larger bundles of intermediate filaments in this layer.

Langerhans cells, star-shaped in structure, are most abundant in this layer of the epidermis. These cells are essentially macrophages, derived from bone marrow, which migrate to the epidermis where they act as outposts of the immune system. They are antigen-presenting cells (APCs), which means they can patrol the epidermis to capture foreign pathogens (antigens), then migrate to lymph tissue where they present the antigen to T cells.

Stratum granulosum

The granular layer is the transition region between the viable and fully differentiated epidermis. This stratum is only several layers of cells thick and is the transition point between the appearance of new cellular components and the programmed destruction of others—a form of programmed cell death. The cells assume a flattened structure in the granular layer and one of their distinguishable features is the accumulation of keratohyalin granules—a dense amorphous material that makes the keratinocyte appear granular.

The major component of the keratohyalin granules is the polyprotein profilaggrin, which is the precursor for the protein, filaggrin. Profilaggrin is essentially a polymer of filaggrin proteins, separated by links. During the transition from a granular to a cornified cell, profilaggrin is converted to filaggrin by proteolysis of the linkages and dephosphorylation of the entire molecule. Filaggrin is an important component of the amorphous phase of the keratinocyte, which aligns KIFs in a direction parallel to the surface of the skin, providing the stratum corneum with a planar cell. Hence the name filaggrin, or filament aggregating protein. K1 and K10 are still present in the stratum granulosum; however, they may undergo proteolysis and phosphorylation to K2 and K11. Keratohyalin granules also contain intermediate filaments and loricrin, a chief component of the cell envelope.

As mentioned previously, lamellar granules can be found in the upper levels of the stratum spinosum. The origin of the lamellar granules is the Golgi apparatus; however, migration occurs first to the periphery of the cell and later to the extracellular space, which usually takes place at the boundary of the stratum granulosum and stratum corneum. Once outside of the cell, the lamellar granules secrete lipids, ultimately forming the lamellae of lipids present in the stratum corneum.

In addition to and following the series of events described thus far in the stratum granulosum, there are several more steps leading to the ultimate transformation of the keratinocyte to a cornified cell. First, the disintegration of ribosomes, mitochondria, and nuclei. In addition to these events, the plasma membrane is no longer able to survive and is replaced by a thick cornified cell envelope. Construction of the cell envelope takes place inside the boundaries of the plasma membrane. Two key proteins in the fabrication of the cell envelope include loricrin, derived from the keratohyalin granules, and involucrin from the cytoplasm. The contents of the cell envelope consist of these two proteins as well as a variety of other proteins, such as small proline-rich proteins, elafin, and envoplakin. The cell envelope is reinforced by epsilon-(gamma-glutamyl)lysine isopeptide cross-links, which are induced by transglutaminases. The resulting membrane is insoluble and impenetrable to polar substances. There are three known transglutaminases, expressed in the stratum granulosum, which carry out distinct functions.

Stratum corneum

At this layer of the epidermis, the cornified cell is present. It is completely void of organelles, filled with intermediate filaments (K1 and K10), and contains the impermeable cell envelope described earlier. Within the stratum corneum, the corneocytes are embedded in a lipid matrix forming the *Bricks and Mortar* structure, analogous to the pattern assumed by bricks within mortar where the corneocytes correspond to the bricks and the lipids to the mortar, as shown schematically in Figure 1.3. The principal lipids in the stratum corneum are ceramides, cholesterol, and free fatty acids. In the lower strata of the epidermis, most of the usual lipids that constitute plasma and organelle membranes, such as phospholipids and cholesterol, can be found.

As already stated, lamellar granules discharge the lipids that constitute the mortar component of the stratum corneum at the boundary of the stratum granulosum and the stratum corneum. The structures of the ceramides found in the stratum corneum are provided in Figure 1.4.[2,3] The latest nomenclature protocol is followed in naming the ceramides.[4] In this system, two to three letters are used as descriptors corresponding to the ceramide base, fatty acid, and the presence of an ester. For example, the base is named accordingly based on its structure: sphingosine (S), 6-hydroxysphingosine (H), and phytosphingosine (P). Secondly, the corresponding designations are utilized for an amide-linked saturated fatty acid (N), alpha-hydroxy acid (A), or omega-fatty acid (O). A third letter is only used in the event that an ester group (E) is present. In addition

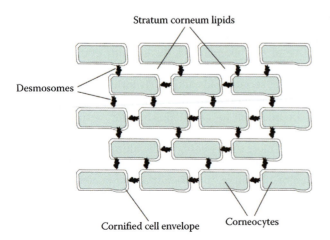

Figure 1.3 Bricks and mortar structure of the stratum corneum.

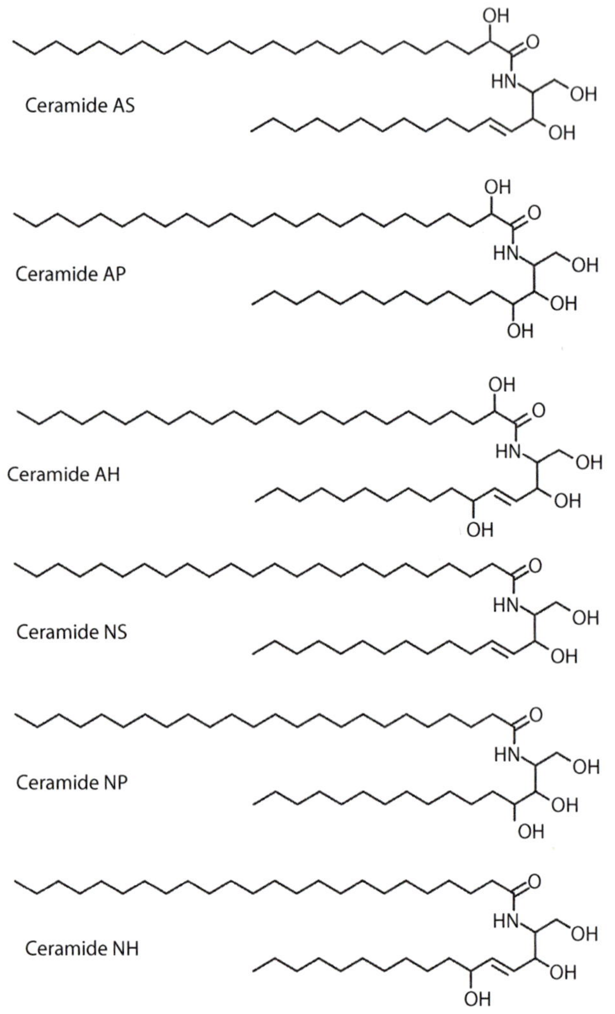

Figure 1.4 Molecular structures of important ceramides found in skin. (Adapted from Michniak-Kohn, B.B. et al., Skin: physiology and penetration pathways, in *Delivery System Handbook for Personal Care and Cosmetic Products*, Rosen, M.R. [Ed.], William Andrew Publishing, Norwich, NY, 77–100, 2005; Harding, C.R. et al., Ceramides and the skin, in *Textbook of Cosmetic Dermatology*, 3rd ed., Baran, R. and Maibach, H.I. [Eds.], Taylor & Francis Group, London, UK, 171–186, 2005.)

to the free ceramides found in the stratum corneum, there are also two—Ceramide OS and Ceramide OH—that are covalently attached to the cell envelope of corneocytes. They are derived from Ceramide EOS and Ceramide EOH. It is believed that the covalently attached ceramides facilitate coalescence of the corneocytes with the free lamellar lipids of the stratum corneum.

The structural arrangement and phase behavior of stratum corneum lipids is a noteworthy topic aimed at giving us a better understanding of the role of lipid organization in mammalian barrier function. In order to explain the stratum corneum's defense against foreign invaders and the impermeability of many molecules, several models were proposed to describe the lamellar organization of stratum corneum lipids. One of the first models—known as the domain mosaic model and proposed by Bo Forslind—suggests that the lipids exist in two phases: a gel (solid) phase and a liquid crystalline phase.[5] Essentially, islands of gel are embedded in a liquid crystalline matrix. As we traverse downward through the stratum corneum, the islands of one lamella will not coincide with those of another—thus making molecular penetration through the stratum corneum, along the liquid crystalline route, a very *tortuous* journey. Other studies, based on X-ray diffraction and electron microscopy experiments, describe the *sandwich* model in which two gel phases (top and bottom), predominantly containing ceramides, form a sandwich around a liquid crystalline phase consisting of cholesterol and free fatty acids.[6,7] There is also a single-phase lipid model that proposes that only one lipid gel phase exists in the stratum corneum.[8] While there are merits to this proposed model, it has stirred some controversy in the field of skin lipid research.[9]

The stratum corneum is often divided into two further lamellar classifications, stratum dysjunctum and stratum compactum, corresponding to the inner and outer portions of the stratum corneum, respectively. Desmosomes, or corneodesmosomes as they are referred to in the stratum corneum, undergo proteolysis in the stratum compactum, which allows corneocytes to be sloughed away from the skin in small sections (possibly individual or small groups of cells) rather than large sheets containing many cells joined together.

The stratum corneum, once considered a *dead* layer of skin, is now a highly respected component of the integument. In addition to its fascinating lipid structure, and the unique properties of corneocytes, there are many active enzymes in the stratum corneum, which carry out various roles to achieve terminal differentiation.

Keratinocyte adhesion and cell junctions

Desmosomes are disc-shape structures that are located on the outside surface of the cell where they serve as cellular junctions that provide a link between adjacent keratinocyte cells. They are connected to the intermediate filaments within the cell and are primarily composed of proteins that come from three different gene families: cadherins, armadillo proteins, and plakins. Molecules from these families are joined together and are located at the surface of the cell (at the cell membrane) and extend to the interior of the cell, where they anchor to intermediate filaments. Inside the cell, intermediate filaments are connected to the plakins. The plakins, located closer to the cell membrane than the intermediate filaments, are connected to proteins from the armadillo family. The cadherins are transmembrane proteins—they cross the cell membrane and are connected to an armadillo protein at its host cell and to another cadherin molecule at a neighboring keratinocyte. Thus, the junction point between two cells begins with the binding of two cadherin proteins and extends into the cytoplasm of each cell, ultimately connecting to intermediate filaments.[10]

Keratinocytes may also be interconnected by tight junctions that are formed at the cell membrane of two cells. This type of connection does not permit the passage of small molecules or ions between the cells, thus preventing the diffusion of these species through the tissue, which is very important for barrier function. Due to the action of the tight junctions, the only pathway for these molecules or ions is to pass through the cell by the normal ion or molecular channels. Tight junctions are constructed of several different types of proteins that anchor the cell membranes of the cells together, most notably proteins from the claudin and occludin families.[11]

Gap junctions are specialized channels between cells that allow the exchange of small molecules and ions between cells. This type of cell signaling allows the cells to communicate and alert each other about their biological condition. As a result, all cells are able to respond to these signals in unison. Gap junctions are composed of proteins that come from two families known as pannexins and connexins to form a supermolecular structure.[12]

Another type of cell junction that provides a strong mechanical linkage between cells are adherens junctions. There are two types of adherens junctions, which differ in their protein structure and organization. One adherens structure is the cadherin-catenin complex, the other a nectin-afadin complex. Both complexes are anchored to keratinocytes by actin filaments located in the cytoplasm of the cell. Overall, adherens junctions provide another form of cellular connectivity, thereby providing mechanical strength for tissue organization.[11]

DERMAL-EPIDERMAL JUNCTION

This region of the skin, also referred to as the basement membrane zone, provides the connection between the dermis and epidermis. It has an extremely important function—not only to provide a good connection between the two layers of skin, but also because it serves as the link between the vascularized dermis and nonvascularized epidermis in which nutrients must pass through to arrive at the epidermis. Often, the dermal-epidermal junction is categorized into four distinct layers: the keratinocyte plasma membrane from the stratum basale along with its associated hemidesmosomes, the lamina lucida, the lamina densa, and the sub-lamina densa fibrillar zone.[13] As can be inferred from their names, the lamina lucida is transparent or lucent when viewed through the electron microscope while the lamina densa is an electron-dense layer. Essentially, these two layers represent the constitutive dermal-epidermal junction.

The overall nature of this zone is far too complex to discuss with any great detail in the present text; however, the reader is encouraged to peruse some of the literature exclusively dedicated to this subject.[13] Nevertheless, we shall at least provide an elementary description of the various components that comprise the junction. As illustrated in Figure 1.5, the lamina lucida provides a connection between the hemidesmosomes of the bottom layer of cells in the stratum basale and collagen in the lamina densa. Typically, a family of glycoproteins, known as the laminins, play an integral role in the structure of basement membranes.

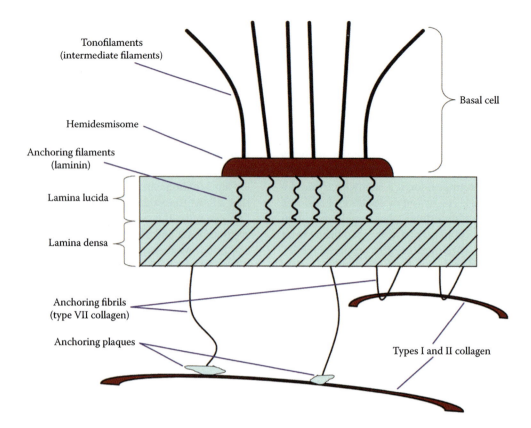

Figure 1.5 The epidermal-dermal junction in skin. (Adapted from Woodley, D.T. and Chen, M., The basement membrane zone, in *The Biology of the Skin*, Freinkel, R.K. and Woodley, D.T. [Eds.], The Parthenon Publishing Group, New York, 133–152, 2001.)

The laminins belong to the type V class of intermediate filaments and consist of several chains that form a cruciform structure. More specifically, it has been established that the laminins constitute most of the lamina lucida and are primarily responsible for the link provided between the hemidesmosomes and the lamina densa. Essentially, they function as anchoring filaments between collagen IV in the lamina densa and the hemidesmosome from the basal cell keratinocyte. In addition to type IV collagen, the lamina densa also contains laminins as well as a proteoglycan specific to the dermal-epidermal junction, heparan sulfate proteoglycan. In addition, there are many minor components that reside in the lamina densa. The sub-lamina densa fibrillar region consists of various anchoring fibrils as well as anchoring plaques.

DERMIS

The dermis of the skin is composed of two distinct regions, namely the papillary dermis and the reticular dermis, and provides the skin with its structural strength. The dermis primarily consists of connective tissue proteins such as collagen and elastic fibers; however, various other components are found as reported in Figure 1.6. In addition, the dermis provides residence for the vascular network in which nutrients from the blood supply are fed to the epidermis via the dermal-epidermal junction. A complex nerve network also resides in the dermis and serves various sensory functions such as touch, pressure, heat, and vibration. Moreover, the appendages of the cutaneous system inhabit the dermis and consist of the nail, pilosebaceous unit, and sudoriferous glands (eccrine and apocrine sweat glands).

The primary cell types present in the dermis include fibroblasts, mast cells, and tissue macrophages (Table 1.2). Fibroblasts are the most abundant cell type and are responsible for the synthesis and structuring of the structural tissue and ground substance. In addition, various cells associated with the immune response are also found in the dermis and are discussed further in the *Skin Immune System* section of this chapter.

The papillary layer receives its name from the dermal papillae, which are finger-like projections of the dermis into epidermis (Figure 1.1). Such a geometric structure provides increased stability for the binding of the dermis and epidermis as well as an increase in the surface area of the papillary layer, which permits greater exchange of nutrients and waste products between the dermis and epidermis.[14] Located just below the dermal-epidermal junction, the papillary layer primarily contains type III collagen, which is arranged into fibrillar bundles. The fibrillar bundles in this layer are smaller than those found in the reticular layer.

The reticular layer of the dermis is bordered above by the papillary layer and below by the hypodermis. Collagen I, which is arranged in large bundles, constitutes the largest population of collagen in this layer. The density of the fibers is much greater in this layer than in the papillary dermis. Collagen is arranged into fibrils or bundles and

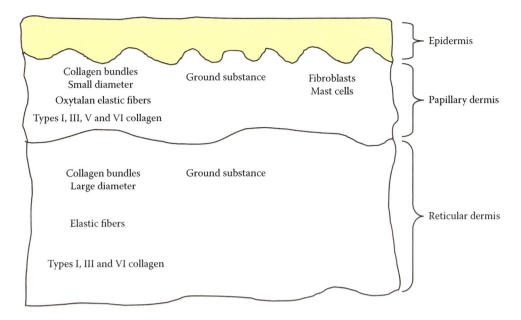

Figure 1.6 Major components of the papillary and reticular dermis.

Table 1.2 Principal dermal cell types.

Cell type	Function
Fibroblasts	Synthesis of structural proteins
Mast cells	Immune system
Macrophages	Immune system
Dermal dendrocytes	Immune system

the elastic fibers are intertwined within this network. Typically, four different types of collagen are present in the dermis and consist of types I, III, V, and VI, but mostly types I and III. Collagen has a polypeptide sequence that follows the scheme, Gly-X-Y, where X and Y correspond to proline and 4-hydroxyproline, respectively. In terms of secondary structure, collagen contains three alpha chains (not to be confused with alpha helices) that are super-twisted (protein tertiary structure) together to provide its fibril structure.[15]

The elastic fibers can be categorized into a fibrillar component (fibrillin) as well as an amorphous component (elastin). Elastic fibers are further classified as: (1) oxytalan fibers—fibers that are lightly coated with elastin; and (2) elaunin fibers—fibers more heavily coated with elastin.

The structural composition of the dermis is not only limited to collagen and elastic fibers, but also to other connective tissue components that are worthy of mention. The ground substance is a gel-like substance that fills all of the interstitial spaces not already filled by collagen, the elastic fibers, dermal cells, or the appendages. The ground substance consists of glycoproteins, glycosaminoglycans, and proteoglycans. There are several predominant glycoproteins in the dermis and these consist of fibronectin, thrombospondin, vitronectin, and tenascin. Typically, the glycoproteins function as surface coatings (sheath) for the fibrillar tissue in the dermis.

Glycosaminoglycans, on the other hand, are polysaccharides made up of repeating units of disaccharides. Those most commonly found in physiology consist of chondroitin sulfate, dermatan sulfate, heparan sulfate, keratan sulfate, heparin, and hyaluronic acid. Typically, glycosaminoglycans form a complex with a protein to form a proteoglycan, which is a subclass of the glycoproteins. An example of such a molecule is provided in Figure 1.7, which contains a hyaluronic acid core with pendant proteins that contain glucosaminoglycan side chains.

CUTANEOUS APPENDAGES

Additional components of the gross anatomical structure of skin consist of the cutaneous appendages: eccrine/apocrine glands, pilosebaceous unit, and the nail unit. The sudoriferous glands aid in controlling body temperature and play a possible role in pheromone signaling. The pilosebaceous unit is composed of the hair follicle and sebaceous gland, which lubricates the mature hair shaft with sebum and antioxidants, bringing them to the surface of skin where they can provide protection. Apocrine glands are also associated with the pilosebaceous unit. Their secretions, mostly composed of lipids and proteins, are also brought to the skin surface by the growing hair fiber.

Eccrine and apocrine glands

Eccrine gland

Eccrine sweat glands cover almost the entire body surface and carry out the physiological function of temperature regulation by evaporative cooling.[16–20] They secrete an ultrafiltrate of plasma, which contains H_2O, inorganic ions (e.g., NaCl, K, etc.), proteins, lactic acid, and urea. Some of the proteins are antimicrobial agents, which play an integral role in the protection of the outermost layer of the skin. Humans typically have two to four million eccrine

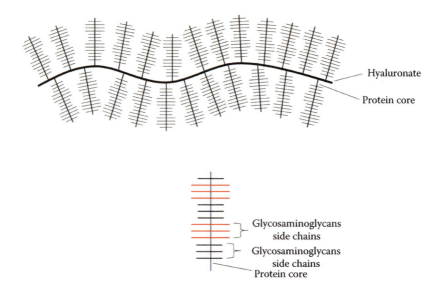

Figure 1.7 Proteoglycan structure. (Adapted from Matthews, C.K. and van Holde, K.E., *Biochemistry*, 2nd ed., Benjamin Cummings, Redwood City, CA, 1996.)

glands, which can output several liters of sweat per day. The number of glands per unit area is greatest on the soles of the feet and hands, and least on the back. The glands are located over the entire body with the exception of the lips, labia minora, clitoris, glans penis, and external auditory canal.[21] Most evolutionary biologists believe that this efficient cooling apparatus evolved in *Homo sapiens* to allow for long periods of strenuous activity, such as chasing prey, and the ability to survive in a variety of climatic conditions. Defective operation of this extraordinary physiological system could lead down the disastrous route of heat exhaustion, heat stroke, hyperthermia, or even death.[22] In addition to its cooling function, the eccrine sweat gland also excretes organic toxins and heavy metals.

The eccrine sweat gland is composed of a secretory coil at its base, located deep in the skin, and a long duct that rises up to the skin surface (Figure 1.8). This duct is further classified as intradermal duct (coiled and straight) and intraepidermal duct, which twists as it makes its way through the epidermis.[20] The secretory coil is the source of fluid secretion and consists of three principal cell types. The dark (mucoid) cells contain dark granules—hence their name—and are located closest to the inner tube of the gland, known as the lumen. The clear (secretory) cells do not directly interface with the lumen, but gain access to the lumen by intercellular canaliculi, located at the interface of two clear cells, which open up into the lumen. Thus, sweat secreted by clear cells enters the lumen by way of the intercellular canaliculum and makes its way from the secretory coil to the duct, and eventually to the surface of the skin. The clear cells of the secretory coil are supported either by an underlying basement membrane or spindle-shaped myoepithelial cells that contain myofilaments—fibrous muscle proteins (Figure 1.9).

Sweat production is initiated by the nervous system (cholinergic mechanism) with the control center located in the hypothalamus. Stimulation of the eccrine gland is then achieved by the neurotransmitter acetylcholine, which is released in the periphery of the gland by associated nerve fibers. In turn, intracellular calcium levels increase, resulting in the opening of K and Cl channels in the clear cell; K channels are located on the basal lateral membrane and Cl channels on the luminal cell membrane (the portion of the membrane in contact with the lumen). As K and Cl are shuttled across the membrane, they must be accompanied by aqueous fluid from the clear cell cytoplasm in order to maintain osmotic balance. Clear cells of the secretory coil are rich in mitochondria and contain the two important transmembrane proteins, Na^+/K^+-ATPase and Na-K-2Cl co-transporter, that allow ion transport across the cell membrane and ultimately play a pivotal role in sweat secretion.

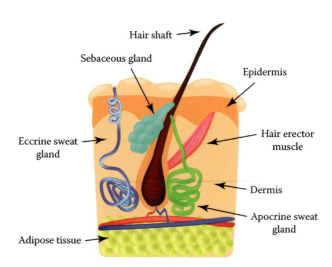

Figure 1.8 Illustration of the pilosebaceous unit along with the sudoriferous glands. Note the anatomical relationship between eccrine and apocrine glands. The apocrine gland is associated with the pilosebaceous unit, while the eccrine gland opens directly to the surface of the skin.

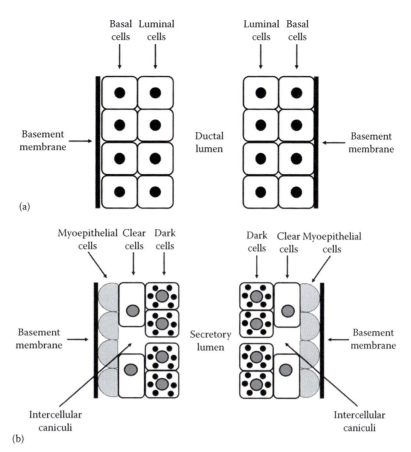

Figure 1.9 Fine structure of the components of the eccrine (a) duct and (b) secretory coil. The secretory coil contains dark cells, which border the secretory lumen and underlying clear cells (no dark dots) that generate sweat. Intercellular caniculi form a reservoir, which bypasses the dark cells to bring sweat to the lumen. At the base of the clear cells (on the side of the myoepithelial cells), mitochondria and the enzyme NA^+/K^+-ATPase are found. The clear cells are supported by underlying myoepithelial cells and a basement membrane.

These ion pumps are located in the portion of the plasma membrane that borders the underlying myoepithelial cells and basement membrane, known as the basolateral membrane, characterized by its highly infolded structure. Na^+/K^+-ATPase functions as a sodium-potassium pump, which transfers the ions in opposite directions across the membrane. On the other hand, Na-K-2Cl co-transporter moves Na, K, and Cl ions across the membrane, all in the same direction. Overall, the net result of all ion transports across the basolateral cell membrane is the activation of Cl channels and the subsequent transfer of Cl ions into the lumen, across the luminal cell membrane. As a result, the luminal cell membrane carries a potential, thereby attracting Na ions, which must be shuttled to the lumen as well; Na ions have to make their way from the basal membrane interstitial region to the lumen via extracellular space.

The duct of the eccrine gland is a tubular structure that begins in the coiled region, followed by a straight, long portion that extends to the surface of the skin. One of the most important functions of the duct is the re-absorption of NaCl and HCO_3^- that is secreted from the lower secretory tubule. This key mechanism prevents the body from entering a state of electrolyte imbalance. Ion recuperation is most effective during slow rates of perspiration and less efficient when the rate of perspiration is high. The duct of the eccrine gland contains two cell types, basal and luminal cells. The luminal cells are located closest to the lumen, while the basal cells provide underlying support. The basal cells are very metabolically active (they have many mitochondria) and contain a cell membrane abundant with Na^+/K^+-ATPase (responsible for the re-adsorption of NaCl). Luminal cells, on the other hand, contain less mitochondria and ATPase. It is believed that luminal cells serve more of a structural role by providing integrity to the duct, which is likely due to the presence of tonofilaments in the region next to the cell membrane closest to the lumen.

Apocrine gland

In contrast to the eccrine gland, the apocrine gland is a larger structure that is associated with the pilosebaceous unit (Figure 1.8). Unlike eccrine glands, which open/secrete sweat directly at the surface of skin, apocrine sweat is secreted onto the hair fiber, just above the sebaceous gland, then makes it way to the surface by following the protrusion of the hair fiber. Therefore, apocrine sweat is milky and viscous, rather than clear and water-like as in the case of eccrine sweat, most likely because it has a different composition and mixes with sebaceous lipids. Apocrine glands are only found in the axillae, perineal region, mammary areolae, scalp, and abdomen.[23] Although the glands are present at birth, they do not become active until puberty. It is believed that the apocrine gland is an antiquated organ that remains from our evolutionary past. Montagna argues this point,

> In the members of the order Primates, to which man, 'the monkeys,' and the apes belong, apocrine glands gradually disappear from the skin of successively higher forms at the same time that eccrine sweat glands take their place.[24]

His conclusion is based on the presence of apocrine glands all over the surface of the body of mammalian species that do not fall into the category of primates. In our distant past, pheromone-like molecules secreted by apocrine glands are believed to have provided warning signals and sexual cues to other individuals. Nevertheless, the odors associated with axillae sweat are due to bacterial waste arising from the decomposition of specific molecules secreted by these glands. Such odors have become a nuisance to societies obsessed with cleanliness and hygiene. As a result, a great deal of effort is expended by the personal care industry to understand the mechanisms behind sweat production and how to prevent it.

The apocrine gland is normally divided into three anatomical components: secretory segment, intradermal duct, and intraepithelial duct.[20] The secretory segment contains two principal cell types: cuboidal/columnar-shaped secretory cells, which border the lumen, and underlying myoepithelial cells. The portion of the cell membrane of the secretory cells facing the lumen contains finger-like projections, known as microvilli. Secretory cells in apocrine glands also contain two distinct types of granules in their cytoplasm, which are distinguished by their size and shape. The duct consists of a double layer of small cuboidal cells. The re-absorption of NaCl by the duct apparatus does not occur in apocrine glands. Further, stimulation of apocrine glands occurs by adrenergic fibers via the release of epinephrine or epinephrine-like (e.g., norepinephrine) neurotransmitters.

Apoeccrine gland

In the late 1980s, Sato and coworkers reported the existence of yet another type of gland, located in the axillae and perineal regions, that possesses characteristics of both eccrine and apocrine glands. While there is some controversy about the time of the apoeccrine's first discovery, most of our current understanding comes from the study of Sato and coworkers.[25] Structurally, the duct of the apoeccrine gland is similar to that found in eccrine glands, while the secretory coil contains portions that share similar characteristics to both apocrine and eccrine glands. Sections of the lumen in the secretory coil differ in diameter. More dilated portions (larger diameter) resemble apocrine glands and contain a single layer of secretory cells. The smaller diameter sections of the secretory coil, characteristic of eccrine gland coils, contain clear cells, dark cells, and intercellular canaliculi. Like their eccrine counterparts, apoeccrine glands have a long duct that extends from the secretory coil to the surface of the skin; it does not open up to the pilosebaceous unit as in the case of apocrine glands. The apoeccrine gland responds to cholinergic and adrenergic stimulation.[23]

Pilosebaceous unit

Within the scientific community, it is often said that human hair is dead tissue. What is really meant by this statement? Well, most biologists will tell you that hair has undergone a process known as differentiation and hardening (keratinization), and its cellular components no longer contain the normal metabolically active organelles, such as the mitochondrion, endoplasmic reticulum, and nucleus. Unfortunately, for this reason many scientists view hair as tissue that is less important. To the contrary, hair is not only a very important biological component of our body, but also an extremely interesting one, from both a practical and scientific perspective. Imagine life without eyelashes. Or, for that matter, an existence without big beautiful eyebrows, which gracefully prevent forehead sebum from seeping into our eyes. Even worse, conjecture a trip to Quebec in the midst of harsh winter without your lush head of hair. On the molecular and morphological level, the biochemistry and physical chemistry of hair are equally fascinating. Let us examine some of these properties and many other facets of hair in the paragraphs that follow.

Hair is a complex, intricate morphological structure that consists of a metabolically active component (hair follicle) and a mature, fully differentiated constituent (hair shaft). The sebaceous gland, which is associated with the fiber, is part of the pilosebaceous unit. There are three types of human hair: lanugo, vellus, and terminal hair. Lanugo hair develops in utero and is shed shortly after birth. Vellus hair consists of small fibers—usually nonpigmented—that cover most of the body, excluding the palm and sole. Terminal hair, on the hand, is usually thick, long, and pigmented (except in the case of subjects who produce little or no pigmentation). Terminal hair can be further classified as primary and secondary terminal fibers. Primary terminal fibers are those from the scalp, eyebrows, and eyelashes. Secondary terminal fibers develop due to hormonal changes. During puberty, high levels of androgens lead to an increase in pubic and axillae hair in both males and females, and an increase in facial, chest, leg, and arm hair in males. Vellus fibers are often replaced by secondary terminal hairs during puberty.

Hair follicle

Our discussion now brings us to an anatomical region of hair that is very alive: the hair follicle. In fact, the cells of this epidermal appendage are among the fastest proliferators in the body. The hair follicle is structurally complex and extends some 2 mm below the skin's basal layers. Its base is the dermal papilla and the overall follicular structure consists of an inner root sheath, outer root sheath, sebaceous gland, and matrix cells responsible for the formation of the mature hair fiber.

The base of the hair follicle is circumfused with nerve fiber endings and capillaries, providing sensation and nourishment. As shown in Figure 1.8, the hair follicle is the base of the pilosebaceous unit and is an invagination of the epidermis into the dermis. The base of the hair follicle is known as the hair bulb, which is the metabolically active portion of the hair fiber (Figure 1.10).[26] At the very bottom of the hair bulb, the dermal papilla protrudes inward into the hair bulb and is lined with matrix cells, which are responsible for the synthesis of the cells that constitute the mature hair shaft. Melanocytes are also located in this region and deposit melanin granules into differentiating cortical cells, which will become part of the mature hair shaft. The portion of the hair follicle in contact with the invaginated epidermis is known as the outer root sheath. It provides a protective coating for most of the hair shaft with the exception of dermal papilla where the matrix cells reside. The outer root sheath is composed of a stratified epithelial layer. The inner root sheath consists of three concentric layers; beginning from the outside going in, they are: Henle, Huxley, and cuticle layer. The Henle layer is a single layer of cuboidal epithelial cells. The Huxley layer—named after the nineteenth century English biologist, Thomas Henry Huxley—contains flattened keratinized cells. The cuticle—not to be confused with the cuticle of the mature hair shaft—borders the outer root sheath (Figure 1.10). Differentiation, or keratinization, takes place in the hair follicle region and results in the production of the mature hair shaft, producing cuticle and cortical cells filled with lipids and keratins and void of metabolically active organelles.

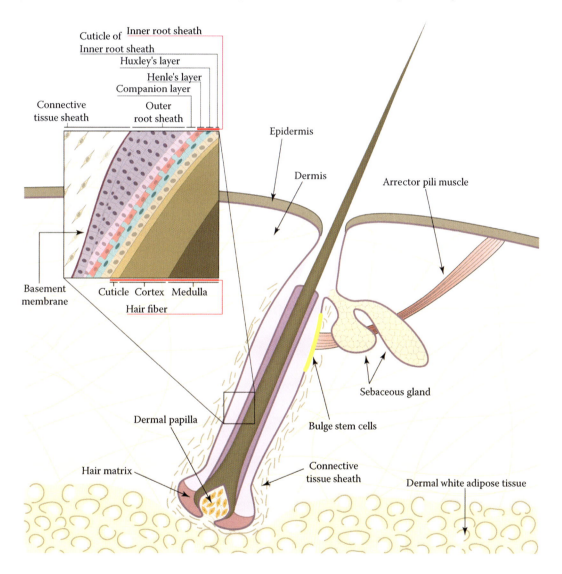

Figure 1.10 Schematic of the hair follicle illustrating the mesenchymal (e.g., connective tissue component, bulge, etc.) and epithelial components (outer root sheath, inner root sheath, hair shaft, etc.), which are separated by a basement membrane. Just above the dermal papilla (not shown in the illustration) reside matrix cells responsible for the growth of the differentiated fiber as well as melanocytes, which deposit melanin granules into the cortex. The hair shaft (i.e., differentiated fiber) consists of three morphological components: cuticle, cortex, and medulla. The epithelial components of the follicle are the outer root sheath and inner root sheath, which are separated by a companion layer. The inner root sheath consists of three layers: cuticle, Huxley's layer, and Henle's layer. (Reprinted with permission from Kiani, M. et al., *ACS Biomat. Sci. Eng.*, 2017, doi:10.1021/acsbiomaterials.7b00072. American Chemical Society.)

The loss of pigmentation in hair is associated with aging processes that occur in the hair follicle. There are a number of factors believed to be responsible for premature hair graying or whitening (canities) including abnormal pH or cysteine levels in melanosomes; possible roles of trace metal ions, vitamin B_{12}, and vitamin D_3; and oxidative stress.[27,28] In fact, the process of melanogenesis, which occurs during the anagen growth phase of the follicle, is a well-known source of oxidative stress, resulting in premature aging and apoptosis. In addition to oxidative stress caused by endogenous sources, there are a number of external factors, including solar radiation, inflammation, and psycho-emotional stress, which can affect the overall redox state and lead to premature aging of the follicle unit and hair graying.[29] Some of the key mechanisms involved include the reduction of catalase expression (an endogenous antioxidant; see Chapter 3) as well as a decrease in the ability to scavenge hydroxyl radicals (see Chapter 2).[30] In addition, high levels of hydrogen peroxide, a reactive oxygen species (see Chapter 2), are found in the hair shaft of graying fibers.[31,32] Overall, melanocytes in hair follicles of individuals with canities are unable to manage high oxidative stress conditions.[33]

Hair shaft

The morphological structure of a mature human hair contains an inner core (cortex) of spindle-shaped cortical cells (5 μm in diameter and 50 μm in length) aligned along the length of the fiber. This is surrounded by overlapping flat cuticle cells that are arranged in a manner analogous to fish scales or shingles (Figures 1.11 and 1.12).[34–38] The fiber

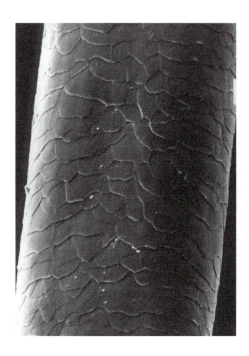

Figure 1.12 Scanning electron micrograph of the intact mature hair shaft illustrating the overlapping cuticle cells on the outermost surface of the fiber.

may also contain a medulla, which is located at the center of the cortex. However, the first thing that usually comes to mind when we think of hair is alpha-keratin, which is located in the cortical cells of the cortex. Most likely,

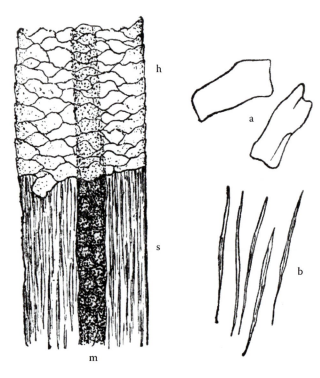

Figure 1.11 Section of a hair shaft: h, hair shaft with cuticles; s, cuticle removed revealing underlying cortex; m, medulla; a, isolated cuticle cells; and b, isolated cortical cells. (Reproduced from Piersol, G.A., *Human Anatomy*, J.B. Lippincott Company, Philadelphia, PA, 1908. With permission.)

this is due to our first introduction to the subject, either in general biochemistry or classic textbooks published on the topic of hair. We envision two strands of slightly different alpha-keratin proteins arranged in an in-phase fashion and twisted together to produce a two-stranded rope (a coiled-coil). Pairs of these associate to produce an anti-parallel offset protein tetramer. By a process, the fine details of which remain to be elucidated, the tetramers associate both longitudinally and laterally to produce a discrete rod of semi-infinite length containing 32 protein chains in its transverse section. This is the *crystalline* part of the hair fiber known as the microfibril (or intermediate filament). Microfibrils (hundreds of them) are embedded in a pseudo-hexagonal array within a cysteine-rich protein matrix to form the keratin macrofibril. Several tens of macrofibrils are packed longitudinally within each cortical cell. The macrofibrils are separated in places by other cellular components such as the effete cell nucleus, melanin pigment granules, and, in places, a thin matrix of protein of low cysteine content (sometimes referred to as *non-keratin*).[39]

In the last two decades, great progress has been made in the elucidation of keratin structure in hair—there are at least fourteen different types of alpha-helical keratins that constitute the crystalline phase of cortical cells in animals.[40] It is universally accepted that the great tensile strength of hair is due to the hierarchal organization of the crystalline phase alpha-keratins. While much attention is owed to alpha-keratin, it is intriguing to understand better the important role played by the amorphous matrix, which is believed to be largely composed of proteins belonging to the family of keratin-associated proteins. Also located in the cortex is a cell membrane complex that separates cortical cells from each other and from the overlaying cuticle cells. The cell membrane complex of the cortex is biologically distinct to that of the cuticle, which is discussed in the following.

While many achievements have been made in ascertaining the internal structure of the hair fiber, there is still room for future discoveries to help explain some of our unanswered questions. Is the highly cross-linked, high-sulfur-containing matrix bestowed with an evolutionary protective role for the crystalline phase alpha-helical keratins that it surrounds? To what extent are the keratin-associated proteins cross-linked with crystalline phase alpha-keratins? Is the intermicrofibrillar matrix the primary target of damaging cosmetic treatments? If so, does this portion of the fiber play an important role in determining overall structural integrity?

Several published reviews describe the morphological and chemical structure of hair;[34,35] however, the description of the cuticle by J. Alan Swift is the most accepted treatise on this subject.[41] Thus, his nomenclature and description of the cuticle will be drawn upon in this text (Figure 1.13). Each cuticle cell, which is *ca.* 0.5 μm thick and 60 μm square, consists of an outer beta layer, epicuticle, A layer, exocuticle, endocuticle, inner layer,

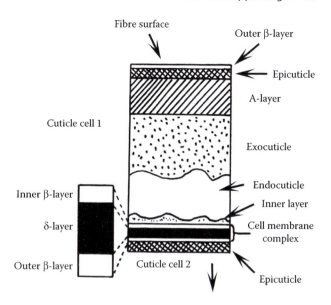

Figure 1.13 Morphological components of the cuticle illustrating the lamellar arrangement of the various layers of the outermost cuticle cell. (From Swift, J.A. and Smith, J.R.: Microscopical investigations on the epicuticle of mammalian keratin fibres. *J Microsc.* 2001. 204. 203–211. Copyright Wiley-VCH Verlag GmbH & Co. KGaA. Reproduced with permission.)

and inner beta layer. These cuticular subcomponents are lamellar and arranged in the order listed earlier from the exterior of the fiber to its interior. The outer and inner beta layers constitute part of what is known as the cell membrane complex, which is unlike most biological phospholipid membranes. It is believed that the outer beta layer, exposed to the surface and to overlying cuticle cells, consists predominantly of 18-methyleicosanoic acid (18-MEA).[42] In addition, the cell membrane complex contains a delta layer, which is the intercellular cement that joins the inner beta layer of one cuticle cell with the outer beta layer of an underlying cuticle cell. The A layer, exocuticle, and inner layer are thought to be proteinaceous in nature and have been shown to be extremely rich in disulfide bonds.[41] The endocuticle, on the other hand, is generally low in cystine, but is also composed of proteinaceous material. Human hair usually contains *ca.* 10 layers of cuticle cells at the root of the fiber; however, this number diminishes along the length of the fiber toward the tip direction.[43] While much has been learned about the cuticle in the last three decades, many questions still perplex us, such as the tertiary structure of the protein constituents that comprise this component of the fiber. Also puzzling is the composition and structural arrangement of the delta layer.[44] Historically, the epicuticle has been a controversial component of the cuticle cell.[44,45] In 1916, von Allwörden demonstrated that membrane-bound sacs may be formed on the surface of hair treated with chlorine water.[44,46] It was not until the atomic force microscope became available as a research tool that the epicuticle was identified as a continuous lamellar layer about 13 nm thick located just above the A-layer and below the outer beta layer.[45]

Sebaceous gland

While the precise role of sebaceous glands in skin has always mystified scientists, it undoubtedly plays an important role in the protection of the hair fiber and surface of the skin. As part of the pilosebaceous unit, the sebaceous gland opens up to the hair follicle canal, secreting its contents onto the surface of the fiber (Figure 1.8). Sebum lipids find their way to the surface and interior of the hair fiber, providing protection to its morphological components by reducing friction and wear. More than likely, lipids in the interior of the fiber probably serve as a reservoir, which are able to exude out onto the surface of the mature hair shaft when surface lipid levels are low. In addition, protection by sebum is conferred to the skin surface in the form of the acid mantle—a low pH film present on the surface of the skin that prevents microbial growth and invasion by foreign pathogens. It also helps protect skin from oxidation and in inflammation, and provides waterproofing properties rendering the skin surface hydrophobic with increased barrier function.[47]

Sebaceous glands can be associated with terminal or vellus hair fibers. In terminal hair, the sebaceous duct opens into the hair follicle canal. In vellus hair, the hair follicle canal and the acini of the sebaceous gland are in close proximity and lead into a principal hair follicle canal. The anatomical distribution of sebaceous glands is unique inasmuch they are not found in the palms of the hands and soles and dorsum of the feet.[48] The size and density of the glands also depend on anatomical location.[49] For example, the facial region contains the largest glands and the highest density of sebaceous glands is found in the scalp, forehead, face, and anogenital region.[50,51] Sex and age are also determinant factors in the size and density of sebaceous glands. The morphological structure of the sebaceous gland consists of several-to-many acini, which contain sebaceous cells. As illustrated in Figure 1.14, the acini are located at the base of the gland and lead into a duct, which eventually makes its way to the hair follicle canal.

The sebaceous cells consist of undifferentiated cells, differentiating cells, and mature cells.[50,51] Just like in the epidermis, cells undergo a differentiation process and progress to successive strata of the acini. The undifferentiated sebaceous cells can be likened to the keratinocytes of the basal layer of the epidermis. They are cuboidal in shape, contain tonofilaments, and are found on the border of the basement membrane zone. Differentiating sebaceous cells are generally located above the undifferentiated cells, do not contain as many tonofilaments, and have lipid vesicles present in their structure. Mature sebaceous cells are large, bulging cells that are at the point of bursting due to the overwhelming abundance of lipid vesicles. Once the cell breaks down, sebum is secreted into the duct (constructed of a stratified squamous epithelium) and makes its way to the pilosebaceous canal. Sebum conditions the hair fiber and is brought to the surface of the skin by the growing fiber. In humans, sebum secretions predominantly consist

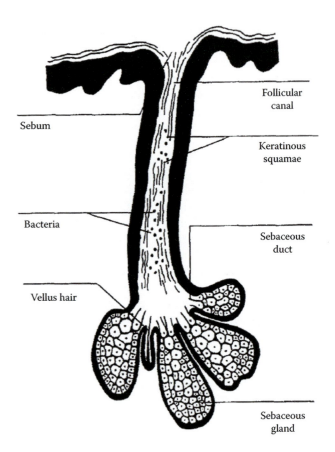

Figure 1.14 The sebaceous follicle. (Reprinted from *J. Am. Acad. Dermatol.*, 32, Leyden, J.J., New understandings of the pathogenesis of acne, S15–S25, Copyright 1995, with permission from Elsevier.)

of triglycerides, wax esters, squalene, free sterols, and sterol esters.[48] Sebum production is controlled hormonally, most notably by androgens and estrogens. Androgens belong to a family of steroid hormones that circulate in the blood and bind to androgen receptors at various locations in the body. They lead to typical anatomical and physiological masculine traits, and also increase the activity and size of sebaceous glands. Testosterone is one of the most common examples of an androgen.

Often conflated, males and females both produce androgens, although much greater quantities are generated by the former group, hence their predominant masculine qualities. In contrast to androgens, estrogens are responsible for many feminine traits and have been shown to decrease sebaceous activity, although there is doubt that physiological levels of estrogens, as opposed to a pharmacologically administered dose, decrease sebum production.[48] One of the most common skin ailments associated with sebaceous glands is acne.[52] It is most prevalent in young men and women (in their 20s), and occurs when colonies of *Propionibacterium acnes* infest the hair follicle concurrently with hyperkeratinization in the follicle and production of sebum.[52] Clinically, this results in the formation of comedones (blackheads and whiteheads), papules, pustules, and nodules.[53]

In the context of antioxidants, much of our interest in sebum and sebaceous glands stems from findings that sebum carries antioxidants to the skin surface.[47,54] Specific antioxidants found include vitamin E and coenzyme Q10.[55,56] Oral and topical administration of these antioxidants leads to greater levels not only in sebum, but also in the stratum corneum.[56] It is believed that antioxidants brought to the skin surface by sebaceous glands may play an integral role in the protection of skin against photodamage and other environmental insults.

The nail unit

Human nail is another extraordinary appendage of the human integument, which carries out many functions in our daily lives. Situated at the distal part (end) on the dorsal side of the digits (fingers and toes), it provides physical protection to the most distal part of our extremities. The nail unit is commonly classified according to several distinct anatomic entities as indicated in the following list and shown in Figure 1.15.[57,58]

1. *Nail body*
   a. *Nail plate*: This is the hard, keratinized portion of the nail unit.
   b. *Lunula*: The lunula is the crescent-shaped, white portion of the nail.
   c. *Eponychium* (*cuticle*): The cuticle is epidermal in nature, borders the lunula, and serves as a superficial transition zone.
   d. *Distal edge*: This refers to the most distal region of the nail plate.
2. *Nail frame*
   a. *Lateral nail fold*: Folded skin structure bordering the sides of the nail plate.
   b. *Proximal nail fold*: Folded skin structure of the skin adjacent to the cuticle.
3. *Matrix*: These are the group of cells responsible for the growth of the nail plate. They provide us with the whitish color observed in the lunula. The nail cells become keratinized and are pushed outward along the nail bed.
4. *Nail support structure*
   a. *Nail bed*: The region that underlies and supports the nail plate.
   b. *Nail mesenchyme*: This is the region between the nail bed and phalangeal bone.
   c. *Phalangeal bone*: Underlying support structure for the nail unit.

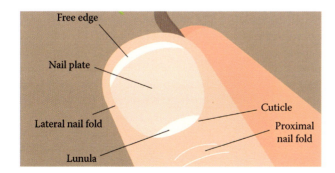

Figure 1.15 Diagram of the nail unit.

The biochemistry of the nail unit is usually described in terms of its keratin composition. Similar to hair, the nail plate contains KIFs that are embedded in a cystine-rich matrix. Overall, the nail unit is composed of 80% hard keratins (similar to those found in hair) and 20% of soft keratins (like those found in skin).[59] Soft keratins (e.g., K1 and K10) are usually expressed in the matrix region of the nail as well as the nail fold. Hard keratins are mostly confined to the nail plate and to the suprabasal regions of the nail bed.[57] While many trace elements are found in the nail (e.g., iron, zinc, and calcium), the lipid composition of the nail is negligible—less than 5% of the total composition.[59]

The role of free radicals and antioxidants in human nail are not immediately apparent by examination of its anatomical structure. To compound matters, very little research has been conducted in the free radical biology of the nail. Nevertheless, there are many consumer products available in the retail market for antioxidant-based treatments of nail. Many of these products focus their attention on antioxidant-rich, oil-based treatments of the nail cuticle. At any rate, it behooves us to gain a better understanding of free radical processes in the nail unit. There have been studies that have shown that we can correlate trace element content of nail—related to antioxidant defense—with mineral and antioxidant consumption.[60] Further, it has been demonstrated that trace elements in nail are inversely associated with inflammatory markers in blood, such as tumor necrosis factor-alpha (TNF-alpha) and the members of the interleukin family (e.g., IL-6, IL-18).[61]

SKIN IMMUNE SYSTEM

The human body is endowed with a rather complex immune system that provides protection from foreign invaders. Typically, the immune system can be categorized into three classes of defense. The first line of defense consists of the components that make up all surfaces of the body that may come in contact with the external environment. The most obvious of these is the skin; however, this also refers to the epithelial tissue that lines the mouth, nose, gastrointestinal tract, lungs, and various other anatomical structures.

Physical barrier to invaders

The morphological nature of the skin and other epithelial tissues prevents easy access for many foreign pathogens. Further, secretions from the skin, including sebum and sweat, render a pH of 3–5 at the skin's surface, thus preventing microbial colonization. Other epithelial tissue, on the other hand, secretes saliva, tears, and mucous, which contain enzymes (e.g., lyzozyme) that destroy bacteria cells.

Innate immune system

When tissues are invaded by foreign substances (pathogens), such as bacteria, viruses, fungi, or parasites, the infected cells are able to communicate their distress through cellular signaling. This leads to mobilization of phagocytic cells, which circulate in the blood stream, and

Table 1.3 Phagocytes present in skin tissues.

Cell type	Function
Neutrophils	These cells represent the largest percentage of all leukocytes.
Eosinophils	Offer protection against parasitic worms.
Basophils	Only represent a small fraction of all leukocytes. Basophils secrete histamine in order to prolong inflammation.
Mast cells	These cells typically reside in tissues. They contain granules of histamine and heparin.
Macrophages	Macrophages are derived from monocytes. They exist as monocytes in the blood stream and transform to macrophages when they migrate to tissues.

migrate to areas of tissue injury where they seek pathogens and destroy them. Typically, phagocytes are white blood cells (leukocytes), which function by engulfing the pathogen and encasing it in a vacuole within its cytoplasm. Table 1.3 contains a list of phagocytes typically found in skin. Of the cell types listed, neutrophils, eosinophils, and basophils belong to the granulocyte class of leukocytes. This cell type reacts very quickly to pathogen invasion, unlike the mast cell, which is slower to mobilize. The mast cell, however, is longer lived than the granulocytes.

In addition to the aggressive action of the phagocytic cells, the body's innate immune system also consists of natural killer cells and antimicrobial proteins. Natural killer cells represent another fast-responding aspect of the innate immune system in which these cells quickly migrate to the infected area and destroy any infected cells by destruction of their plasma membrane. As indicated by the name, antimicrobial proteins seek microbes and either destroy them or prevent further proliferation. There are two groups of proteins that constitute the antimicrobial proteins, namely the complement proteins and interferons.

The inflammatory response to tissue infection or injury is a very complex process that involves the cell types described earlier and numerous signaling cascades. Inflammation can be characterized as redness, swelling, elevated temperature, and pain to the infected area. Cellular signaling from the infected cells or the foreign invaders induces the inflammatory response. Through a process of vasodilation, vasoconstriction, and vascular permeability, the blood vessels can control the amount of blood, hence white blood cells, which migrate to the infected area. Vasodilation occurs in order to increase the amount of blood that arrives at the tissue. Vasoconstriction, which occurs on the other side of the tissue relative to the flow of blood, prevents blood from leaving the localized area. Thus, more blood flows into the site due to vasodilation and less blood leaves the site due to vasoconstriction. During this process, the vascular permeability of the capillaries near the injured site increases, allowing blood to exude out of the capillaries and into the tissue resulting in edema (swelling) and elevated temperature. Moreover, the swelling causes pressures on local nerves resulting in the sensation of pain at the infected area. In summary, we can see that the body's natural immunologic defense is to increase the supply of blood to a region under duress. This in turn permits more nutrients, clotting proteins, oxygen, leukocytes, and antibodies to enter the infected area.[14] In addition, the inflammatory response prevents the pathogens from spreading to other regions of the body. There are also occasions when the body's response to foreign pathogens is more delocalized. This occurs when body temperature reaches elevated levels, commonly referred to as fever, in response to invasion by microorganisms. The body's temperature is controlled by neurons in the hypothalamus. Through cellular signaling a fever may be induced by leukocytes, which excrete pyrogens, molecules capable of inciting a change in the body temperature.

Adaptive immune system

The innate immune system, already discussed, represents the body's initial response to pathogen invasion. However, in many cases the pathogen is a molecule that the immune system is not familiar with and a more complex response is necessary. Specialized cells of the immune system, called lymphocytes, circulate in the blood and are located in the spleen, lymph nodes, and lymph. When a foreign invader is encountered, this results in cellular signaling, from either the pathogen or affected cells to the lymphocytes, ultimately generating an immune response. The specific response is due to an antigen, which is a foreign molecule (typically a protein) from the invading bacteria, viruses, fungi, and parasites. The antigen is presented to lymphocytes by cells referred to as antigen presenting cells (APCs), such as Langerhans cells. Lymphocytes are classified into two major groups, either T cells or B cells. T cells can be further categorized as helper T cells or cytotoxic T cells.

The adaptive immune system is typically classified into two types of immune response depending on the nature of its course. The humoral immune response occurs when free antigen activates B cells resulting in the manufacture of antibodies, which are then able to circulate in the blood. In contrast, the cell-mediated immune response does not involve the expression of antibodies but does depend on the action of helper T cells. Figure 1.16 provides a diagrammatic overview of both immune responses as well as the communication between the two routes via cellular signaling. As seen in the figure, the primary feature of the humoral response is the direct interaction of a free antigen with a B cell, which contains a surface receptor capable of binding the antigen. In fact, the surface receptor of the B cell is an antigen receptor (immunoglobulin). Once antigen binding has taken

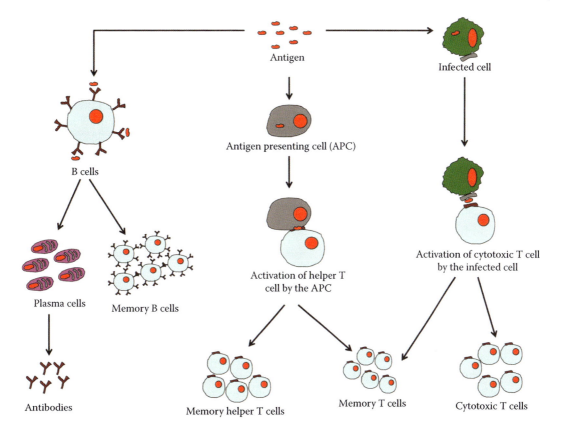

Figure 1.16 Summary and interrelationships between the innate and adaptive immune systems. (Adapted from Marieb, E.N., *Human Anatomy & Physiology*, 7th ed., Benjamin Cummings, Menlo Park, CA, 2006.)

place, the B cell expresses the appropriate antibody. It is important to bear in mind that only B cells are capable of expressing antibodies. This gives rise to the proliferation of memory B cells as well as plasma cells. The memory B cells can be utilized for future encounters with the same antigen. The plasma cells, on the other hand, circulate through the blood and secrete antibodies to fight off antigens in the system.

In the cell-mediated immune response, there are two major pathways that can be followed. First, a cell that is infected with an antigen can present the antigen on the surface of its plasma membrane with the help of a Class I Major Histocompatibility Complex (Class I MHC) protein. The infected cell is then able to interact with a cytotoxic T cell in which a bridge is formed between the two cells by the antigen, Class I MHC protein, and the receptor on the surface of the cytotoxic T cell. This results in the activation of the cytotoxic T cell, which renders it capable of initiating an attack on infected cells, ultimately leading to apoptosis. A second pathway in the cell-mediated immune response that may be followed occurs when a pathogen is engulfed by an APC, such as a macrophage. Once the APC digests the pathogen, protein fragments can be brought to the plasma membrane surface of the APC by a Class II Major Histocompatibility Complex (Class II MHC) protein. The APC can then bind to a helper T cell in which a bridge is formed between the APC and helper T cell by the Class II MHC protein and the antigen. The outcome of such an interaction is the activation of the helper T cell resulting in proliferation of helper T cells and memory T cells.

An extremely important aspect of the adaptive immune system, not shown in Figure 1.16, is the connection provided not only between the humoral and cell-mediated immune responses, but also among the two pathways within the cell-mediated system. This occurs through cellular signaling, commonly with proteins from the cytokine family. For example, helper T cells secrete specific cytokines such as interleukin-2 (IL-2), which helps B cells to differentiate into plasma cells. In addition, IL-2 secreted by helper T cells also assists cytotoxic T cells in transforming from inactive cells to active killers. Further, during phagocytosis by the APC it secretes interleukin-1 (IL-1), which is received by the helper T cell and aids in the activation of IL-2 production.

Important features of the skin immune system

The outermost surface of the skin serves as the first line of immunological defense. Colonies of flora, embedded on the surface of skin, prevent foreign pathogens from gaining access to the body's internal elements. In addition, sebum and stratum corneum lipids maintain a low pH, which is less favorable for the colonization of certain harmful bacteria. Other immediate defense mechanisms in skin consist of the mobilization of various immune cells, as previously discussed. The launch of signaling proteins, such as cytokines and chemokines, or antimicrobial peptides may also form part of the skin's first response. Keratinocytes can mount an immune response through the secretion of the antimicrobial peptide beta-defensin or the many inflammatory cytokines, such as TNF-alfa, IL-1, IL-6, IL-8, and IL-10. Phagocytes, such as macrophages, also play an extremely important role in the skin immune system. They contain receptors on the cell surface that can identify distinguishing molecular markers on the surface of bacteria and fungi. Toll-like receptors fall in the category of one such class of receptors. As already mentioned, Langerhans cells also carry out an essential function in the skin immune system. After capturing antigens in the epidermis, they migrate to lymph tissue where they present antigen to T cells, which launch a full immune response. An illustration of inflammatory response initiated by the skin immune system as a result of UV irradiation, which can cause photoimmunosuppression, or exposure to foreign pathogens is shown in Figure 1.17.[62] As demonstrated in the figure, there is a great deal of complexity in the communication between keratinocytes, fibroblasts, immune cells (T cells, B cells, and leukocytes), and Langerhans cells.

CONCLUDING REMARKS

This chapter has attempted to cover some of the fundamental concepts involving the structure and function of skin. The skin is a very intricate structure that maintains homeostasis through a variety of mechanisms. Epidermal cells (keratinocytes) undergo differentiation to produce stratified epithelial layers, resulting in a stratum corneum that prevents TEWL (from inside the body to outside in the environment) and the invasion of foreign pathogens. The macromolecules that constitute the dermis provide the skin with its unique mechanical properties. These consist of collagen, elastin, and other molecules that comprise the ground substance—the material found in extracellular space. The dermis also houses a vascular network that nourishes the skin. The epidermis and dermis are connected together by a fine protein fiber network, predominantly made of collagens and laminins. We also present concepts related to the anatomy and physiology of skin appendages, such as sudoriferous glands (eccrine/apocrine), the pilosebaceous unit, and the nail unit. In addition, skin carries out an extremely important role in immunity. In addition to resident immune cells, e.g., keratinocytes and Langerhans cells, other immune cells can be deployed to the skin to ward off attack by foreign invaders. As we will find throughout this text, all of the morphological components of skin described in this chapter are involved in free radical and antioxidant processes.

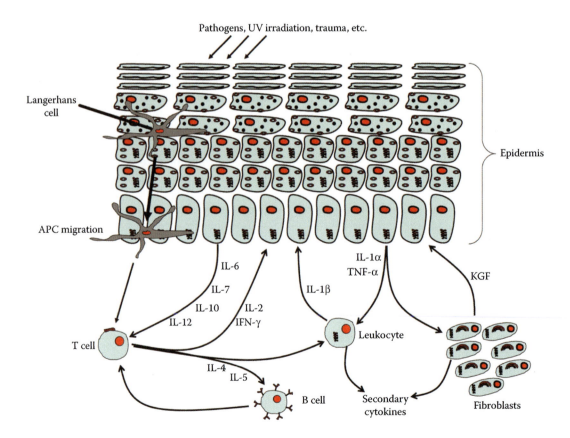

Figure 1.17 Cellular signaling during the inflammatory response. (Adapted from Rich, B.E. and Kupper, T.S., *Curr. Biol.*, 11, R531–R534, 2001.)

REFERENCES

1. Chu DH et al. The structure and development of skin. In: Freedberg IM, Eisen AZ, Wolff K, Austen KF, Goldsmith LA, Katz SI (Eds.). *Fitzpatrick's Dermatology in General Medicine*. I, 6th ed. New York: McGraw-Hill; 2003, pp. 58–88.
2. Michniak-Kohn BB et al. Skin: Physiology and penetration pathways. In: Rosen MR (Ed.). *Delivery System Handbook for Personal Care and Cosmetic Products*. Norwich, NY: William Andrew Publishing; 2005, pp. 77–100.
3. Harding CR et al. Ceramides and the skin. In: Baran R, Maibach HI (Eds.). *Textbook of Cosmetic Dermatology*, 3rd ed. London: Taylor & Francis Group; 2005, pp. 171–86.
4. Motta S et al. *Biochim Biophys Acta*. 1993;1182:147–151.
5. Forslind B. *Acta Derm Venereol*. 1994;74:1–6.
6. Bouwstra JA et al. *J Lipid Res*. 2001;42:1759–1770.
7. Wertz PW. Integral lipids of hair and stratum corneum. In: Jollès P, Zahn H, Höcker H (Eds.). *Formation and Structure of Human Hair*. Basel, Switzerland: Birkhäuser Verlag; 1997, pp. 227–238.
8. Norlén L. *J Invest Dermatol*. 2001;117:830–836.
9. Bouwstra J A et al. *J Invest Dermatol*. 2002;118:897–898.
10. Green KJ, Simpson CL. *J Invest Dermatol*. 2007;127:2499–2515.
11. Niessen CM. *J Invest Dermatol*. 2007;127:2525–2532.
12. Mese G et al. *J Invest Dermatol*. 2007;127:2516–2524.
13. Woodley DT, Chen M. The basement membrane zone. In: Freinkel RK, Woodley DT (Eds.). *The Biology of the Skin*. New York: The Parthenon Publishing Group; 2001. pp. 133–152.
14. Marieb EN. *Human Anatomy and Physiology*, 7th ed. Menlo Park, CA: Benjamin Cummings; 2006.
15. Matthews CK, van Holde KE. *Biochemistry*, 2nd ed. Redwood City, CA: Benjamin Cummings; 1996.
16. Sato K. *Rev Physiol Biochem Pharmacol*. 1977;79:51–131.
17. Sato K et al. *J Am Acad Dermatol*. 1989;20:537–563.
18. Groscurth P. Anatomy of sweat glands. In: Kreyden OP, Böni R, Burg G (Eds.). *Hyperhidrosis and Botulin Toxin in Dermatology: Current Problems in Dermatology*. Basel, Switzerland: Karger; 2002.
19. Munger BL. *J Biophys Biomed Cytol*. 1961;11:385–402.
20. Saga K. *Progr Histochem Cytochem*. 2002;37:323–386.
21. Hurley HJ. The eccrine sweat glands: Structure and function. In: Freinkel RK, Woodley DT (Eds.). *The Biology of the Skin*. New York: The Parthenon Publishing Group; 2002, pp. 47–76.
22. Goldsmith LA (Ed.). *Physiology, Biochemistry, and Molecular Biology of the Skin*. New York: Oxford University Press; 1991.
23. Quinton PM et al. Structure and function of human sweat glands. In: Laden K (Ed.). *Antiperspirants and Deodorants*. New York: Marcel Dekker; 1999, pp. 17–57.
24. Montagna W. *J Soc Cosmet Chem*. 1963;14:641–652.
25. van der Putte SCJ. *Am J Dermatopathol*. 1994;16:23–30.
26. Kiani M et al. The hair follicle: An underutilized source of cells and materials for regenerative medicine. *ACS Biomat Sci Eng*. 2017; Article ASAP. doi:10.1021/acsbiomaterials.7b00072.
27. Sehrawat M et al. *Pigment Int*. 2017;4:7–12.
28. Trüeb R. *Int J Trichology*. 2009;1:6–14.
29. Arck P et al. *FASEB J*. 2006;20:1567–1569.
30. Shi Y et al. *PLoS One*. 2014;9(4):e93589.
31. Wood J et al. *FASEB J*. 2009;23:2065–2075.
32. Schallreuter K et al. *Pigment Cell Melanoma Res*. 2011;24:51–62.
33. Tobin D. *Curr Probl Dermatol*. 2015;47:128–138.
34. Robbins CR. *Chemical and Physical Behavior of Human Hair*, 5th ed. Berlin: Springer-Verlag; 2012.
35. Jollès P et al. *Formation and Structure of Human Hair*. Basel, Switzerland: Birkhäuser Verlag; 1997.
36. Forslind B, Lindberg M. *Skin, Hair, and Nails: Structure and Function*. New York: Marcel Dekker; 2004.
37. Bouillon C, Wilkinson J. *The Science of Hair Care*. Boca Raton, FL: CRC Press; 2005.
38. Piersol GA. *Human Anatomy*. Philadelphia, PA: J.B. Lippincott Company; 1908.
39. Swift JA. The description of the microfibrils and macrofibrils as well as their arrangement in the matrix was contributed by J. Alan Swift. 2008.
40. Powell BC, Rogers GE. The role of keratin proteins and their genes in the growth, structure and properties of hair. In: Jollès P, Zahn H, Höcker H (Eds.). *Formation and Structure of Human Hair*. Basel, Switzerland: Birkhäuser Verlag; 1997.
41. Swift JA. The structure and chemistry of human hair. In: Evans T, RR Wickett (Eds.). *Practical Modern Hair Science*. Carol Stream, IL: Allured; 2012. pp. 1–37.
42. Jones LN, Rivett DE. *Micron* 1997;28:469–485.
43. Garcia ML, et al. *J Soc Cosmet Chem*. 1978;29:155–175.
44. Wolfram L. *J Am Acad Dermatol*. 2003;48:S106–S114.
45. Swift JA, Smith JR. *J Microsc*. 2001;204:203–211.
46. von Allwörden K. *Z Angew Chem*. 1916;29:77–88.
47. Zouboulis CC et al. *Exp Dermatol*. 2008;17:542–551.
48. Strauss JS et al. Sebaceous glands. In: Goldsmith LA (Ed.). *Physiology, Biochemistry, and Molecular Biology of the Skin*. I. New York: Oxford University Press; 1991, pp. 712–740.
49. Botek AA, Lookingbill DP. The structure and function of sebaceous glands. In: Freinkel RK, Woodley DT (Eds.). *The Biology of the Skin*. New York: The Parthenon Publishing Group; 2001, pp. 87–100.
50. Montagna W, Parakkal PF. *The Structure and Function of Skin*. New York: Academic Press; 1974.
51. Leyden JJ. *J Am Acad Dermatol*. 1995;32:S15–S25.
52. Smith KR, Thiboutot DM. Sebaceous gland lipids: Friend or foe? *J Lipid Res*. 2008;49:271–281.
53. Liao DC. *J Fam Practice*. 2003;52(1):43–51.
54. Thiele JJ, Weber SU, Packer L. *J Invest Dermatol*. 1999;113:1006–1010.
55. Passi S et al. *Free Radic Res*. 2002;36:471–477.
56. Passi S et al. *Biofactors*. 2003;18:289–297.

57. Levit EK, Scher RK. Basic science of the nail unit. In: Freinkel RK, Woodley DT (Eds.). *The Biology of the Skin*. New York: The Parthenon Publishing Group; 2001, pp. 101–112.
58. de Berker D, Forslind B. The structure and properties of nails and periungual tissues. In: Forslind B, Lindberg M (Eds.). *Skin, Hair, and Nails*. New York: Marcel Dekker; 2004, pp. 377–390.
59. Tosti A, Piraccini BM. Biology of nails. In: Freedberg IM, Eisen AZ, Wolf K, Austen KF, Goldsmith LA, Katz SI (Eds.). *Fitzpatrick's Dermatology in General Medicine. I*. New York: McGraw-Hill; 2003, pp. 159–163.
60. Ovaskainen M-L et al. *Am J Clin Nutr*. 1993;57:662–665.
61. Puchau B, et al. *Biol Trace Elem Res*. 2010;133:304–312.
62. Rich BE, Kupper TS. *Curr Biol*. 2001;11:R531–R534.

Free radicals in biology

> All radicals are not oxidants.
> And all oxidants are not radicals.
>
> —William A. Pryor
> *Natural Antioxidants in Human Health and Disease*

The evolution of life on Earth traces an anaerobic environment to an aerobic environment. The consequences of living in an oxygen-rich atmosphere, *ca.* 21% O_2, results in some negative outcomes, especially in terms of oxidation or the generation of free radicals. For example, free radical damage is believed to be involved in or responsible for a number of diseases, including cancer, cardiovascular disease, Parkinson's disease, Alzheimer's disease, cataracts, and diseases of the immune system.[1] In biological species, the onset of free radical damage occurs when free radicals are produced in the healthy cell. This results in molecular damage to cellular components, such as lipids, proteins, and DNA, eventually leading to a damaged cell and, finally, disease state or cell death. Free radical damage in tissues can be caused by exposure to ultraviolet (UV) radiation, ozone, smoke, and certain drugs. As the outermost protective organ of the body, the skin continuously finds itself in contact with such dangerous elements. In addition, there are many processes that occur in mammalian biology that produce free radicals. Two endogenous examples of free radical sources consist of the mitochondrial electron transport chain and the inflammatory process, which is part of our immune response to ward off foreign pathogens. Chemically, the formation of free radicals may occur as the result of covalent bond scission, an electron transfer reaction (Fe, Cu, Mn, etc.), or lipid peroxidation. This chapter will explore the various topics related to free radical mechanisms that occur in biological systems. In particular, the various radical species that an organism may encounter, the sources of radicals, and the types of reactions they are likely to be involved in will be thoroughly reviewed.

TERMINOLOGY

The reader is advised to bear in mind the following defined terminology while progressing through this chapter, and to refer back to it as needed:

Radical: An atom or molecule with one or more electrons that are not paired together in an orbital. Radicals can be neutral, positively charged, or negatively charged. Often a radical is defined as a species that contains an odd number of electrons.[2]

Free radical: A radical that has moved from the original vicinity where it was created.[3]

Covalent bond: Two electrons with opposite spins that share the same orbital.

Oxidation: The addition of oxygen, or the withdraw of hydrogen, or the withdrawal of electrons with or without the withdrawal of protons.[4]

Reduction: The withdrawal of oxygen, or the addition of hydrogen, or the addition of electrons, with or without the addition of protons.[4]

REACTIVE OXYGEN AND NITROGEN SPECIES

Typically, when free radical species in human physiology are discussed, this usually refers to reactive oxygen species (ROS) and reactive nitrogen species (RNS). Table 2.1 contains a list of some of the most common ROS and RNS found in biology. For clarity, the radical and nonradical species for each class have been grouped separately. In addition, the table also includes another class of reactive species that involves sulfur. Typical sulfur-containing molecules include proteins or enzymes, as well as some low molecular weight compounds, such as glutathione (Chapter 3). An in-depth discussion of the different types of ROS and RNS is provided in the subsections that follow.

Table 2.1 ROS, RNS, and other species involved in the free radical chemistry of biological organisms.

Reactive oxygen species	Reactive nitrogen species	Miscellaneous
Free Radicals		
Superoxide ($O_2^{\bullet-}$)	Nitric oxide ($NO^{\bullet}$)	Thiyl ($RS^{\bullet}$)
Hydroxyl ($HO^{\bullet}$)	Nitrogen dioxide ($NO_2^{\bullet}$)	Hydrogen ($H^{\bullet}$)
Alkoxyl ($RO^{\bullet}$)		
Peroxyl ($RO_2^{\bullet}$)		
Hydroperoxyl ($HO_2^{\bullet}$)		
Nonradicals		
Singlet oxygen ($^1O_2$)	Peroxynitrite (ONO_2^-)	Thiol (RSH)
Hydrogen peroxide (H_2O_2)	Peroxynitrous acid (ONO_2H)	
Alkyl peroxides (RO_2H)	Nitronium cation (NO_2^+)	
Ozone (O_3)	Nitrosyl cation (NO^+)	
Nitrosyl cation (NO^+)	Nitrosyl anion (NO^-)	
Hypochlorous acid (HOCl)	Dinitrogen trioxide (N_2O_3)	
	Dinitrogen teroxide (N_2O_4)	
	Nitrous acid (HNO_2)	
	Nitrosothiol (RSNO)	
	Alkyl peroxynitrite (RO_2NO)	

Hydroxyl radical (HO·)

The hydroxyl radical (HO·) is considered the most deleterious radical encountered in biological systems due to its high reactivity. Its reaction with a substrate is only limited by its ability to maneuver (diffusion-controlled) and it is considered to be a nonselective radical. The two most common routes for the formation of HO· are the Fenton reaction or homolytic bond scission by UV irradiation. The production of HO· by the Fenton reaction relies on the presence of an Fe^{2+} salt and hydrogen peroxide (H_2O_2).

$$Fe^{2+} + H_2O_2 \rightarrow Fe^{3+} + HO^- + HO^· \quad (2.1)$$

Reaction 2.1 is a very well-known reaction that was first observed by Fenton in the late 1800s. In the 1930s, Haber, Wilstätter, and Weiss were working in this area and were able to elucidate subsequent mechanisms associated with the original Fenton reaction. The ensuing reactions came to become known as the Haber–Weiss cycle.[5]

$$HO^· + H_2O_2 \rightarrow H_2O + O_2^{·-} + H^+ \quad (2.2)$$

$$O_2^{·-} + H^+ + H_2O_2 \rightarrow H_2O + O_2^{·-} + H^+ \quad (2.3)$$

Another source of HO· is the absorption of UV irradiation by H_2O_2 and results in a homolytic scission reaction yielding two hydroxyl radicals.

$$H-O-O-H \xrightarrow{h\nu} 2HO^· \quad (2.4)$$

In general, the HO· is able to react with various species by three different pathways. First, HO· can abstract a proton from the substrate, usually a C–H bond.

$$HO^· + R-H \xrightarrow{h\nu} H_2O + R^· \quad (2.5)$$

Secondly, HO· can also oxidize metals as a result of the transfer of an electron from the metal to the radical. As shown in Reaction 2.6, this yields water and a higher valence state of the metal.

$$M^{n+} + HO^· \rightarrow M^{n+1} + H_2O \quad (2.6)$$

Last, HO· can participate in an addition reaction to a double bond.

$$HO^· + \overset{\diagdown}{\underset{\diagup}{C}}=\overset{\diagup}{\underset{\diagdown}{C}} \longrightarrow OH-\overset{|}{\underset{|}{C}}-\overset{|}{\underset{|}{C}}^· \quad (2.7)$$

Superoxide anion ($O_2^{·-}$)

Despite its name, the superoxide anion ($O_2^{·-}$) is a far less reactive radical species than HO·; however, it can also be dangerous, because it can participate in further reactions resulting in the formation of HO·. Biological sources of $O_2^{·-}$ include phagocytotic cells, such as those described in Table 1.3 in Chapter 1, in which the cells experience a *respiratory burst* during the immune response and their oxygen consumption is greatly increased.[6] During this process the formation of $O_2^{·-}$ is catalyzed by the enzyme, nicotinamide adenine dinucleotide phosphate (NADPH) oxidase, and NADPH is utilized as a source of electrons.

$$2O_2 + NADPH \rightarrow NADP^+ + H^+ + 2O_2^{·-} \quad (2.8)$$

Additional enzymes also catalyze the formation of $O_2^{·-}$. One that receives a great deal of attention in the literature is xanthine oxidase, an enzyme discussed in Chapter 3 with regard to the metabolism of purines to uric acid. In addition, $O_2^{·-}$ is formed when certain molecules undergo autoxidation in the presence of O_2. Some examples of these compounds consist of reduced flavin mononucleotide, reduced flavin adenine dinucleotide (FAD), L-DOPA, adrenalin, noradrenalin, dopamine, and so on (see Appendix 2).[7] Heme-containing proteins, such as hemoglobin and myoglobin, are also responsible for the release of $O_2^{·-}$. It is believed that during the process of O_2 binding to the coordinated Fe^{2+} atom of a heme group, an occasional $O_2^{·-}$ escapes from the transition state.[7] More than likely, the principal source of $O_2^{·-}$ in biological systems is probably the mitochondrial electron transport chain (see the section of this chapter on endogenous sources of free radicals). As electrons are passed from one complex to another along the electron transport chain, an occasional electron is leaked from one of the complexes and is able to react with O_2, leading to the formation of $O_2^{·-}$. As stated, $O_2^{·-}$ itself is not very lethal; however, it can lead to the formation of HO·. Since $O_2^{·-}$ is metabolized (Chapter 3) by superoxide dismutase to H_2O_2, it can further undergo the Fenton reaction, ultimately leading to the production of HO·. This proceeds by Reaction 3.1 in Chapter 3, in which two radicals of $O_2^{·-}$ react with two protons, resulting in the production of H_2O_2 and O_2. A second fate for $O_2^{·-}$ is its involvement in a reaction similar to the Fenton reaction in which $O_2^{·-}$ oxidizes a metal, typically Fe^{3+} or Cu^{2+}, which is then capable of reducing H_2O_2 and producing HO·.

$$Cu^{2+} + O_2^{·-} \rightarrow Cu^+ + O \quad (2.9)$$

$$Cu^+ + H_2O_2 \rightarrow Cu^{2+} + HO^- + HO^· \quad (2.10)$$

These reactions are known as the Haber–Weiss reactions.

Singlet oxygen ($^1O_2$)

Singlet oxygen ($^1O_2$) is an excited state species of ground state molecular oxygen (O_2). In contrast, the O_2 that we breathe every day and takes part in aerobic metabolism is a diradical triplet species. This can be attributed to an electron located on each oxygen molecule of O_2, in which case both electrons are degenerate (equal in energy) and have the same spins; however, they are in distinct orbitals since they are located on different atoms. In contrast,

$^1O_2$ is not a radical and arises as a high-energy state of O_2 in which the two unpaired electrons of O_2 are paired together in the same orbital. The formation of $^1O_2$ occurs in the presence of a photosensitizer, which is a chromophore that absorbs light and is excited to a higher energy level—an excited state. The energy absorbed by the photosensitizer can then be transferred to an adjacent molecule of O_2, allowing the photosensitizer to return to its ground state and the O_2 molecule to transform into its excited state species, $^1O_2$. There are two possible singlet states for O_2, $^1\Delta g$ or $^1\Sigma g^+$, with the former being the most predominant species found and what is referred to throughout this text.

Once the excited state species has been reached, that is, $^1O_2$, there are two fates for the dissipation of energy. $^1O_2$ can be quenched by another molecule inasmuch as its energy can be transferred to another species, resulting in the migration of $^1O_2$ back to the ground state (O_2) and the species receiving the energy transfer entering into an excited state. A second destiny for $^1O_2$ is to undergo reactions with compounds containing conjugated systems of double bonds, such as carotenoids and fatty acids. These types of reactions usually result in addition of the oxygen atoms to the substrate, resulting in the formation of hydroperoxides or endoperoxides.[7]

Alkoxyl (RO·), peroxyl (RO₂·), and hydroperoxyl (HO₂·) radicals

Due to their involvement in deleterious lipid peroxidation reactions, the alkoxyl and peroxyl radicals are often referred to as lipid alkoxyl (RO·) and lipid peroxyl (RO₂·) radicals, respectively. As shown in Chapter 5—dedicated to the topic of lipid peroxidation—the $RO_2^\bullet$ radical is formed as a result of the reaction between a carbon-centered radical and O_2. Further, $RO_2^\bullet$ can abstract a proton from a substrate, typically a polyunsaturated fatty acid, giving rise to a lipid hydroperoxide (ROOH) (Chapter 5). A common biological fate of ROOH is the reaction with a transition metal.[7] For example, ROOH may react with either one of the oxidation states of iron, resulting in the formation of $RO_2^\bullet$ or $RO^\bullet$:

$$ROOH + Fe^{3+} \to RO_2^\bullet + Fe^{2+} + H^+ \quad (2.11)$$

$$ROOH + Fe^{2+} \to RO^\bullet + Fe^{3+} + OH^- \quad (2.12)$$

Hence, the presence of transition metals adversely affects the homeostasis of the cell by contributing to the regeneration of radical species.

The simplest form of $RO_2^\bullet$ is when R is equal to H—the hydroperoxyl radical ($HO_2^\bullet$). This species is in fact the protonated form of $O_2^{\bullet-}$; however, the presence of $HO_2^\bullet$ from this source in biological tissues is very minute, because the pKa of dissociation is low (≈ 4.8).[7] Hence:

$$HO_2^\bullet \rightleftharpoons H^+ + O_2^{\bullet-} \quad (2.13)$$

Hydrogen peroxide (H₂O₂)

As can be seen throughout this text, H_2O_2, like other ROS, is a normal byproduct of aerobic metabolism. Endogenous sources of H_2O_2 include various enzymes, the mitochondrial electron transport chain, the respiratory burst by phagocytes, the cytochrome P-450 family of enzymes, and peroxisomes. Enzymatic sources of H_2O_2 include superoxide dismutase, xanthine oxidase, D-amino oxidase, and urate oxidase.[7] The latter two of this group are present in peroxisomes—small cellular organelles responsible for eliminating toxins from the cell, as well as beta-oxidation of fatty acids and decomposition of amino acids. As a result of these peroxisomal processes, H_2O_2 is formed. The production of H_2O_2 by the electron transport chain and respiratory burst stem from the formation of $O_2^{\bullet-}$ by these processes, which is dismutated by superoxide dismutase to H_2O_2.

In turn, H_2O_2 can be decomposed by enzymes, such as catalase, present in peroxisomes, or glutathione peroxidase, usually found in the cytoplasm or mitochondrion. In vivo, H_2O_2 is not very reactive and is considered to be a weak oxidizing and reducing agent; however, it is considered to be toxic at cellular concentrations of 10–100 μM.[7] Unlike $O_2^{\bullet-}$, H_2O_2 can cross lipid bilayer membranes, which can be dangerous if it escapes from an organelle and is able to react with a transition metal, such as Fe^{2+}, yielding the extremely reactive $HO^\bullet$ radical (see the section that discussed $HO^\bullet$ earlier).

In addition, H_2O_2 can also cause cellular damage by deactivating thiol (RSH) and heme-containing proteins by reacting with these sites. To conclude, H_2O_2 can be decomposed by UV irradiation, which serves as yet another source for the formation of $HO^\bullet$.

$$H_2O_2 + h\nu \to 2HO^\bullet \quad (2.14)$$

Hypochlorous acid (HOCl)

As part of the inflammatory response, H_2O_2 and $O_2^{\bullet-}$ are produced by activated leukocytes, such as neutrophils. Also presented at the site of infection by the same cells is the heme-containing enzyme myeloperoxidase, which catalyzes the reaction between H_2O_2 and chlorine to yield hypochlorous acid (HOCl):

$$H_2O_2 + Cl^- \to HOCl \quad (2.15)$$

HOCl—which, by the way, is the active ingredient in household bleach—is considered to be the most abundant and powerful oxidant produced by the leukocytes. The primary oxidation targets of HOCl are RSH groups, ascorbate, tryptophan residues, and urate.[8] HOCl can also execute chlorination reactions—wreaking havoc on the tyrosine residues of proteins, pyrimidine bases of DNA, unsaturated lipids, and cholesterol.[7]

Ozone (O₃)

The existence of ozone (O_3) in nature has come to serve two distinct functions. On the one hand, the presence of O_3 in the stratosphere provides a protective layer for earth-dwelling species against the extremely harmful effects of UVC and some UVB radiation from the Sun. In contrast, O_3 that is present at ground level in the troposphere can be detrimental to the livelihood of mammalian species as it may act as an oxidant at the surface of the skin and in the respiratory system. A well-known degradation pathway for unsaturated fatty acids and lipids is a process known as Criegee ozonation, where O_3 adds to double bonds to form a Criegee ozonide (Figure 2.1), which contains a peroxide bond that may decompose to form radicals.[9] Other possible routes to radical formation as a result of O_3 exposure are electron-transfer reactions ultimately leading to the formation of $HO^{\bullet}$.[9]

$$R + O_3 \rightarrow R^{\bullet+} + O_3^{\bullet-} \qquad (2.16)$$

$$O_3^{\bullet-} + H^+ \rightarrow O_2 + HO^{\bullet} \qquad (2.17)$$

R represents electron donor species such as RSHs, amines, and phenolic compounds. In proteins, the amino acids cysteine, tryptophan, tyrosine, histidine, and methionine fall into this category and are known targets of O_3.[7] It has also been well established that O_3 in aqueous solutions may interact with the carbonyl oxide, also leading to $HO^{\bullet}$ formation.[9]

Reactive nitrogen species

In addition to ROS, RNS have evolved as an important class of radical species in biology. The simplest molecule from this group, nitric oxide ($NO^{\bullet}$), is believed to play many roles in human physiology and biochemistry. For example, useful roles of $NO^{\bullet}$ include its participation in vasodilation and neurotransmission. Alternatively, $NO^{\bullet}$ is released by phagocytes during the immune/inflammatory response where it serves as a combatant of pathogens,

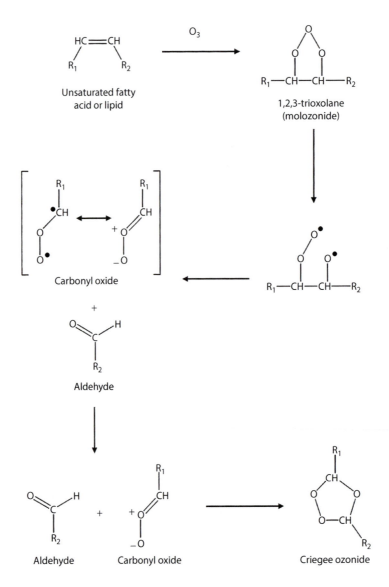

Figure 2.1 Criegee ozonation of unsaturated molecules.

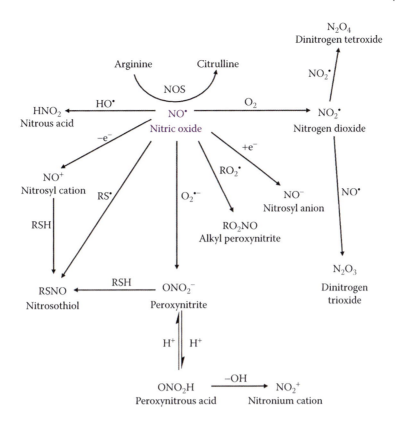

Figure 2.2 RNS in biological systems. (Adapted from Acworth, I. et al., The analysis of free radicals, their reaction products, and antioxidants, in Baskin, S. and Salem, H. [Eds.], *Oxidants, Antioxidants, and Free Radicals*, Taylor & Francis Group, Washington, DC, 23–77, 1997.)

which threaten cellular homeostasis. The complexity of the relationship between $NO^{\bullet}$ and other RNS is demonstrated in Figure 2.2.[10]

First, please note that the synthesis of $NO^{\bullet}$ is a result of the enzymatic conversion of arginine to citrulline (Appendix 2) in the presence of O_2 and NADPH.[11] The enzymes responsible for this reaction belong to the family $NO^{\bullet}$ synthases. While Figure 2.2 may be a simplified diagram with respect to the overall RNS chemistry, it illustrates the formation of other RNS and ROS from $NO^{\bullet}$, which may be more deleterious to cellular viability than $NO^{\bullet}$ itself. For example, while $NO^{\bullet}$ may serve several positive functions, the creation of nitrogen dioxide ($NO_2^{\bullet}$) and peroxynitrite (ONO_2^-) almost always leads to injury.[12] A full discussion of the role played by RNS in human biology is beyond the scope of the current discussion; however, it is the author's intention to provide the reader with a general commentary on this subject. For a more thorough review of this subject matter the reader is referred to several comprehensive publications specifically devoted to RNS.[13–17]

Thiyl radicals ($RS^{\bullet}$)

As stated in other sections of this text, sulfur containing proteins and low molecular weight sulfur compounds, such as glutathione, play an important and crucial role in the endogenous antioxidant network that helps to maintain cellular homeostasis. In fact, RSHs play a dual role in which they can serve as antioxidants or are capable of becoming free radical species. For example, RSH can react with other radicals, such as $HO^{\bullet}$ and $RO_2^{\bullet}$, to yield thiyl radicals ($RS^{\bullet}$). In addition, $RS^{\bullet}$ can be formed by the reaction of RSH with transition metals, such as Fe^{3+} or Cu^{2+}, or by the cleavage of a disulfide bond in either proteins or reduced glutathione. As a result of $RS^{\bullet}$ formation, other free radical species may be formed and antioxidants may be depleted.

FREE RADICAL REACTIONS

In general, there are three types of reactions in relation to biological free radical chemistry. These are briefly reviewed in the subsections that follow and consist of atom abstraction, electron transfer, and radical addition reactions. These reactions often take place during free radical-related processes, such as lipid peroxidation. In fact, examples of atom abstraction, radical addition reactions, and homolytic bond cleavage are observed in lipid peroxidation processes. Please see Chapter 5 for a thorough discussion of lipid peroxidation.

Atom abstraction

This type of reaction usually takes place between a radical species ($A^{\bullet}$) and a molecule containing a covalently bound hydrogen atom.

$$A^{\bullet} + RH \rightarrow AH + R^{\bullet} \qquad (2.18)$$

Electron transfer

Electron transfer reactions usually take place between metal ions; however, as indicated in Chapter 3 they are also very common with enzyme cofactors such as nicotinamide adenine dinucleotide (NADH), FAD, glutathione, and so forth.

$$A^{\bullet-} + B \rightarrow A + B^{\bullet-} \quad (2.19)$$

Radical addition

In this type of reaction, the radical species can either add to a double bond (Equation 2.20) or, alternatively, two radicals may combine to form a covalent bond together (Equation 2.21).

$$A^{\bullet} + \underset{R}{\overset{H}{C}}=\underset{R}{\overset{H}{C}} \longrightarrow \underset{R}{\overset{A}{C}}-\underset{R}{\overset{\bullet}{C}} \quad (2.20)$$

$$A^{\bullet} + A^{\bullet} \rightarrow A_2 \quad (2.21)$$

ENDOGENOUS SOURCES OF FREE RADICALS

As part of normal aerobic metabolism, free radicals are continuously produced in the body. For example, oxidative phosphorylation, via the mitochondrial electron transport chain, is the primary source of cellular energy in the form of adenosine triphosphate (ATP). Unfortunately, due to an occasional leak in the transport chain free radical species may be liberated in the cell. It is estimated that 1%–3% of the mitochondrial intake of O_2 each day is converted to ROS.[18] Further, during the inflammatory response phagocytes are deployed, which destroy foreign pathogens by generating free radical species. Free radicals are also produced during the metabolism of xenobiotic compounds in which byproducts of the degradation reactions are often ROS. Many cellular enzymatic processes also yield ROS or RNS, whether it is by mistake or as part of the inflammatory response. Finally, free transition metals in the cytoplasm, such as those discussed in preceding sections, can be involved in the Fenton or Haber–Weiss reactions ultimately producing $HO^{\bullet}$. For illustration, Figure 2.3

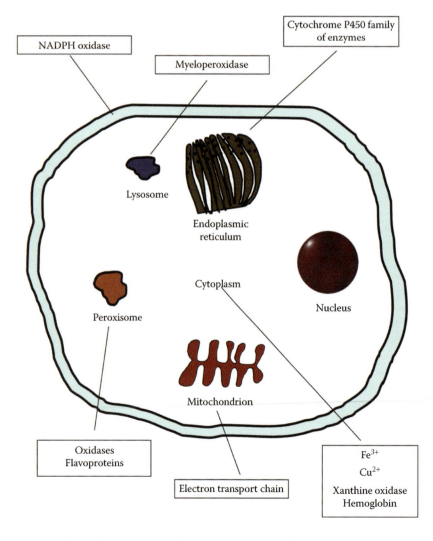

Figure 2.3 Cellular sources of free radicals. (Adapted from Kehrer, J. and Smith, C., Free radicals in biology: Sources, reactivities, and roles in the etiology of human diseases, in Frei, B. [Ed.], *Natural Antioxidants in Human Health and Disease*, Academic Press, San Diego, CA, 1994.)

contains a rudimentary schematic of the cell and some of the possible sources of ROS or RNS.

Mitochondrial electron transport chain

The electron transport chain is found in the inner mitochondrial membrane of eukaryotic cells and consists of a series of proteolipid complexes. It is likely one of the most important energy harnessing processes in biochemistry. In general, electrons are passed along the electron transport chain within the membrane, resulting in proton pumps at several of the complexes in which protons are shuttled from within the mitochondrial matrix across the inner membrane and into the intermembrane space. As a result, the [H$^+$] is greater in the intermembrane space than in the matrix of the mitochondrion. Consequently, proton motive force is garnered from this series of events and is utilized to synthesize ATP, the basic source of energy for the cell.

As shown in Figure 2.4, there are five protein complexes that constitute the mitochondrial electron transport chain. Electrons are passed from complex to complex by molecules such as coenzyme Q (Chapter 3) and cytochrome c (Appendix 2). As a result of electron transfer, protons are transferred at several of the complexes from the mitochondrial matrix to intermembrane space. The resulting concentration gradient causes protons to be funneled back to the mitochondrial matrix via Complex V, known as ATP synthase (F_0F_1), providing the energy necessary to synthesize ATP.

The electron transport chain is known to be an endogenous source of free radicals, as it can sometimes leak electrons. It is believed that electron leakage is in fact the release of $O_2^{\cdot-}$, which is thought to occur most frequently at Complexes I and III in the transport chain. The source of $O_2^{\cdot-}$ in Complex I is still a controversial subject; however, in Complex III it is believed to result from the autoxidation of the ubisemiquinone anion (UQ$^{\cdot-}$) radical.[19]

In addition, the mitochondrion is also believed to be a large source of H_2O_2.[20] Since $O_2^{\cdot-}$ can be dismutated to H_2O_2, and further, H_2O_2 can serve as a potential source for HO$^{\cdot}$, this can be very detrimental for cellular viability. For further reading on the subject of free radical production in mitochondria, the reader is referred to several reviews that have been written on this topic.[19–21]

Phagocytic cells

As discussed in Chapter 1, part of the body's immune response consists of the deployment of phagocytes (neutrophils, monocytes, etc.) in response to pathogen invasion. In order to kill bacteria, viruses, and infected cells, phagocytes produce a number of ROS and RNS. In fact, the immune cells experience a respiratory burst in which their O_2 consumption greatly increases, which ultimately leads to the development of $O_2^{\cdot-}$. The conversion of O_2 to $O_2^{\cdot-}$ is catalyzed by NADPH oxidase, which requires the presence of NADPH. Further, $O_2^{\cdot-}$ can undergo reactions that convert it first to H_2O_2, which as mentioned previously can diffuse across the organelle membrane and into the cytoplasm where it can be converted to the extremely reactive HO$^{\cdot}$. In addition, phagocytes are also known to produce HOCl and NO$^{\cdot}$. While the aim of the ROS or RNS is to destroy the foreign pathogen, often healthy cells also experience some form of damage as a result of the inflammatory response.

Peroxisomes

Similar to lysosomes, peroxisomes are organelles that rid the cell of toxins. Further, peroxisomes contain enzymes, which are capable of transferring hydrogen from selected substrates to oxygen, often resulting in the formation of H_2O_2—hence, the name peroxisome. Also, peroxisomes are equipped with the enzyme, catalase, which decomposes H_2O_2 to O_2 and H_2O. During the process of H_2O_2 decomposition, catalase also oxidizes other substrates, for

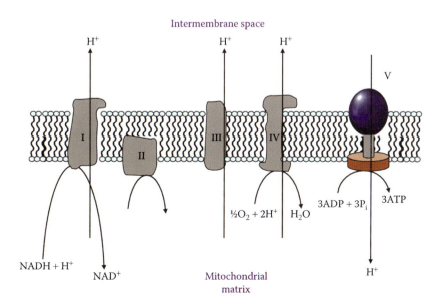

Figure 2.4 Electron transport chain located in the inner mitochondrial membrane.

example, alcohol, which are considered cellular toxins. In addition to other metabolic processes, a very important role played by peroxisomes is the beta-oxidation of long-chain fatty acids. Throughout the processes described earlier, it is conceivable that H_2O_2 could easily diffuse through the peroxisome membrane and into the cytoplasm, where it would be likely to encounter either iron or copper, thereby resulting in the Fenton reaction and ultimately leading to the formation of HO·.

Endoplasmic reticulum

The enzymes that are part of the Cytochrome P450 family play an essential role in the removal of toxins from the body. They are heme-containing proteins that are mostly present in the endoplasmic reticulum. The cytochrome P450 molecules typically act by hydroxylating xenobiotic substances, such as drugs and carcinogens, which makes the toxin more soluble and thus secretable by the organism. Often, byproducts of xenobiotic metabolism result in free radical species, which can compromise cellular homeostasis.

Heme proteins

Proteins that contain a prosthetic heme group, such as hemoglobin or myoglobin, are capable of binding O_2 to the coordinated iron atom of the porphyrin ring. Due to electron delocalization, the bound oxygen can sometimes be converted to $O_2^{·-}$.[7]

Enzymatic sources

In general, enzymes can be sources of free radicals as they are often involved in electron transfer reactions, which occasionally result in the leakage of electrons.[2] In addition, various enzymes that serve roles as oxidases can potentially be sources of free radical species. Several examples include:

D-amino acid oxidase: This enzyme is responsible for the eradication of unwanted amino acids in the cell.
Xanthine oxidase: As part of purine metabolism, the degradation of hypoxanthine to xanthine and xanthine to uric acid is achieved by xanthine oxidase (Chapter 3).
Nitric oxide synthase: Actually, this is a family of enzymes that is responsible for the synthesis of NO·.
Myeloperoxidase: During phagocytosis (already discussed) this enzyme is responsible for the formation of HOCl.
NADPH oxidase: As a membrane-bound protein, this enzyme participates in the production of $O_2^{·-}$ during phagocytosis.

Transition metals

Often, metals such as iron or copper serve as enzyme cofactors or they participate in electron transfer reactions in vivo. As mentioned throughout this text, the presence of free iron and copper in the cell can be deleterious to cell viability as these two metals are able to participate in the Fenton reaction, which results in the formation of HO·. In order to ward off such reactions, the cell is equipped with proteins that are able to sequester ions, thus preventing an ensuing oxidative cascade.

CONCLUDING REMARKS

The field of free radicals in biology has exploded in the last 30 years as evidenced by numerous publications in this area.[22–29] This chapter attempts to cover some of the basic technical aspects of free radical biology; however, one should be aware that only a general introduction to the subject is provided. A more thorough introduction can be found in the contemporary, yet classic, text by Halliwell and Gutteridge.[30]

REFERENCES

1. Ames B. Foreword. In: Frei B (Ed.). *Natural Antioxidants in Human Health and Disease*. San Diego, CA: Academic Press; 1994.
2. Pryor W. The role of free radical reactions in biological systems. In: Pryor W (Ed.). *Free Radicals in Biology. 1*. New York: Academic Press; 1976, pp. 1–49.
3. Kehrer J, Smith C. Free radicals in biology: Sources, reactivities, and roles in the etiology of human diseases. In: Frei B (Ed.). *Natural Antioxidants in Human Health and Disease*. San Diego, CA: Academic Press; 1994.
4. Clark W. *Oxidation-Reduction Potentials of Organic Systems*. Baltimore, MD: Williams & Wilkins; 1960, p. 6.
5. Koppenol W. *Redox Rep*. 2001;6:229–234.
6. Bensasson R et al. *Excited States and Free Radicals in Biology and Medicine: Contributions from Flash Photolysis and Pulse Radiolysis*. Oxford: University Press; 1993.
7. Halliwell B, Gutteridge J. *Free Radicals in Biology and Medicine*, 4th ed. Oxford: University Press; 2007.
8. Winterbourn C. *Toxicology*. 2002;181–182:223–227.
9. Pryor W. *Am J Clin Nutr*. 1991;53:702–722.
10. Acworth I et al. The analysis of free radicals, their reaction products, and antioxidants. In: Baskin S, Salem H (Eds.). *Oxidants, Antioxidants, and Free Radicals*. Washington, DC: Taylor & Francis Group; 1997, pp. 23–77.
11. Mathews C et al. *Biochemistry*, 4th ed. Upper Saddle River, NJ: Prentice Hall; 2012.
12. Halliwell B, Aruoma O. Free radicals and antioxidants: The need for in vivo markers of oxidative stress. In: Aruoma O, Cuppett S (Eds.). *Antioxidant Methodology: In Vivo and In Vitro Concepts*. Champaign, IL: AOCS; 1997, pp. 1–22.
13. Darley-Usmar V et al. *FEBS Lett*. 1995;369:131–135.
14. Dedon P, Tannenbaum S. *Arch Biochem Biophys*. 2004;423:12–22.
15. Patel R et al. *Biochim Biophys Acta*. 1999;1411:385–400.
16. Tamir S, Tannenbaum S. *Biochim Biophys Acta*. 1996;1288:F31–F36.
17. MacMicking J et al. *Annu Rev Immunol*. 1997;15:323–350.
18. Batandier C et al. *J Cell Mol Med*. 2002;6:175–187.
19. Ježek P, Hlavatá L. *Int J Biochem Cell Biol*. 2005;37:2478–2503.
20. Cadenas E, Davies K. *Free Rad Biol Med*. 2000;29:222–230.
21. Brand M et al. *Free Radic Biol Med*. 2004;37:755–767.

22. Frei B (Ed.). *Natural Antioxidants in Human Health and Disease.* San Diego, CA: Academic Press; 1994.
23. Moslen M, Smith C (Eds.). *Free Radical Mechanisms of Tissue Injury.* Boca Raton, FL: CRC Press; 1992.
24. Pryor W. *Free Radicals in Biology.* Vol. 1. New York: Academic Press; 1976.
25. Pryor W. *Free Radicals in Biology.* Vol. 2. New York: Academic Press; 1976.
26. Pryor W. *Free Radicals in Biology.* Vol. 3. New York: Academic Press; 1977.
27. Pryor W. *Free Radicals in Biology.* Vol. 4. New York: Academic Press; 1980.
28. Pryor W. *Free Radicals in Biology.* Vol. 5. New York: Academic Press; 1982.
29. Pryor W. Free radicals and lipid peroxidation: what they are and how they got that way. In: Frei B (Ed.). *Natural Antioxidants in Human Health and Disease.* San Diego, CA: Academic Press; 1994, pp. 25–62.
30. Halliwell B, Gutteridge J. *Free Radicals in Biology and Medicine*, 5th ed. Oxford: University Press; 2015.

The skin's endogenous antioxidant network

> Such terms as free radicals, antioxidants, and oxidative stress have experienced an almost inflationary use in the lay press and thus raised enormous interest in the public.
>
> —Jens Thiele and Peter Elsner
> *Oxidants and Antioxidants in Cutaneous Biology*

The epidermal antioxidant network consists of a complex defense system against oxidative stress in which the function of one antioxidant often supplements or regenerates another antioxidant. These important antioxidants consist of detoxication enzymes and small-molecule antioxidants, which can be further characterized as water-soluble and lipid-soluble antioxidants. In the case of the enzymes, each one contains a cofactor, which carries out the antioxidant activity—usually by electron transfer reactions that neutralize reactive oxygen species (ROS). The behavior of small-molecule antioxidants is partially determined by the solubility—either lipid- or water-soluble. Lipid-soluble antioxidants are found in cell membranes and other lipid-rich regions—for example, embedded in the lipid lamellar structures of the stratum corneum. One would expect to find most water-soluble small antioxidants in the cytosol; however, keep in mind that many free radical reactions also take place at interfaces. In general, small-molecule antioxidants can act as preventive antioxidants or radical-scavenging antioxidants (Figure 3.1).[1] Preventive antioxidants keep radicals from forming in the first place, while radical-scavenging antioxidants prevent the initiation of free radical chain reactions or they stop free radical chain reactions from propagating. Nevertheless, when antioxidants are not able to prevent free radical damage, the organism, or in this case the skin, is found in a state of oxidative stress leading to disease, cancer, or aging.

ENZYMATIC ANTIOXIDANTS

The endogenous enzymatic antioxidants in skin consist of superoxide dismutases (SODs), catalase, glutathione (GSH) peroxidase, NAD(P)H:Quinone reductase, and the thioredoxin (Trx) system, which catalyze the breakdown or consumption of compounds capable of initiating oxidation reactions. As already noted, the antioxidant enzymes are often referred to as detoxication enzymes. Typically, detoxication refers to those enzymes capable of metabolizing a diverse range of drugs and toxins.

Superoxide dismutases

SODs [EC 1.15.1.1] are metalloenzymes that catalyze the decomposition of superoxide anions ($O_2^{\cdot-}$), resulting in the formation of hydrogen peroxide (H_2O_2) and molecular oxygen (O_2).

$$2H^+ + O_2^{\cdot-} + O_2^{\cdot-} \rightarrow H_2O_2 + O_2 \quad (3.1)$$

There are three distinct forms of SOD found in mammalian tissues, which can be characterized by their physiological location. A dimeric form of the enzyme exists, which contains Cu^{2+} and Zn^{2+} at the active site, and is found in the cytoplasm and nucleus (Cu, Zn-SOD). There is also a tetrameric form of the enzyme that is found in the mitochondrion and contains Mn^{3+} at its active site (Mn-SOD).[2] In addition, there is an extracellular form of the SOD that also contains Cu^{2+} and Zn^{2+} at its active sites (EC-SOD). Table 3.1 contains a brief description of each enzyme in terms of its most common classification as well as an alternate naming sequence, the molecular mass (MM), the number of subunits, and the physiological location. In the case of each enzyme, the subunits are homogenous. EC-SOD is a glycoprotein that contains a domain capable of binding to the glycosaminoglycans, heparin, and heparan sulfate, as well as type I collagen, which are thought to serve as an anchor for the enzyme.[3,4] Proteolytic cleavage of EC-SOD's binding domain allows the enzyme to be secreted into intercellular space. Thus, it is the only species able to metabolize the $O_2^{\cdot-}$ anion outside of the cell.

Cu, Zn-SOD and Mn-SOD are structurally unique, not only in terms of the catalytically active ions, but also the protein secondary structure. As shown in Figure 3.2, Mn-SOD contains many more alpha-helices than Cu, Zn-SOD, which is more abundant in beta-sheets. Likewise, EC-SOD is equally distinct and only shares the commonality with Cu, Zn-SOD of utilizing Cu^{2+} and Zn^{2+} for its catalytic activity. In addition, mechanistic actions that take place in the active site during catalysis are different for each enzyme. However, aside from their differences, all of the SODs share the same course of action and outcome for deactivation of $O_2^{\cdot-}$. During the conversion of $O_2^{\cdot-}$, the active site ions in each enzyme are converted from an oxidized state (Cu^{2+} and Mn^{3+}) to a reduced state (Cu^+ and Mn^{2+}) then back to an oxidized state.[5]

$$SOD_{oxid} + O_2^{\cdot-} + H^+ \rightarrow SOD_{red} + O_2 \quad (3.2)$$

$$SOD_{red} + O_2^{\cdot-} + H^+ \rightarrow SOD_{oxid} + H_2O_2 \quad (3.3)$$

As shown in Equations 3.2 and 3.3, this phenomenon occurs by a two-step process in which one $O_2^{\cdot-}$ anion is bound to the enzyme in conjunction with a proton followed by the subsequent release of O_2. Second, another $O_2^{\cdot-}$ anion is bound by the enzyme along with another proton, ultimately leading to the generation of H_2O_2.

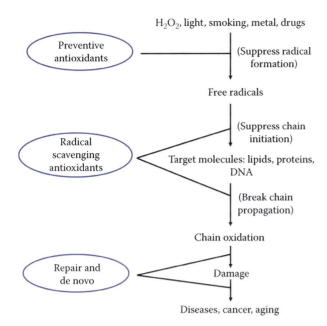

Figure 3.1 Defense systems against oxidative damage. (Adapted from Rangarajan, M. and Zatz, J.L., *J. Cosmet. Sci.*, 50, 249–279, 1999.)

Table 3.1 Superoxide dismutases found in mammalians.

Enzyme	Alternate name	MM (kDa)	Subunits	Location
Cu, Zn-SOD	SOD1	32	Dimeric	Cytoplasm, nucleus
Mn-SOD	SOD2	96	Tetrameric	Mitochondrion
EC-SOD	SOD3	135	Tetrameric	Extracellular

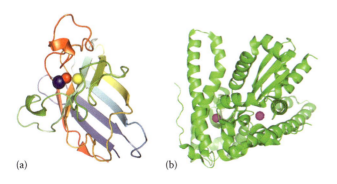

Figure 3.2 Structures of two of the SODs found in humans. (a) Cu, Zn-SOD where Cu = blue sphere, (b) Mn-SOD—purple spheres = Mn.[6] Three-dimensional coordinates for structures were obtained from the Protein Data Bank (Cu, Zn-SOD—1B4T; Mn-SOD—1N0J).[2,7] Protein structures were drawn using the PyMOL Molecular Graphics System, Version 1.3, Schrödinger, LLC.

As we shall see in the following subsections, H_2O_2 can further be metabolized by other enzymatic antioxidants that constitute the skin's endogenous antioxidant system. One additional point, yet to be addressed, is the activity of Zn^{2+} in both Cu, Zn-SOD and EC-SOD. In general, Zn^{2+} is not directly involved with catalytic activities of these molecules; however, it is essential for protein structure.[6]

Catalase

The decomposition of H_2O_2 is enzymatically controlled by catalase [EC 1.11.1.6], which is a four-subunit protein (*ca.* 240 kDa) that is found in most eukaryotic cells. In fact, catalase is located in peroxisomes, which are organelles found in all eukaryotes whose primary function is to purge toxins present in the cell. The overall reaction catalyzed by catalase consists of the decomposition of two H_2O_2 molecules into water and O_2.

$$2H_2O_2 \rightarrow 2H_2O + O_2 \quad (3.4)$$

As illustrated in Figure 3.3, each subunit of catalase contains an active site with a heme-Fe^{3+} (ferric) group, which is directly involved with the catalysis. The reaction proceeds via a two-step sequence consisting of an initial step where Fe^{3+} reduces H_2O_2, resulting in the production of H_2O as well as an intermediate species (referred to as Compound I). The heme group iron binds with oxygen, resulting in the $Fe^{4+}=O$ (oxoferryl) species in conjunction with a free radical delocalized on the pi orbital system of the porphyrin ring. During the second and final step of the reaction, Compound I reacts with a second H_2O_2 by oxidation, resulting in the formation of H_2O and the liberation of the oxoferryl species as H_2O. This is demonstrated by the two-step reaction shown in the following.[8]

$$H_2O_2 + \text{Catalase-Fe}^{3+} \rightarrow \text{Compound I (Fe}^{4+}) \quad (3.5)$$

$$\begin{aligned}\text{Compound I (Fe}^{4+}) + H_2O_2 \rightarrow \\ \text{Catalase-Fe}^{3+} + H_2O + O_2\end{aligned} \quad (3.6)$$

In addition to the heme group, the structural motif in Figure 3.3 illustrates additional components of catalase as well as essential features of its tertiary structure. The structure shown in Figure 3.3 is one subunit of catalase. The heme group is surrounded by a beta-barrel and helical domain, rendering a very hydrophobic core for the active site. The threading arm provides the connection between monomers by looping through the wrapping loop of another subunit.[9] Nicotinamide adenine dinucleotide phosphate (NADPH) is also present at a position adjacent to the active site, where it protects the heme group and has been shown to prevent the formation of an inactive form of catalase called Compound II, which would not permit the successful completion of the second step of the reaction shown in Equation 3.6.[10]

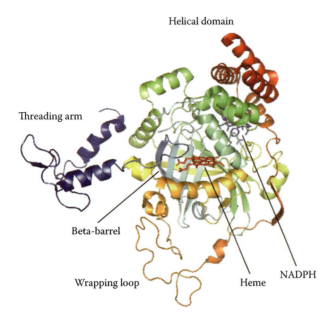

Figure 3.3 Structure of one subunit of catalase. See Appendix 2 for the structure of NADPH and Figure 3.21 for the heme group structure. Three-dimensional coordinates for structures obtained from the Protein Data Bank (1DGB—human erythrocyte catalase).[9] Protein structures were drawn using the PyMOL Molecular Graphics System, Version 1.3, Schrödinger, LLC.

Glutathione peroxidase

In addition to catalase, H_2O_2 can also be metabolized by GSH peroxidase [EC 1.11.1.9], a selenium-dependent enzyme typically found in the cytoplasm of most mammalian cells. Selenium is incorporated into the protein structure as a selenocysteine group and is present at the active site in each of the four subunits of the protein. Selenocysteine is structurally equivalent to cysteine except the sulfur in cysteine is replaced by selenium. The presence of selenocysteine is illustrated in Figure 3.4, in which two of the four subunits of GSH peroxidase are shown. The catalytic activity of GSH peroxidase depends on the cofactor GSH, which provides reducing equivalents for the enzyme. As shown in Figure 3.5, GSH peroxidase catalyzes the decomposition of H_2O_2 and fatty acid hydroperoxides with the concurrent cystine bond formation between two GSH molecules. GSH is a tripeptide of glutamic acid, cysteine, and glycine. A proposed mechanism for the catalytic cycle of GSH peroxidase is shown in Figure 3.6.[11] It is believed that the native enzyme form (E-Se-H) reacts with a peroxide (ROOH) yielding a selenic acid form of the enzyme (E-Se-OH). Further, reaction of E-Se-OH with GSH produces an intermediate selenyl sulfide adduct (E-Se-S-G) in which the GSH is bound to the selenium ion. The selenyl sulfide adduct can react with another molecule of GSH, yielding oxidized GSH (GSSG), in which the two GSH units are linked by a disulfide bond, and the original enzyme (E-Se-H).

In order to maintain an adequate supply of GSH in the cells, the oxidized form of GSH is reduced back to GSH in

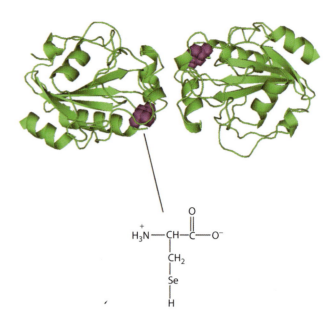

Figure 3.4 Structure of two subunits of GSH peroxidase.[12] Selenocysteine is shown in purple. Three-dimensional coordinates for structures obtained from the Protein Data Bank (1GP1—selenoenzyme GSH peroxidase). Protein structures were drawn using the PyMOL Molecular Graphics System, Version 1.3, Schrödinger, LLC.

the presence of the enzyme, GSH reductase. This proceeds by a reaction that is dependent on reducing power from NADPH.[8]

$$GSSG + NADPH + H^+ \rightarrow 2GSH + NADP^+ \quad (3.7)$$

The NADPH provided for the execution of this reaction comes from the pentose phosphate pathway, which is an alternative metabolic pathway to the citric acid cycle for the metabolism of glucose.

Thus far, we have referred to GSH peroxidase as a single entity. In fact, GSH peroxidase actually represents a family of isozymes and can be categorized as selenium-dependent or selenium-independent. The catalytic activity of the most well-known enzymes from this family depends on the presence of a selenium atom, which is incorporated into the active site of the protein as a selenocysteine group. In mammalians, there are four major types of selenium-containing GSH peroxidases: classical, gastrointestinal, plasma, and phospholipid GSH peroxidase. Up to now, only the classical form of GSH peroxidase, also known as GPX-1, has been discussed. Table 3.2 contains a list of the four major selenium-dependent GSH peroxidases along with their molecular weights, cellular location, and the substrates that they metabolize. GPX-1 and GPX-4 are expressed ubiquitously throughout the body, while GPX-2 and GPX-3 are expressed in the gastrointestinal tract and plasma, respectively.[13]

NAD(P)H:Quinone reductase

Quinones are aromatic molecules that contain two ketone groups. They can easily undergo reduction by the

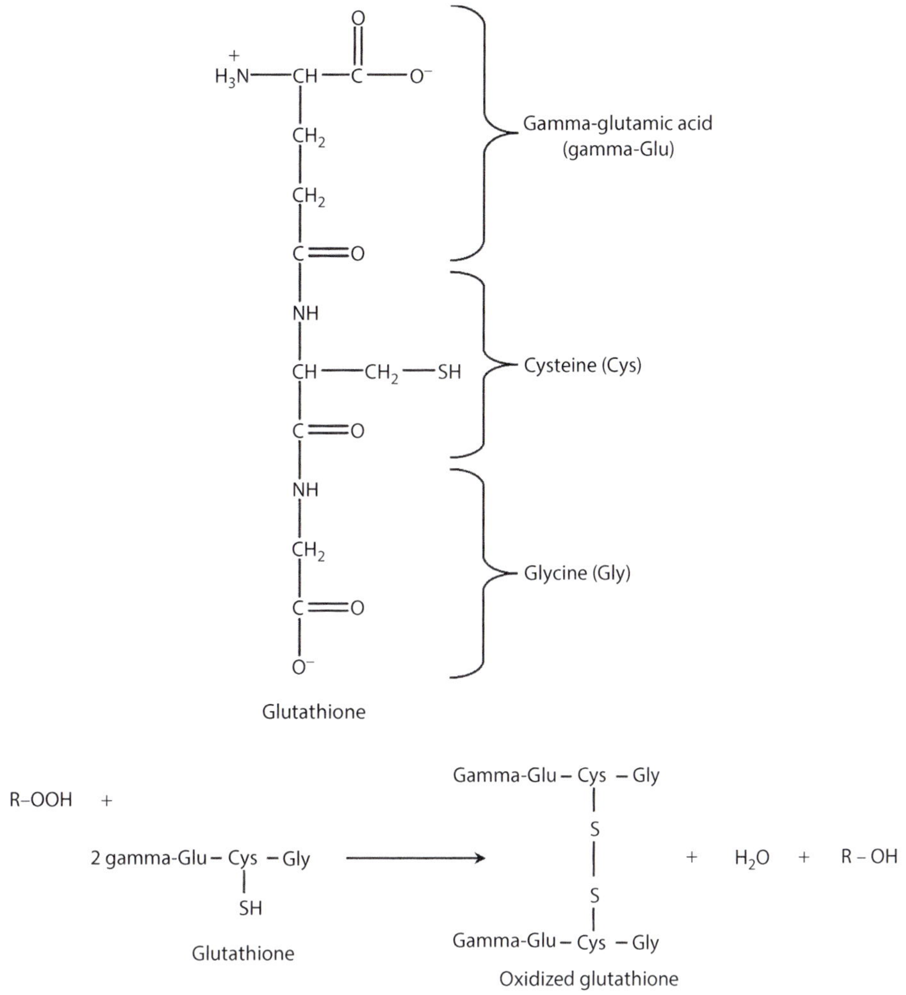

Figure 3.5 Structure of GSH and its reaction with peroxides, which is catalyzed by GSH peroxidase.

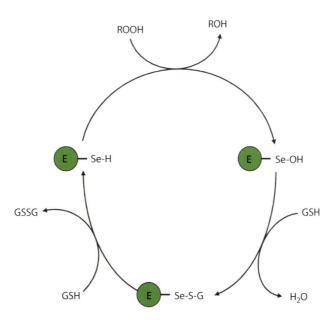

Figure 3.6 Proposed mechanism of GSH peroxidase activity. E-Se-H: selenol enzymatic form; ROOH: peroxide; ROH: alcohol; E-Se-OH: selenic acid enzymatic form; GSH: gluthathione; E-Se-S-G: selenyl sulfide adduct enzymatic form; GSSG: oxidized GSH. (Adapted from Mugesh, G. et al., *J. Am. Chem. Soc.*, 123, 839–850, 2001.)

Table 3.2 Selenium-dependent GSH peroxidases in mammalians.

Name	Alternate name	Sub-units	MM (kDa)	Site of action	Substrates
GPX-1	Classical GPX	Tetramer	22	Cytosolic	H_2O_2 & FA hydroperoxides
GPX-2	Gastrointestinal GPX	Tetramer	24	Cytosolic	H_2O_2 & FA hydroperoxides
GPX-3	Plasma GPX	Tetramer	25	Extracellular	Cholesterol hydroperoxides
GPX-4	Phospholipid GPX	Monomer	19	Cytosolic, mitochondrial	Phospholipid hydroperoxide

Source: Lackner, K.L. and Blankenberg, S., *Ital. Heart J.*, 5, 169–172, 2004.
Abbreviations: GPX = glutathione peroxidase; FA = fatty acid; MM is provided per sub-unit.

addition of one electron, forming a semiquinone radical, which can deleteriously affect cell viability (Figure 3.7). Further, addition of another electron results in the formation of the more stable species, hydroquinone, which can then be excreted by the body. Endogenous examples of quinones consist of Vitamin K1 (phylloquinone), a blood clotting agent, or coenzyme Q (ubiquinone), which is part of the electron transport chain in the mitochondrial membrane. Exogenously, quinines can be introduced to the body as drugs, especially chemotherapy agents, in which case they are referred to as xenobiotics. Quinones often undergo a one-electron reduction reaction, which is catalyzed by flavoproteins and utilizes an electron from either nicotinamide adenine dinucleotide (NADH) or NADPH. This leaves the radical semiquinone species free to engage in deleterious reactions if it is not further reduced to hydroquinone. Semiquinone radicals are considered dangerous as they are able to undergo redox cycling, a process in which a molecule is reduced, leaving it with a free electron that then reacts with oxygen, resulting in the formation of $O_2^{\cdot-}$. This leads to an accumulation of $O_2^{\cdot-}$ in the cell, which by itself is not that dangerous, though it can react with H_2O_2 in the presence of transition metals, resulting in the highly reactive hydroxyl radical ($HO^{\cdot}$), whose reactivity is only determined by diffusivity.

The conversion of highly reactive quinones and quinoneimines to more stable hydroquinones is enzymatically catalyzed by NAD(P)H:quinone reductase [EC 1.6.5.5], which is also known as DT-diaphorase. It is a homodimer (*ca.* 31 kDa per monomer) that contains the cofactor, flavin adenine dinucleotide (FAD). The enzyme functions by performing a two-electron reduction of its substrate in which it utilizes either NADH or NADPH as a source of electrons. The structure of NAD(P)H:quinone reductase is shown in Figure 3.7, where the FAD cofactor can be seen buried within the enzyme's tertiary structure. FAD is not covalently attached to the enzyme; however, it remains tightly bound during the catalytic process. The proposed mechanism for this process is provided in Figure 3.8, which is initiated by entry of NADH or NADPH at the active site where it donates a proton to the FAD portion of the enzyme.[15,16] This is followed by a sequence of mechanisms at the FAD site, which is influenced by neighboring amino acid moieties. Eventually, reduction of the quinone occurs from a one-electron reduction reaction, leaving the semiquinone radical. This is followed by a subsequent one-electron transfer reaction, yielding the stable form of the molecule, hydroquinone. In addition to its ability to convert quinones to hydroquinones, NAD(P)H:quinone reductase can also neutralize quinoneimines and azo dyes. Another essential function of this enzyme is to regenerate vitamin E quinone and ubiquinone back to their antioxidant active forms, vitamin E and ubiquinol (Figure 3.9).

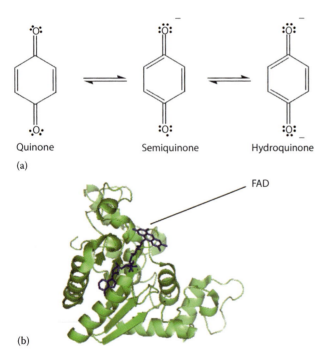

Figure 3.7 (a) Conversion of quinone to semiquinone to hydroquinone by a two-step two-electron reduction. (b) Structure of one subunit of NAD(P)H:quinone reductase. Three-dimensional coordinates for structure (1D4A—human NAD(P)H-quinone oxidoreductase) obtained from the Protein Data Bank.[14] Protein structure was drawn using the PyMOL Molecular Graphics System, Version 1.3, Schrödinger, LLC. See Appendix 2 for the structure of FAD.

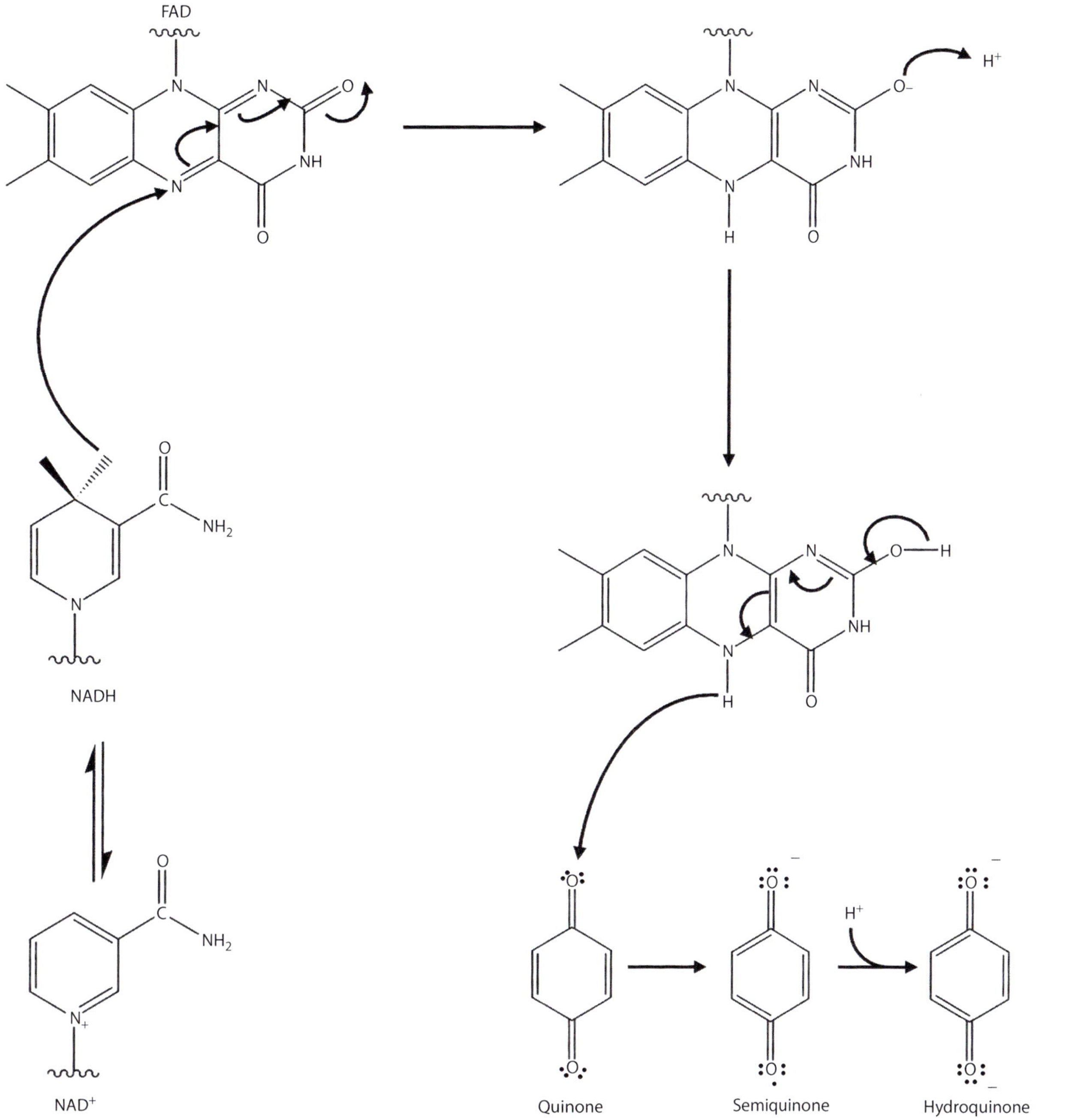

Figure 3.8 Mechanism for the two-electron reduction of quinone by NAD(P)H:quinone reductase. Only part of the FAD portion of the enzyme is shown. See Appendix 2 for the entire structure of FAD and NADH. (Adapted from Li, R. et al., *Proc. Natl. Acad. Sci. USA*, 92, 8846–8850, 1995.)

The thioredoxin system

Another important component of the endogenous antioxidant system is the Trx system.[17] It consists of two protein structures, Trx and Trx reductase (TrxR), which work in concert, resulting in antioxidant activities as well as the influence of other cellular functions. TrxR is often likened to GPX, as it is also a thiol redox system, and belongs to a family of enzymes known as the pyridine nucleotide oxidoreductases. However, similar to NAD(P)H:quinone reductase (discussed in the preceding section), TrxR is an avoprotein that contains four subunits (*ca.* 55–65 kDa per monomer), in which each subunit contains an active site with the amino acid, selenocysteine, and FAD. Trx is a small one-subunit protein (*ca.* 12 kDa) found in most tissues of the body. Further, TrxR utilizes NADPH for reducing equivalents, in which an electron is transferred first to FAD then to the enzyme (TrxR). As indicated in the scheme provided in Figure 3.10a, this action results in the cleavage of a disulfide bond in TrxR. The enzyme then donates an electron to its substrate, Trx, resulting in the reformation of a disulfide

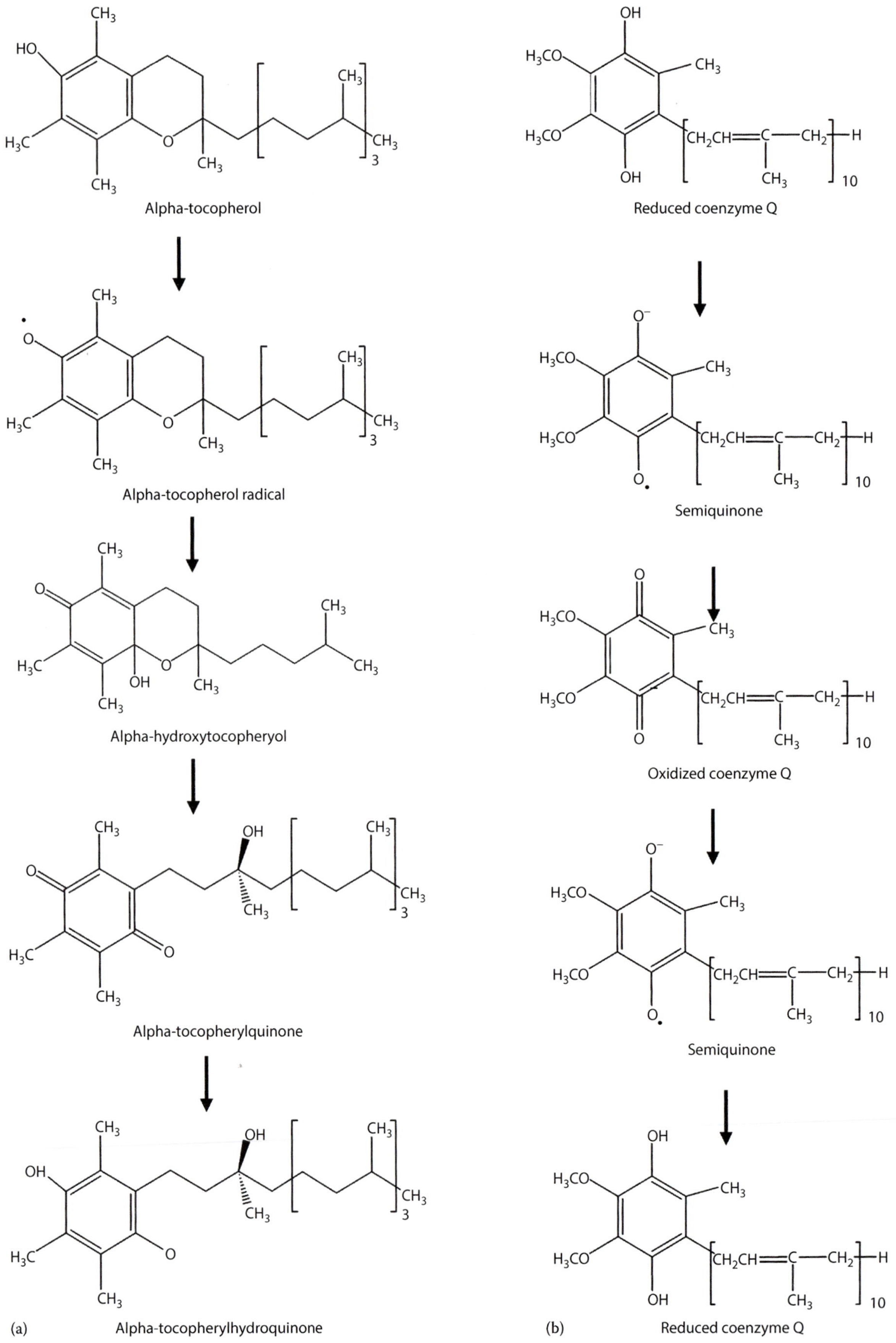

36 The skin's endogenous antioxidant network

Figure 3.9 Reduction of (a) alpha-tocopherylquinone and (b) oxidized coenzyme Q by NADP:quinone reductase.

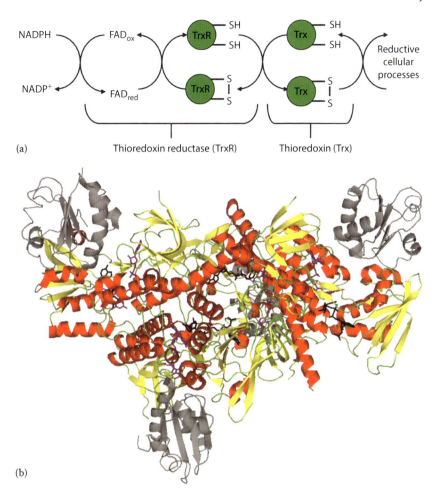

Figure 3.10 (a) Catalytic activity of the Trx system and (b) Structure of TrxR—Trx complex. The red and yellow ribbons are TrxR. The grey ribbons represent Trx molecules. The purple sticks = FAD and the black sticks = the NADP+ ANALOG, AADP+. Three-dimensional coordinates for structure (1F6M) obtained from the Protein Data Bank. Protein structure was drawn using the PyMOL Molecular Graphics System, Version 1.3, Schrödinger, LLC. ([a] Adapted from Lennon, B.W. et al., *Science*, 289, 1190–1194, 2000. With permission.)

bond in TrxR and the cleavage of a disulfide bond in Trx. The structure of the four subunit enzyme, TrxR, along with four Trx molecules, each interacting with a subunit, is shown in Figure 3.10b. In the figure, TrxR is shown in yellow and gold, while Trx is colored gray. Also shown is FAD (purple sticks) and NADP+ (black sticks). In fact, the analog 3-aminopyridine adenine dinucleotide phosphate (AADP+) is shown instead of NADP+; however, the principal is the same.

The Trx system exhibits antioxidant behavior and influences other cellular function in several ways (Figure 3.11).[18,19] First, TrxR itself can utilize substrates other than Trx. For example, antioxidants (e.g., ascorbic acid and lipoic acid) in their oxidized state may be regenerated to their active form by TrxR. When TrxR utilizes Trx as a substrate, Trx is then free to provide reducing equivalents to various enzymes such as Trx peroxidase, which catalyzes the decomposition of H_2O_2 to H_2O. Another example of Trx activity includes its interaction with the enzyme ribonucleotide reductase, which catalyzes the reduction of

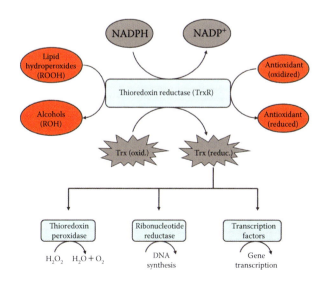

Figure 3.11 Cellular functions of TrxR and Trx. (Adapted from Mustacich, D. and Powis, G., *Biochem. J.*, 346, 1–8, 2000.)

ribonucleotides to deoxyribonucleotides, ultimately regulating DNA synthesis. In addition, Trx serves as a regulator for transcription factors, which serve as cofactors for the enzymes responsible for the transcription of DNA to RNA. Moreover, similar to NAD(P)H:quinone reductase, it is believed that TrxR also plays a role in the regeneration of coenzyme Q as well as the reduction of other quinones.[20,21]

SMALL-MOLECULE ANTIOXIDANTS

Water-soluble antioxidants in skin include ascorbic acid, uric acid, and GSH, while lipid-soluble antioxidants consist of alpha-tocopherol, coenzyme Q, and beta-carotene. These antioxidants function by various mechanisms, which are discussed in detail in the subsections that follow. In addition, the antioxidant role of melanin, which is the primary pigment in skin and hair, is also of paramount importance in terms of its free radical-scavenging capabilities and its role in the endogenous antioxidant network.

L-Ascorbic acid (vitamin C)

While many mammals are able to biosynthesize ascorbic acid, humans fall into that small category of species deficient of an enzyme required for the synthesis of vitamin C. Therefore, it is an essential vitamin or ingredient that must be obtained from other food sources. Dietary deficiency of vitamin C can lead to scurvy, a disease that used to be common in sailors during colonial exploratory times due to the absence of fresh fruits and vegetables during extended periods at sea. Vitamin C is the L-enantiomer of ascorbic acid. The structure of L-ascorbic acid ($AscH_2$) and its oxidation products are shown in Figure 3.12. Essentially, the structure of $AscH_2$ consists of a lactone ring containing an ene-diol group. Both of the hydroxyl groups in the ene-diol are ionizable, and $AscH_2$ is able to undergo a two-electron oxidation. At physiological pH (ca. pH 7.4), the anionic form of the molecule, referred to as ascorbate ($AscH^-$), is the most predominant form of the antioxidant found. It is this structure that circulates through the blood and other tissues to exert its antioxidant activity. In addition to its antioxidant properties, $AscH^-$ is also an important cofactor for many enzymes. Key examples include proline hydroxylase and lysine hydroxylase, which are involved in collagen synthesis, as well as dopamine-beta-hydroxylase, which catalyzes the conversion of dopamine to noradrenaline.

As shown in Figure 3.12, oxidation of $AscH^-$ results in the generation of the ascorbate radical ($Asc^{\cdot-}$), known as semidehydroascorbate, which is a very stable free radical due to the delocalization of the electron in the pi-conjugated system. In addition, $Asc^{\cdot-}$ is known to undergo a disproportionation reaction in which two of the radical species yield one mole each of $AscH^-$ and dehydroascorbate (DHA).

$$2 Asc^{\cdot-} \rightarrow AscH^- + DHA \qquad (3.8)$$

Thus, for every two $AscH^-$ molecules depleted one is regenerated so that it may participate in further antioxidant protection. The other product of the disproportionation reaction is DHA, which is unstable and can rapidly decompose to other degradation products that interfere with enzymatic processes of the cell. Another fate of DHA is to be regenerated reductively to $AscH^-$ by the enzyme DHA

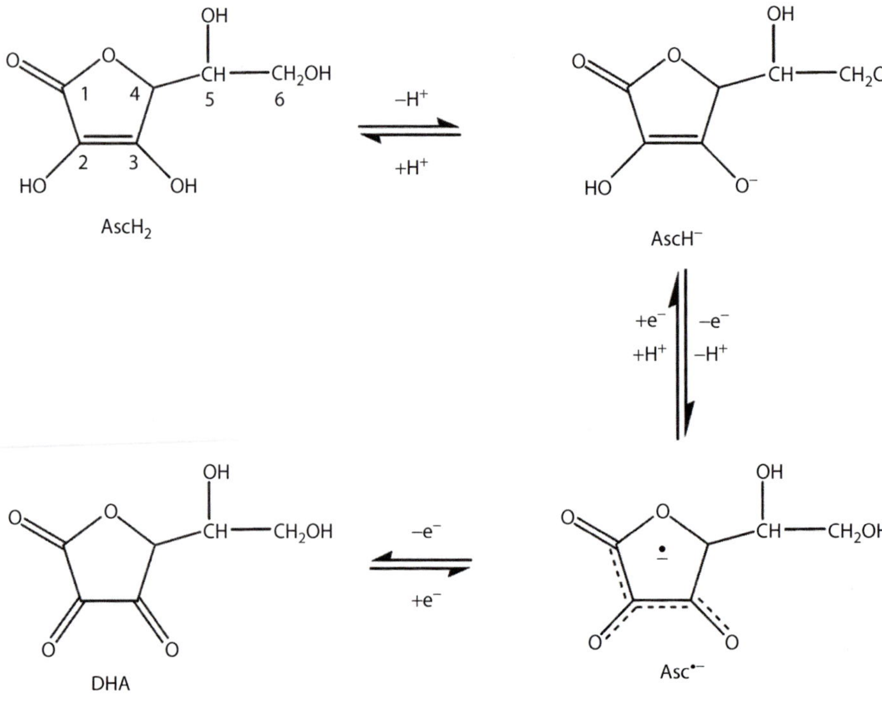

Figure 3.12 Structure of L-ascorbic acid and related structures. $AscH_2$ = ascorbic acid, $AscH^-$ = ascorbate, $Asc^{\cdot-}$ = semidehydroascorbate, DHA = dehydroascorbate.

reductase. The action of this enzyme is dependent on the available pool of GSH, as it is required as an electron donor.

AscH$^-$ is a very powerful water-soluble antioxidant that is a reducing agent. AscH$^-$ is well known for its role in scavenging $O_2^{\cdot-}$, HO$^\cdot$, lipid peroxyl radical (ROO$^\cdot$), singlet oxygen ($^1O_2$), and thiyl radical (RS$^\cdot$). It is also known to scavenge pollutants, such as ozone (O_3) and nitrogen dioxide ($NO_2^\cdot$). In addition, AscH$^-$ plays an integral role in the regeneration of alpha-tocopherol from the alpha-tocopheryl radical (see Figure 3.15 in the *Glutathione* section of this discussion). Thus, it helps maintain membrane integrity by maintaining a replenished pool of vitamin E.

Uric acid

With pKa values of 5.4 and 10.3, uric acid exists in the deprotonated form at physiological pH and hence is typically referred to as urate. As shown in Figure 3.13, uric acid tautomerizes between an enol and keto form. The enol form of the molecule contains a hydroxyl group able to dissociate into the ionic form, urate. In vivo, uric acid is synthesized as a result of purine nucleotide metabolism (Figure 3.14).[22] One route is the enzymatic degradation of adenosine monophosphate (AMP) eventually forming hypoxanthine, which is converted to xanthine in the presence of H_2O, O_2, and the enzyme, xanthine oxidase. Likewise, guanosine monophosphate (GMP) undergoes a similar process and is converted to xanthine without first forming hypoxanthine. Please note that Figure 3.14 does not contain the intermediate steps that take place between AMP and hypoxanthine, as well as GMP and xanthine. In primates, uric acid is the final product of purine metabolism and is excreted in the urine. In some individuals, uric acid excretion is impaired, resulting in the accumulation of insoluble sodium urate crystals in the bodily fluids. This condition, which is known as gout, results in painful inflammation of the joints.

As an antioxidant, urate is able to react with HO$^\cdot$, $^1O_2$, and ROO$^\cdot$. In addition, urate is known to react with $NO_2^\cdot$ and O_3 as well as with the non-free radical species hypochlorous acid (HOCl).[8] Further, urate is a known chelator of copper and iron, which probably prevents these metals from taking part in deleterious reactions.

Glutathione

One of the activities of GSH has already been discussed in the section on GSH peroxidase. In that capacity, GSH serves as a cofactor and is utilized for its ability to donate an electron to the substrate that GPX acts upon. As already shown in Figure 3.5, the structure of GSH is composed of the tripeptide sequence gamma-glutamyl-cysteinyl-glycine. As mentioned previously, two molecules of GSH participate in the reaction catalyzed by GPX and become cross-linked via a disulfide bond as a result of the reduction reaction. The resulting species, oxidized GSH, can be reduced back to its original form by the enzyme GSH reductase at the expense of NADPH (see Equation 3.7). In addition to a cofactor role, GSH can also directly react with free radicals, such as HO$^\cdot$, alkoxyl radical (RO$^\cdot$), and ROO$^\cdot$.[23]

$$\text{HO}^\cdot, \text{RO}^\cdot, \text{ or ROO}^\cdot + \text{GSH} \rightarrow \\ \text{H}_2\text{O, ROH, or ROOH} + \text{GS}^\cdot \quad (3.9)$$

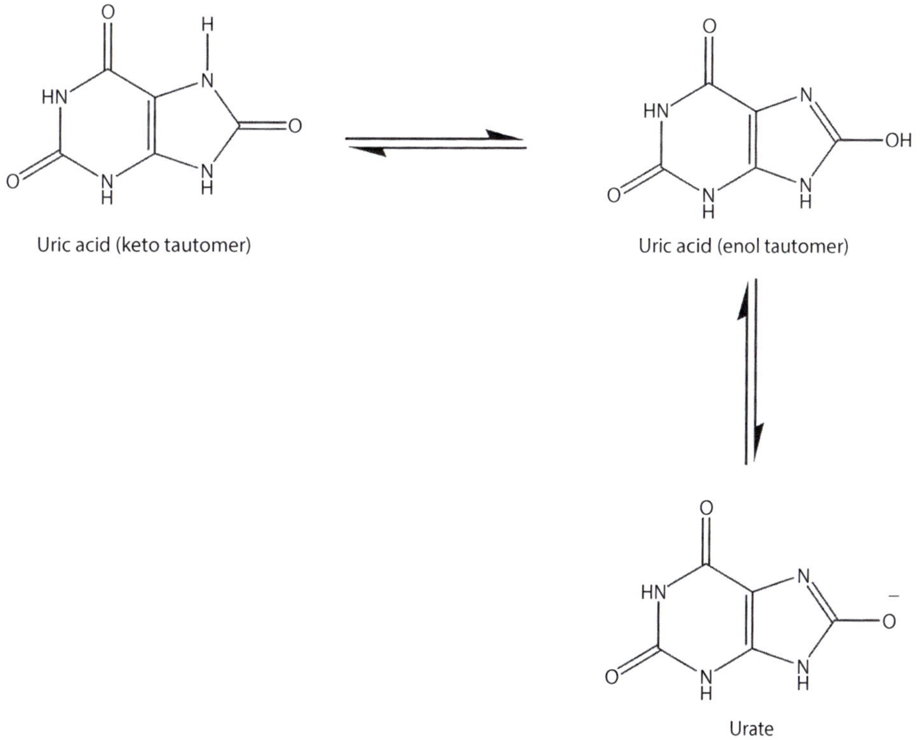

Figure 3.13 Structures of uric acid-related structures.

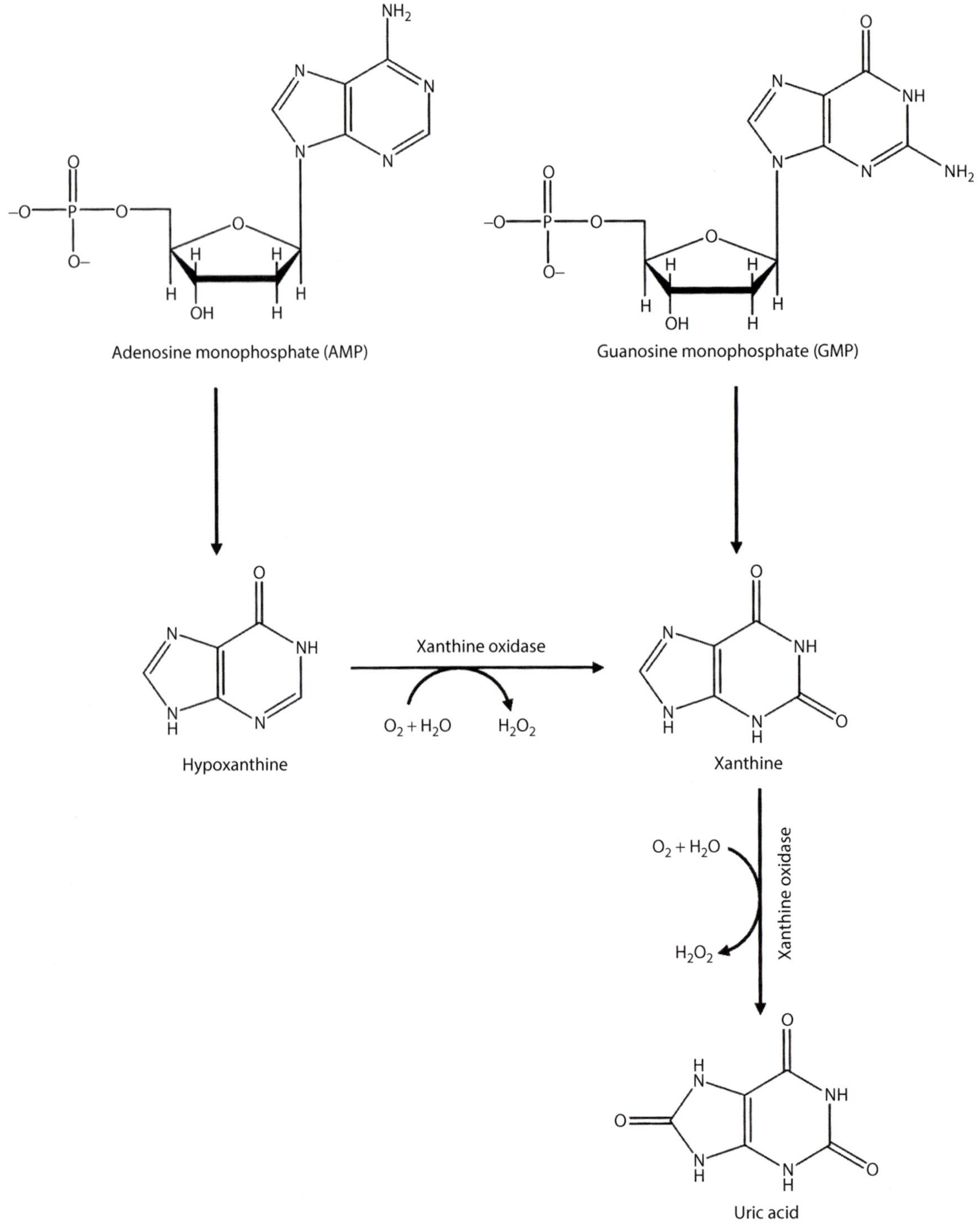

Figure 3.14 Purine nucleotide metabolism resulting in the formation of uric acid. (Adapted from Mathews, C. et al., *Biochemistry*, 4th ed., Prentice Hall, Upper Saddle River, NJ, 2012.)

The expected fate of the resulting glutathiyl radical is that it reacts with another molecule of itself, yielding GSSG. However, other outcomes are likely as well, especially the reaction of glutathiyl radical with the ionized form of GSH. At physiological pH only a very small amount of GSH is expected to be ionized since it has a pK_a of 9.2.[8]

$$GSH \rightleftharpoons GS^- + H^+ \quad (3.10)$$

Thus, we would expect to only see small amounts of GS$^-$ present in the tissues. Even with low concentrations of ionized GSH, it is very likely that free GS$^\cdot$ can react with GS$^-$:

$$GS^- + GS^\cdot \rightarrow GSSG^{\cdot -} \quad (3.11)$$

The oxidized GSH radical (GSSG$^{\cdot -}$) is then able to react with O_2, resulting in the formation of $O_2^{\cdot -}$.[8] As shown in Figure 3.15, other activities of GSH include

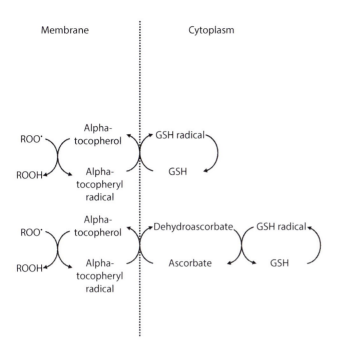

Figure 3.15 Regeneration of alpha-tocopherol and ascorbate by GSH. (Adapted from Acworth, I.N. et al., The analysis of free radicals, their reaction products, and antioxidants, in *Oxidants, Antioxidants, and Free Radicals*, Baskin, S.I. and Salem, H. [Eds.], Taylor & Francis Group, Washington, DC, 23–77, 1997.)

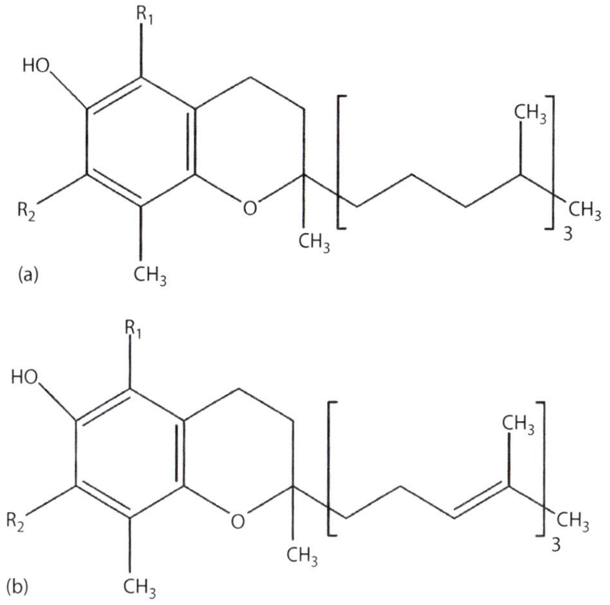

the antioxidant regeneration of alpha-tocopherol and ascorbate from their oxidized forms.[23]

Vitamin E

As a major fat-soluble vitamin, vitamin E has received a great deal of attention in academic literature pertaining to human health and disease. It is typically found in lipid bilayer membranes and lipoproteins. Normally, low-density and high-density lipoproteins serve as transporters of cholesterol in human blood plasma and their oxidation leads to life-threatening disease such as atherosclerosis. In terms of biological localization, vitamin E is mostly found in the mitochondrion and endoplasmic reticulum. Vitamin E is a known scavenger of $^1O_2$, $O_2^{•-}$, and $HO^•$; however, its most noted role is in the scavenging of $ROO^•$. In this capacity, vitamin E impedes radical damage at the initiation and propagation stage of the lipid peroxidation cascade.

The designation vitamin E has become synonymous with its most well-known and abundant stereoisomer, alpha-tocopherol. In fact, vitamin E represents a family of compounds composed of the different isomeric forms of tocopherols and tocotrienols. The basic structures for both the tocopherols and tocotrienols are shown in Figure 3.16. Each structure contains a chromanol ring with a long alkyl side chain (phytyl tail), rendering it lipid-soluble. The primary difference between these two classes of compounds is the structure of the aliphatic chain. In contrast to the tocopherols, which contain a phytyl tail, the tocotrienols contain a double bond next to the pendant methyl group at

Figure 3.16 Structures of the various isomers of vitamin E: (a) tocopherols and (b) tocotrienols.

three different locations along the alkyl chain. The designation for the four different isomeric forms of the tocopherols and tocotrienols is also provided in Figure 3.16, indicating that the alpha-isomer contains a total of three methyl groups on the chromanol ring, the beta- and gamma-isomers two, and the delta-isomer one. The vitamin E forms are further classified into their various geometrical stereoisomers. R and S are used to indicate the position of the methyl groups along the phytyl tail. This designation refers to the position of the first three methyl groups, and not the fourth one, along the side chain of the molecule, in which case each methyl group can be the R or S isomer. All of the vitamin E forms found in nature are the RRR stereoisomer. Synthetic forms, on the other hand, contain a mixture of enantiomers. As an example, alpha-tocopherol itself can have up to eight stereoisomers: RRR, RSR, RSS, RRS, SRR, SRS, SSR, and SSS.

As already mentioned, the most noteworthy function of vitamin E is its role in the inhibition of lipid peroxidation as the major chain-breaking antioxidant. This is mainly due to its high reactivity towards $ROO^•$ ($k = 10^6 M^{-1}s^{-1}$) as compared to the lower reactivity of $ROO^•$ with other lipids ($k = 10^2 M^{-1}s^{-1}$).[8] An example of the free radical-scavenging ability of alpha-tocopherol is provided in Figure 3.17 where it reacts with a $ROO^•$, resulting in the formation of the alpha-tocopheryl radical. Further, another $ROO^•$ can be neutralized by reacting with an alpha-tocopheryl radical

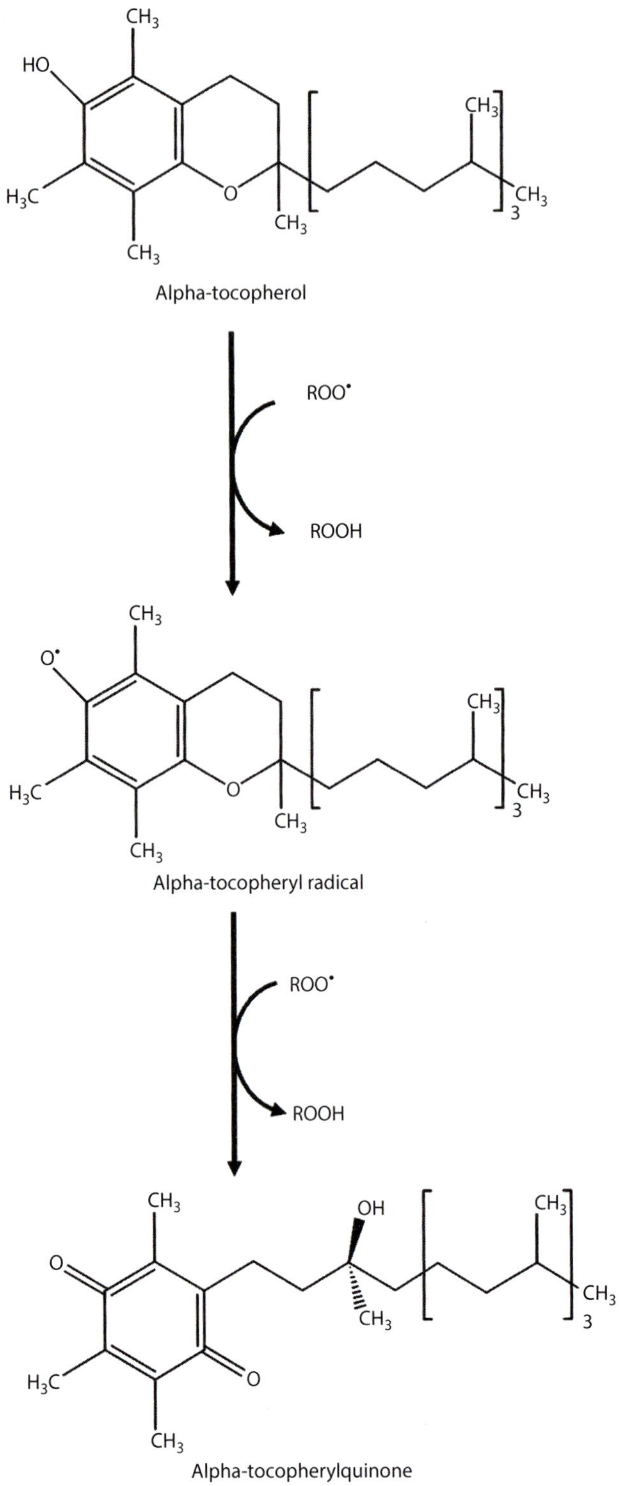

42 The skin's endogenous antioxidant network

Figure 3.17 The role of alpha-tocopherol in the inhibition of lipid peroxidation.

and forming alpha-tocopherylquinone. Thus, one molecule of alpha-tocopherol is able to eliminate two ROO• radicals, making this antioxidant very unique.

Coenzyme Q

Perhaps the most well-known function of coenzyme Q is its role as an electron carrier in the mitochondrial electron transport chain. As a lipid-soluble antioxidant, it is present in plasma membranes, organelle membranes, and, to some extent, in low-density lipoproteins. As illustrated in Figure 3.18, coenzyme Q belongs to the ubiquinone class of molecules and is characterized by its long isoprenoid tail, allowing it to anchor itself into membranes. The oxidized form of the molecule is also known by the name ubiquinone-10, where the number ten represents the number of isoprene groups present in the structure of the molecule. The reduced form of coenzyme Q, also known as ubiquinol, is the most capable form of the molecule to exert antioxidant protection. Like vitamin E, coenzyme Q acts as free radical scavenger of ROO•, thereby preventing lipid peroxidation. In addition, coenzyme Q can react with the

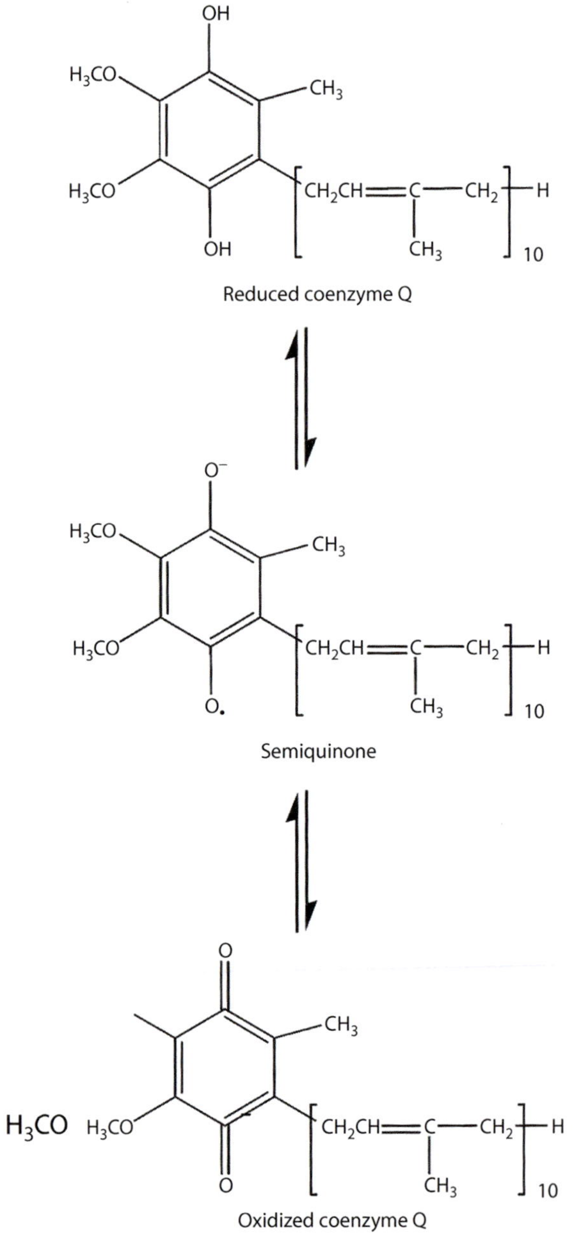

Figure 3.18 The structure of the reduced and oxidized forms of coenzyme Q and its intermediate radical form.

tocopheryl radical, thereby regenerating the viable form of alpha-tocopherol.

Carotenoids

Compounds from this class are not synthesized in vivo and are typically obtained in the diet from plant sources and fruits. More than 600 carotenoids have been identified in nature; however, the most well-known is beta-carotene.[24,25] They generally have strong absorption in the visible region of the electromagnetic spectrum and are therefore natural pigments that exhibit an array of colors. As just one example, the yellow and orange colors present in sunflowers can be attributed to the presence of beta-carotene, which has a maximum absorption of ~450 nm. This results in the absorption of much of the blue light in the spectrum and the reflection of yellow, orange, and red bands of light. Some of the most common carotenoids, listed in Figure 3.19, are characterized by a long chain that contains an extensive system of conjugation. Human skin contains a variety of carotenoids, which can easily be probed using Raman spectroscopy and provide an overall status of antioxidant capacity.[26]

Most carotenoids exert their antioxidant action by quenching triplet-state sensitizers, quenching $^1O_2$, and scavenging ROO•s. Porphyrins and flavins, which are abundant in the human body, can act as triplet-state sensitizers. They abstract a proton or electron from another molecule, resulting in the formation of free radicals, or react with O_2 in its ground state to yield $^1O_2$. As an example, a carotenoid can quench $^1O_2$ by absorbing energy from it, resulting in a triplet-state carotenoid.

$$^1O_2 + \text{Carotenoid} \rightarrow O_2 + \text{Carotenoid}* \quad (3.12)$$

$$\text{Carotenoid}* \rightarrow \text{Carotenoid} + \Delta \quad (3.13)$$

The excited carotenoid easily dissipates energy, in the form of heat, to the surrounding solvent. Due to their highly conjugated systems, carotenoids stabilize their excited states through resonance and delocalization.[27] The same mechanism takes place for the quenching of triplet-state sensitizers. On the other hand, the interaction between a carotenoid and peroxyl radical operates by a different mechanism; however, the details are still uncertain. As demonstrated in Figure 3.20, it is believed that the carotenoids trap free radicals by forming a free radical complex in which the electron is delocalized over its conjugated structure.[28]

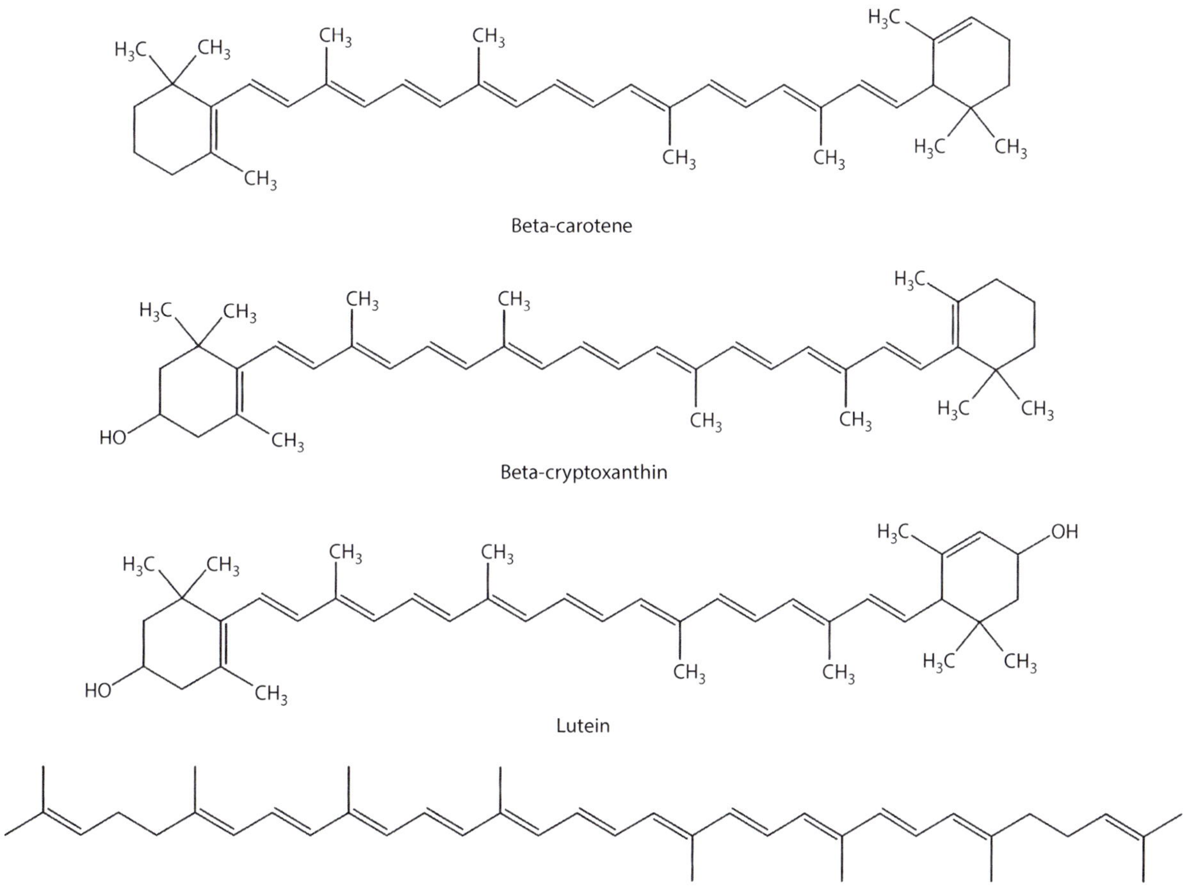

Figure 3.19 Structures of some common carotenoids.

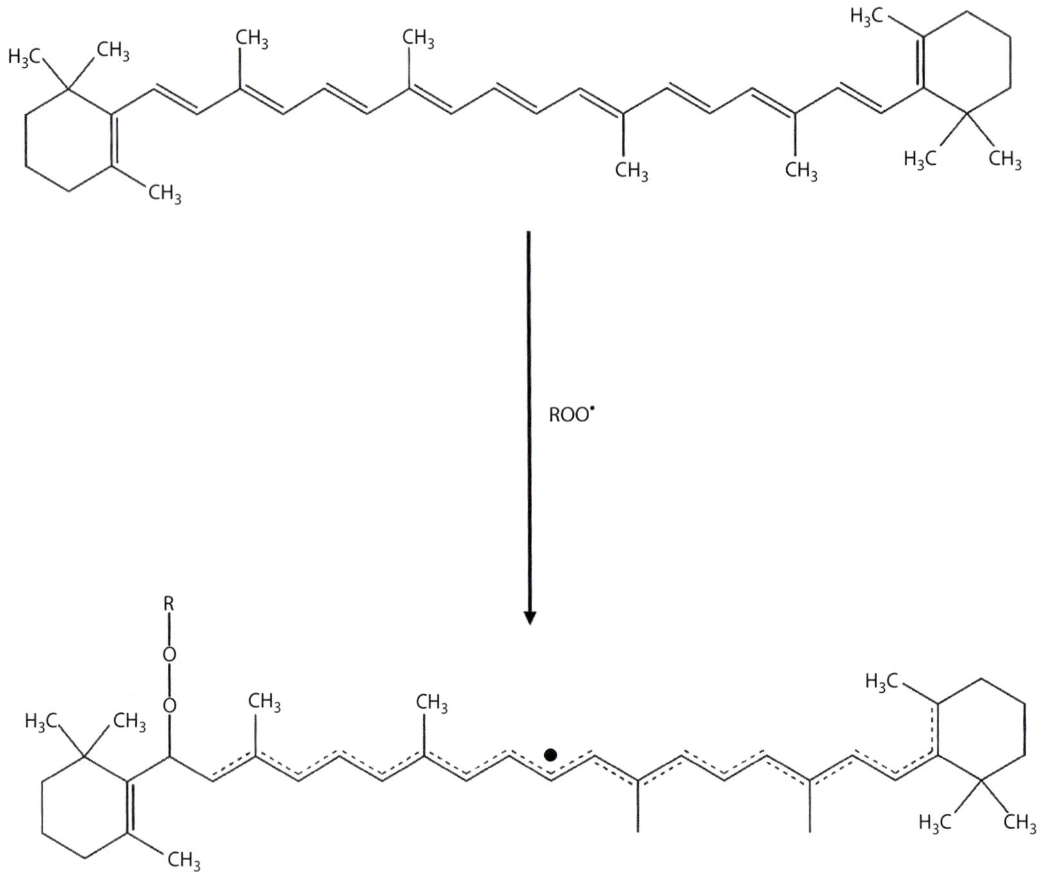

Figure 3.20 Mechanism for free radical trapping by beta-carotene. (Adapted from Burton, G.W., *Science*, 224, 569–573, 1984.)

Bilirubin

Hemoglobin is responsible for the transfer of oxygen from the lungs to myoglobin in the tissues via the blood stream. It is a four-subunit protein in which each subunit contains a heme group with iron at its core, which coordinates with O_2. Catabolism of heme (when blood cells are destroyed) is catalyzed by heme oxygenase, resulting in the formation of biliverdin, which is further broken down to bilirubin by the enzyme biliverdin reductase (Figure 3.21).[29]

Bilirubin has a characteristic yellowish color, such as that observed in an old bruise.[30] In recent years, much interest has arisen in the elucidation of the mechanisms related to the activity of hemoxygenase-1 in skin, especially its role as an anti-inflammatory mediator and anti-apoptotic agent.[31] In fact, evidence indicates that hemeoxygenase-1 is a key factor in UVA-induced immunoprotection.[32] Many years ago, bilirubin was relegated to the role of a lipid-soluble waste product. This reputation stemmed from the involvement of bilirubin and its degradation products in excretion and their association with the yellow color in urine, brown color of feces, and the yellowish tone of skin resulting from jaundice. However, in the last couple of decades the antioxidant properties of bilirubin have been elucidated. Studies have shown a prominent role for bilirubin in the scavenging of peroxyl radicals.[33] Unfortunately, its activity in skin has yet to be fully understood or appreciated.

Melatonin

Melatonin is a circadian rhythm-regulating hormone that provides us with an internal clock based on its blood concentration levels. It is the metabolic product of tryptophan and is responsible for the onset of sleepiness experienced after eating turkey—a tryptophan-rich substance—on Thanksgiving day. Melatonin (Figure 3.22) also carries out functions as an antioxidant. It can engage in free radical scavenging, facilitate the activity of antioxidant enzymes, prevent the endogenous production of radicals in the mitochondrion, and help to make other antioxidants more efficacious.[34] In skin, melatonin plays an important role in the hair growth cycle, hair pigmentation, and regulation of melanoma.[35] Moreover, it acts as an antioxidant in skin and suppresses UV-induced damage.[36,37] In addition to being an endogenous antioxidant synthesized in skin, it also offers promise in treatment protocols from exogenous topical applications.[37]

MELANINS

As discussed in Chapter 1, melanocytes are specialized cells capable of synthesizing melanin, which is a pigment responsible in part for the color of our skin and hair.

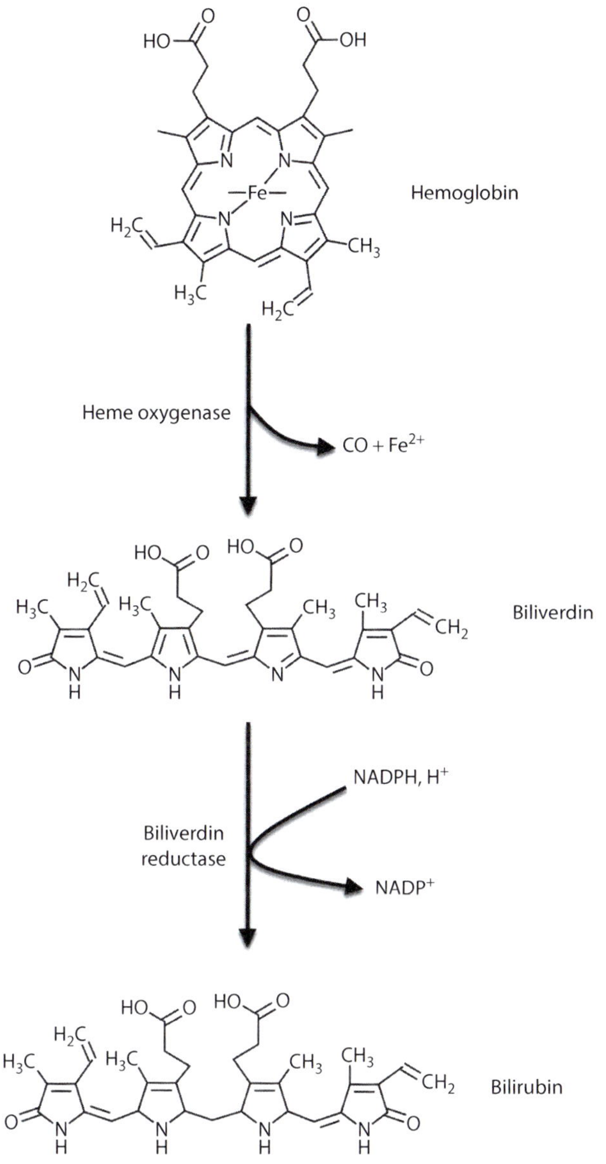

Figure 3.21 Degradation of heme to bilirubin. (Adapted from Abraham, N. and Kappas, A., *Pharmacol. Rev.*, 60, 79–127, 2008.)

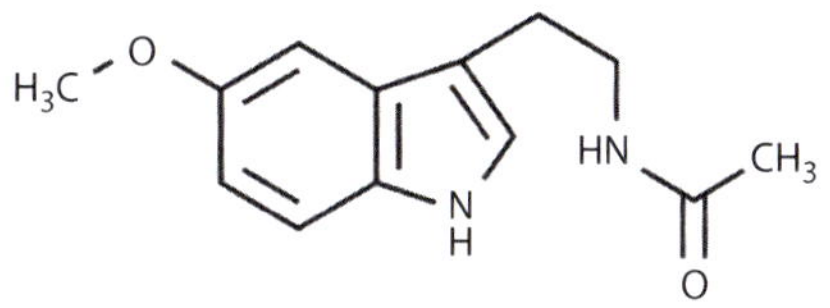

Figure 3.22 Structure of melatonin.

Molecules of melanin are packed in cellular organelles known as melanosomes. In the epidermis of skin, melanosomes are transferred from melanocytes to keratinocytes in order to provide protection to the nucleus, hence DNA, of these cells. In the mature hair shaft, melanin exists as granules in the cortex protecting the keratin intermediate filaments, which confer the fiber with its great tensile strength.

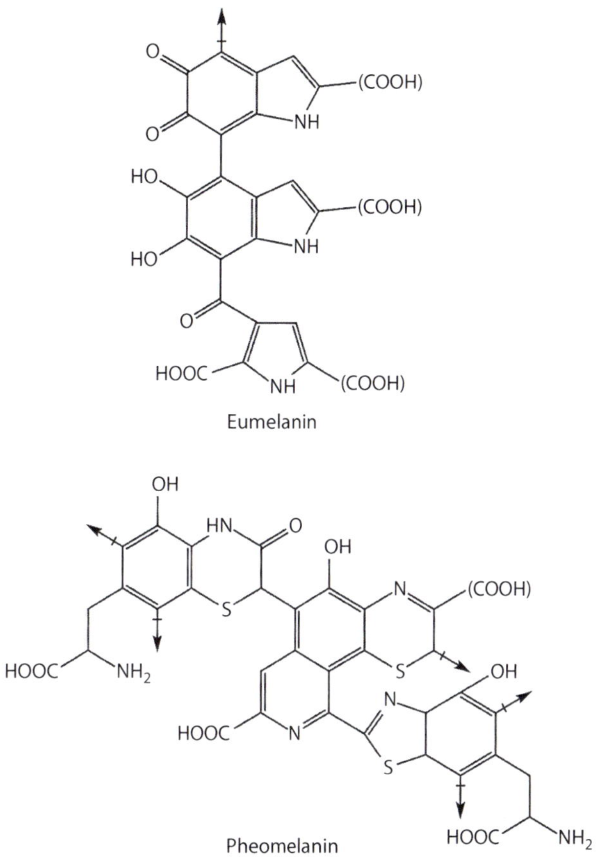

Figure 3.23 Structure of eumelanin and pheomelanin as proposed by Ito and Wakamatsu. (Adapted from Ito, S. and Wakamatsu, K., Chemistry of melanins, in *The Pigmentary System*, Nordlund, J.J. et al. [Eds.], Wiley-Blackwell, Malden, MS, 2006.)

There are two types of biological melanin present in skin and hair: eumelanin and pheomelanin (Figure 3.23).[38] Eumelanin is responsible for dark color pigmentation and results in brown and black tones. Pheomelanin, on the other hand, is a red and yellow pigment and is more predominantly found in fair-skinned individuals, e.g., individuals with red hair contain greater quantities of pheomelanin than eumelanin. The synthesis of both types of melanin begins with the aromatic amino acid tyrosine in a reaction that is catalyzed by the enzyme, tyrosinase. This results in the formation of 3,4-dihydroxyphenylalanine (DOPA) which further undergoes conversion to dopaquinone. At this point, two separate reaction pathways proceed for the synthesis of eumelanin and pheomelanin (see Appendix 2 for a schematic of melanin synthesis).

With its highly conjugated structure, melanin is a highly efficient absorber of UV and visible light with an absorption profile that is extremely high at low wavelengths (UV region) and decreases monotonically with increasing wavelengths into the visible region of the electromagnetic spectrum.

There are various sites present in the polymeric structure of melanin that contain free electrons able to participate in free radical reactions. Our current scientific understanding indicates that these radical sites can serve as reaction centers for other free radical species, and so melanin is often referred to as a free radical sink. Further, it is believed that through this process melanosomes are capable of trapping free radicals within their organelle structure, prohibiting further diffusion throughout the cell.

There has been a lot of exciting research in recent years in the area of melanocyte biology and the elucidation of the physical and chemical properties of melanin.[39,40] Eumelanin is considered the principal photoprotective agent and antioxidant of the skin, while pheomelanin is often faulted as a photosensitizer susceptible to solar radiation. The relative quantities of eumelanin and pheomelanin present are thought to determine the pro-oxidant and antioxidant properties. There has been a lot of controversy about the pro-oxidant versus antioxidant properties of melanin; however, many of these studies demonstrate the effect in vitro in conditions that are not found in normal physiologically conditions.[39] Recent research has also shed light on the importance of the molecular structure of eumelanin and pheomelanin on their light absorption, antioxidant, and redox behavior.[40] Essentially, the degree of decarboxylation in the overall melanin structure affects these key properties.

OTHER NOTABLE ENDOGENOUS ANTIOXIDANTS

So far we have discussed many antioxidants whose role in skin has been extensively studied. There are several other important endogenous antioxidants worth mentioning, namely: ferritin, L-carnitine, alpha-lipoic acid, and metallothioneins.[41]

Ferritin

Ferritin is a 24-subunit globular protein responsible for iron storage in the cell. Free iron in the cell can be toxic and produce free radicals via Fenton-type reactions. Therefore, ferritin plays an integral role in cellular homeostasis. More specifically related to skin, evidence suggests that ferritin is activated as part of a defense mechanism during UV exposure.[42–44]

L-Carnitine

Responsible for the transport of fatty acids from the cytosol of the cell to the mitochondrion, L-carnitine is also essential for antioxidant activity, especially the prevention of membrane lipid peroxidation. Its role as an endogenous antioxidant in skin is rarely discussed in the literature. However, the use of L-carnitine in topical compositions has been more forthcoming.[45]

Alpha-lipoic acid

Alpha-lipoic acid is an extremely important antioxidant in human physiology.[46] While it is a known endogenous antioxidant, its distribution in skin tissue and cells has not been a recurring theme in the literature. Its mechanism of action and use in topical applications for skin are thoroughly discussed in Chapter 8.

Metallothioneins

Metallothioneins are a group of low molecular weight proteins abundant with cysteine residues. They are important regulators of cell growth and proliferation, and due to their sulfur-containing residues are able to bind trace elements such as cadmium, mercury, platinum, and silver, thereby protecting cells from heavy metal toxicity. In terms of their antioxidant action, metallothioneins are known combatants of $HO^{\bullet}$.[47] Several studies were carried out to investigate its behavior in skin, illustrating an essential role for metallothionein in preventing UVB-induced injury.[48–50]

ANTIOXIDANT LEVELS AND DISTRIBUTION IN SKIN

Several texts offer information about the levels and activity of antioxidants present in skin; what follows is a brief summary of their findings.[51–53] In general, the antioxidant activity in the epidermis is greater than that found in the dermis. As an example, a possible explanation for the fivefold increase in ascorbate epidermal concentrations as compared to the levels in the dermis may be due to the increased utilization of this molecule for the synthesis of collagen and elastin in the dermis.[52] In addition, the levels of small-molecule antioxidants in skin seem to be much higher than enzymatic antioxidants, with the exception of catalase, the Trx system, and NAD(P)H:quinone reductase, which also exhibit significant levels of activity. In comparison with other body tissues, such as heart, liver, or brain, the activity of SOD and GPX are lower in skin.[53]

Overall, the levels of ascorbate, urate, alpha-tocopherol, and coenzyme Q are relatively high in skin.[53] Twice as much GSH is found in the epidermis than in the dermis; however, the ratio of GSSG/GSH is four times higher in the dermis than the epidermis.[53] Thus, the epidermis is either much more efficient at maintaining the level of GSH, or GSH utilization is much greater in the dermis than the epidermis. In regard to carotenoids, the most common ones found in skin include carotenes (alpha-, beta-, and gamma-), lycopene, lutein, and zeaxanthin.[54] They are obtained in the diet and found distributed in the dermis and epidermis. Carotenoids find their way to the epidermis by way of adipose tissue (where they are stored), blood, or lymph. In addition, they may be secreted by sweat or sebaceous glands.[26] At any rate, carotenoids play an important role in the protection of skin from the elements. The anatomical distribution of antioxidants may also vary from one site to the next. For example, Darvin and coworkers were able to discern distinct distributions of carotenoids in several tested anatomical locations including palm, forehead, and volar forearm.[55] Their studies were conducted in vivo on human subjects with Raman spectroscopy. Overall, clinical studies indicate that the levels of endogenous antioxidants are greatly influenced by both diet and exposure to stress.[56]

CONCLUDING REMARKS

As the outermost organ of the body, skin constantly finds itself in contact with the elements, including UV light and other damaging species, which cause the formation of free radical species. In order to combat such threats, skin contains a powerful antioxidant defense system consisting of structurally complex enzymes as well as small molecules, such as alpha-tocopherol and L-ascorbic acid, which help protect the skin from oxidative stress. In order to protect skin from oxidative stresses, it seems logical that when the human organism's own antioxidant defense mechanism becomes overwhelmed, supplementation or topical treatment with antioxidants can be a beneficial approach. In fact, numerous studies have focused on the enhanced protective effects offered to skin by fortification with exogenous antioxidants. Chapter 8 will discuss treatment of skin with key antioxidants that have been proven to be efficacious in repeated studies.

REFERENCES

1. Rangarajan M, Zatz JL. *J Cosmet Sci.* 1999;50:249–279.
2. Miriyala S et al. *Biochim Biophys Acta.* 2012;1822:794–814.
3. Petersen SV et al. *J Biol Chem.* 2004;279:13705–13710.
4. Adachi T et al. *Arch Biochem Biophys.* 1992;297:155–161.
5. Miller A. *Curr Opin Chem Biol.* 2004;8:162–168.
6. Johnson F, Giulivi C. *Mol Aspects Med.* 2005;26:340–352.
7. Hart PJ et al. *Biochemistry.* 1999;38:2167–2178.
8. Halliwell B, Gutteridge JMC. *Free Radicals in Biology and Medicine*, 5th ed. Oxford, UK: University Press; 2015.
9. Putnam CD et al. *J Mol Biol.* 2000;296:295–309.
10. Kirkman HN et al. *J Biol Chem.* 1987;262:660–666.
11. Mugesh G et al. *J Am Chem Soc.* 2001;123:839–850.
12. Epp O et al. *Eur J Biochem.* 1983;133:51–69.
13. Lackner KL, Blankenberg S. *Ital Heart J.* 2004;5:169–172.
14. Faig M et al. *Proc Natl Acad Sci USA.* 2000;97:3177–3182.
15. Li R et al. *Proc Natl Acad Sci USA.* 1995;92:8846–8850.
16. Zhou Z et al. *Biochemistry.* 2003;42:1985–1994.
17. Lennon BW et al. *Science.* 2000;289:1190–1194.
18. Mustacich D, Powis G. *Biochem J.* 2000;346:1–8.
19. Nordberg J, Arnér ESJ. *Free Radic Biol Med.* 2001;31:1287–1312.
20. Cenas N et al. *J Biol Chem.* 2004;279:2583–2592.
21. Xia L et al. *J Biol Chem.* 2003;278:2141–2146.
22. Mathews C et al. *Biochemistry*, 4th ed. Upper Saddle River, NJ: Prentice Hall; 2012.
23. Acworth IN, McCabe DR, Maher TJ. The analysis of free radicals, their reaction products, and antioxidants. In: Baskin SI, Salem H (Eds.). *Oxidants, Antioxidants, and Free Radicals.* Washington, DC: Taylor & Francis Group; 1997, pp. 23–77.
24. Olson JA, Krinsky NI. *FASEB.* 1995;9:1547–1550.
25. Stahl W, Sies H. *Mol Aspects Med.* 2003;24:345–351.
26. Darvin M et al. *Molecules.* 2011;16:10491–10506.
27. Handelman GJ. Carotenoids as scavengers of active oxygen species. In: Cadenas E, Packer L (Eds.). *Handbook of Antioxidants.* New York: Marcel Dekker; 1996, pp. 259–314.
28. Burton GW, Ingold KU. *Science.* 1984;224:569–573.
29. Abraham N, Kappas A. *Pharmacol Rev.* 2008;60:79–127.
30. Hughes V et al. *J Clin Pathol.* 2004;57:355–359.
31. Xiang Y et al. *BioScience Trends.* 2011;5:239–244.
32. Tyrell R, Reeve V. *Prog Biophys Mol Biol.* 2006;92:86–91.
33. Stocker R et al. *Science.* 1987;235:1043–1046.
34. Reiter R et al. *Acta Biochim Pol.* 2003;50:1129–1146.
35. Slominski A et al. *Endocrine.* 2005;27:137–148.
36. Fischer T, Elsner P. *Curr Probl Dermatol.* 2001;29:165–174.
37. Slominski A et al. *FASEB J.* 2005;19:176–194.
38. Ito S, Wakamatsu K. Chemistry of melanins. In: Nordlund JJ, Boissy RE, Hearing VJ, Oetting W, King RA, Ortonne J-P (Eds.). *The Pigmentary System.* Malden, MS: Wiley-Blackwell; 2006.
39. Micillo R et al. *Int J Mol Sci.* 2016;17:746.
40. Denat L et al. *J Invest Dermatol.* 2014;134:1512–1518.
41. Rizzo A et al. *Adv Exp Med Biol.* 2010;698:52–67.
42. Applegate L et al. *J Invest Dermatol.* 1998;111:159–163.
43. Pourzand C et al. *Proc Natl Acad Sci USA.* 1999;96:6751–6756.
44. Orino K et al. *Biochem J.* 2001;357:241–247.
45. Fox L et al. *Skin Pharmacol Physiol.* 2011;24:330–336.
46. Moini H et al. *Toxicol Appl Pharmacol.* 2002;182:84–90.
47. Thirumoorthy N et al. *World J Gastroenterol.* 2007;13:993–996.
48. Oord J, Ley M. *Arch Dermatol Res.* 1994;286:62–68.
49. Hanada K. *J Dermatol Sci.* 2000;23(Suppl 1):S51–S56.
50. Wang W et al. *Clin Exp Dermatol.* 2004;29:57–61.
51. Chaudhuri RK. Role of antioxidants in sun care products. In: Shaath NA (Ed.). *Sunscreens: Regulation and Commercial Development.* Boca Raton, FL: Taylor & Francis Group; 2005, pp. 603–638.
52. Thiele JJ, Dreher F. Antioxidant defense systems in skin. In: Elsner P, Maibach HI (Eds.). *Cosmeceuticals and Active Cosmetics: Drugs versus Cosmetics. Cosmetic Science and Technology, 27,* 2nd ed. Boca Raton, FL: Taylor & Francis Group; 2005, pp. 37–88.
53. Vessey DA. The cutaneous antioxidant system. In: Fuchs J, Packer L (Eds.). *Oxidative Stress in Dermatology.* New York: Marcel Dekker; 1993, pp. 81–103.
54. Stahl W, Sies H. *Biochim Biophys Acta.* 2005;1740:101–107.
55. Darvin M et al. *Exp Dermatol.* 2009;18:1060–1063.
56. Jung S et al. *Skin Pharmacol Physiol.* 2014;27:293–302.

Effects of solar radiation, air pollution, and artificial blue light on the skin

> The Sun is such a familiar companion that many people forget that sunlight is a prerequisite for life on Earth.
>
> —Elli Kohen, René Santus, and Joseph G. Hirschberg
> *Photobiology*

The world as we know it would not be possible without the presence of the Sun. It gives life to just about every imaginable thing we come into contact with on a daily basis. At the same time, we are susceptible to sun damage. The amount of solar radiation reaching the Earth's surface depends on latitude, altitude, time of day, season, and atmospheric conditions.[1] As the body's first defense against the elements, skin is frequently exposed to the Sun's emitted electromagnetic radiation. As a result, several conditions may develop within the skin, including photoaging, photoimmunosuppression, and photocarcinogenesis.

Photoaging results in the degradation and deformation of connective tissue in the dermis, which changes the overall mechanical properties and appearance of skin. Exposure to ultraviolet (UV) radiation may also result in a compromised immune system manifested as photoimmunosuppression, also known as UV-induced immune suppression. Photoimmunosuppression is closely interrelated with photocarcinogenesis, the gravest disease state of skin. This discovery was first made when it was observed that transplanted tumors grow in immune suppressed subjects and are not able to grow in normal subjects. In any event, all of these processes begin at the molecular level with chromophoric absorption of light. In some cases, direct absorption of UVB light by deoxyribonucleic acid (DNA) leads to genetic mutations. In others, free radical mechanisms are fully responsible for many of the other disease states of the skin. For example, absorption of UVA light by a sensitizer results in the generation of reactive oxygen species (ROS) capable of damaging DNA, proteins, or lipids. This chapter provides an overview of the light reactions that occur in skin and the resulting disease states, along with a discussion of the molecular mechanisms responsible for such phenomena, beginning with light absorption.

In the last decade, there has been a significant amount of work dedicated to understanding the effects of visible and infrared light on the skin. Such reactions proceed through photosensitization reactions ultimately resulting in the production of ROS that damage connective tissue of the dermis, and may have implications beyond.

The ramifications of exposure of the skin to air pollution are another important area in skin health. In the following sections, we provide a comprehensive discussion of the effects of various components of air pollution: oxides (nitrogen oxides and sulfur oxides), ozone (O_3), particulate matter (PM), polycyclic aromatic hydrocarbons, tobacco smoke, and volatile organic compounds (VOCs). In addition, we discuss the consequences of artificial blue light exposure on the skin and attempt to provide the reader with a balanced look at this emerging area.

INTERACTION OF LIGHT WITH SKIN

The interaction of light with skin consists of reflection, scattering, and absorption. In terms of reflection, depending on the local geometry of the skin surface only a small fraction of the incident light undergoes reflection (Figure 4.1). However, anywhere from 93% to 96% of the incident light may be scattered or absorbed by endogenous chromophores.[2] The next section discusses the various chromophores present in skin and their respective contributions to skin's absorbance profile. Also, solar radiation penetrates the dermis and may be scattered by the resident collagen fibers, thereby affecting the overall depth of penetration and, thus, the chromophoric absorption.[2]

As the outermost organ of the body, the skin is in constant contact with solar radiation. UV, visible, and infrared radiation reaching the surface of the Earth interact with the integument (Figure 4.2). In terms of biological insult, UV light is of particular concern due to the potentially damaging biochemical reactions that may result. UV light is often further categorized into its component

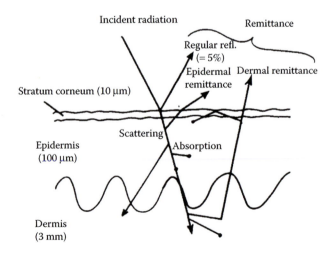

Figure 4.1 Interaction of light with the skin. (Reprinted from *J. Invest. Dermatol.*, 77, Anderson, R.R. and Parrish, J.A., The optics of human skin, 13–19, Copyright 1981, with permission from Elsevier.)

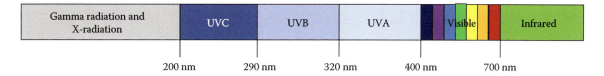

Figure 4.2 Electromagnetic spectrum.

parts as UVA (320–400 nm), UVB (290–320 nm), and UVC (200–290 nm). Wavelengths less than 290 nm (UVC) are filtered by O_3 present in the stratosphere. Wavelengths of light greater than 290 nm reach the surface of the Earth and interact with the skin in various manners. Historically, UVB was known to be very detrimental to the integrity of the skin as it is directly absorbed by nucleic acid bases, resulting in DNA mutations. In addition, due to UVB's higher energy rays, more research was conducted investigating its deleterious effects on skin. On the other hand, the amount of UVA that reaches the Earth's surface is much greater than that of UVB. Thus, it has been recognized that the role played by UVA in damage to the skin is also of substantial concern. In fact, in more recent years the deleterious effects of UVA have been realized and it is now well recognized that exposure to UVA results in photosensitization reactions in skin, leading to free radical damage. Moreover, while sunburn (erythema) is principally caused by UVB radiation, pigmentation changes, photoaging, photoimmunosuppression, and photocarcinogenesis result from exposure to both UVB and UVA radiation. In recent years, it has been recognized that visible and near-infrared radiation also cause free radical processes in the skin. Evidence has shown that high doses of light in this region can cause considerable damage as manifested by erythema, oxidative stress, DNA damage, and photoaging.[1,3,4]

An important aspect regarding the interaction of light with skin is an understanding of the skin penetration capabilities of the different segments of the electromagnetic spectrum. Figure 4.3 provides a diagram of the layers of skin and the penetration of various types of electromagnetic radiation into these layers.[5] Based on the diagram, we can see that depending on the wavelength of light, the penetration depth within the skin varies. For example, longer wavelength light such as that found in the visible region of the spectrum is able to penetrate deep into the dermis. On the other hand, UVA radiation typically manages to make its way to the mid- to upper-layers of the dermis while UVB is limited to the epidermis. When taken into this perspective, we can gain a better understanding of the interaction of light with the various components of skin. For example, since UVB typically only penetrates as deep as the epidermis, we would expect this type of light to affect epidermal cells, especially keratinocytes, since they are the most abundant cells present. Further, UVB interacts with nucleic acid bases and aromatic amino acids. Thus, we

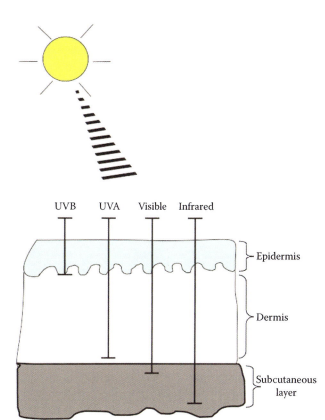

Figure 4.3 Penetration of solar radiation into the skin. (Adapted from Kohen, E. et al., *Photobiology*, Academic Press, San Diego, CA, 1995.)

shall expect that UVB radiation is most damaging to the DNA and cellular proteins present in keratinocytes. In fact, after melanosome synthesis by melanocytes, these organelles are deposited into adjacent basal layer keratinocytes, where they confer protection to the mitotic cells by surrounding the nucleus.

CHROMOPHORES IN SKIN

There is a plethora of chromophores present in human skin, ranging from cellular DNA to hemoglobin present in the vascular network.[2,6–8] These molecules absorb electromagnetic radiation in the UVB, UVA, and visible region of the spectrum. Table 4.1 contains a list of the most common chromophores found in skin along with pertinent information, such as the absorption maxima and molar absorptivity values, as well as the anatomical or cellular

Table 4.1 Selected chromophores present in skin.

Classification	Chromophore	λ_{max}	ε_{max} (10^{-3})(L mol^{-1} cm^{-1})	Location
Nucleotides[a]	AMP	259[9]	15.4	Nucleus and mitochondrion of epidermal and dermal cells
	GMP	252[9]	13.7	
	CMP	271[9]	9.1	
	UMP	262[9]	10.0	
	GMP	267[9]	10.2	
Amino acids[a]	Tryptophan	280[9]	5.6	Cellular and structural proteins
	Tyrosine	275[9]	1.42	
	Phenylalanine	257[9]	0.197	
	Cystine			
Pigment molecules	Eumelanin[b]	UV/visible		Epidermis
	Pheomelanin[b]	UV/visible		Epidermis
	Lipofuscins			
	Beta-carotene[b]	visible		
Porphyrin related compounds	Hemoglobin	visible		Vascular vessels in the dermis
	Oxyhemoglobin	visible		
Cofactors[a]	NAD(P)H	340[10]	6.222	See text
	Flavins (FMN+, FAD+)	300–500		See text
Cross-linking amino acids	Pyridine derivatives	UVA		ECM proteins
	Quinones	UVA/UVB		
	Pterines	UVA		See text
	7-Dehydrocholesterol			Dermis/epidermis
	trans-Urocanic acid	UVA/UVB		Stratum corneum

[a] Appendix 2
[b] Chapter 3 (See for structures)

location. The first group of molecules outlined in the table is the nucleotides—the building blocks of nucleic acids. In general, the absorption maximum for DNA is reported at 260 nm, which is an overlap of the contributions of the various nucleotides resulting in a composite absorption spectrum. Figure 4.4 contains absorption spectra for DNA and other chromophores present in skin.

The second class of compounds shown in Table 4.1 is the chromophore-containing amino acids. In general, cellular proteins produce an absorption maximum at 280 nm, which results from a combination of absorption from the amino acids, tryptophan, tyrosine, and phenylalanine. Absorption at lower wavelengths can result due to high concentrations of cystine; however, its molar absorption coefficient is much less than the aromatic amino acids. In addition to proteins and nucleic acids, pigment molecules in skin, such as the melanins, are broad spectrum absorbers. Moreover, lipofuscin granules, which are composed of lipid and protein oxidation products, can also be found in skin.[10,11] They are present in many tissues; however, in skin they are responsible for what are commonly referred to as liver spots. Several heme-containing molecules are found in the arterial vessels of the dermis, which absorb visible light. The deoxygenated and oxygenated forms of hemoglobin have slightly shifted absorption maxima as shown in Figure 4.4b, which are either a reddish (oxygenated) or bluish (deoxygenated) color. Bilirubin—a hemoglobin degradation product—is also found in the blood and is yellowish in color.

As seen in Chapter 3, coenzymes (cofactors) play an integral role in the redox chemistry of the cell. They are often responsible for many of the biosynthetic reactions involving electron transfer in which they exist as auxiliary groups within the enzyme. Enzyme cofactors, such as nicotinamide adenine dinucleotide (NADH) or nicotinamide adenine dinucleotide phosphate (NADPH), are involved in oxidation-reduction reactions in which they are able to interconvert from the oxidized form (NAD$^+$ or NADP$^+$) to the reduced state (NADH or NADPH)—a one-electron reduction process without a stable intermediate state. The only structural difference between the two coenzymes is the presence of a phosphate moiety in NADPH; thus, both molecules have identical photochemical properties. The oxidized form of the cofactor absorbs light in the UVA region with λ_{max} = 340 nm. Furthermore, NAD$^+$ and NADP$^+$ fluoresce at 445 nm when excited at 340 nm.[12] Other cofactors include the flavins (flavin mononucleotide [FMN] and flavin adenine dinucleotide [FAD]), which are derived from vitamin B$_2$, also known as riboflavin. Both flavins exist as cofactors in enzymes and are further able to undergo two-electron reduction reactions. In the reduced form, FMNH$_2$ or FADH$_2$, the cofactors do not absorb visible light. However, in the protonated semiquinone form both FMNH or FADH have an absorption maximum

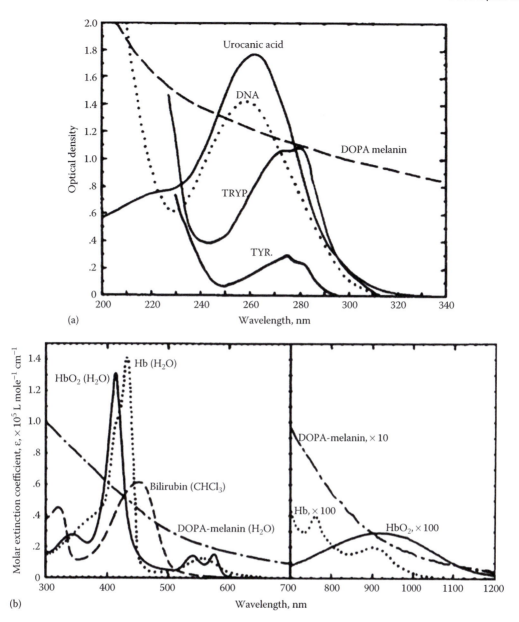

Figure 4.4 Absorption spectra of major chromophores in skin in the (a) UV and (b) visible regions of the electromagnetic spectrum. (Reprinted from *J. Invest. Dermatol.*, 77, Anderson, R.R. and Parrish, J.A., The optics of human skin, 13–19, Copyright 1981, with permission from Elsevier.)

at 560 nm. In the fully oxidized form, λ_{max} = 450 nm for FMN and FAD. Figure 4.5 provides absorption spectra for the oxidized and reduced species of NAD^+/NADH and FMN/FMNH; however, it is noteworthy that the same spectral details apply for $NADP^+$/NADPH and FAD/$FADH_2$, respectively.[13]

Elastin, found in the dermis, provides skin with elastic properties. Cross-links exist within the protein structure that help to maintain its elastic nature, preventing indefinite extension of the elastic fibers. The cross-links are formed between lysine residues with the amino acid desmosine (Figure 4.6) and its isomer, isodesmosine. Due to the pyridinium ring in desmosine and isodesmosine, absorption occurs in the UVB and UVA region of the spectrum, lending to its ability to act as a photosensitizing agent. Similarly, cross-linking of collagen in the dermis is due to the amino acid, pyridinoline, which displays similar photochemical behavior as the desmosine isomers (Figure 4.6). Further, as a result of UV-induced damage, advanced glycation end products are produced in the extracellular matrix (ECM). This results in cross-links that are produced by pyridinium compounds, such as glycol-aldehyde pyridine. Other pyridine containing compounds are found in skin, many of which may act as photosensitizing agents by absorbing UVA radiation.[7,8]

In addition to the chromophores already mentioned, there are several compounds categorized under the heading miscellaneous in Table 4.1. These include quinones, which is a class of compounds that share the common structural feature of an aromatic ring containing two

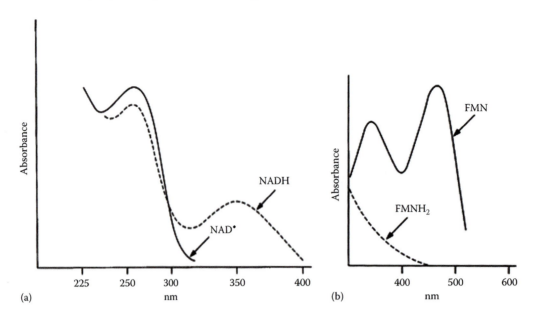

Figure 4.5 Absorption spectra of (a) NAD+/NADH and (b) FMN/FMNH. (From Boyer, R.F., *Modern Experimental Biochemistry*, Benjamin/Cummings, Redwood City, CA, 1993. Reprinted with permission from Pearson Education, Copyright 1993.)

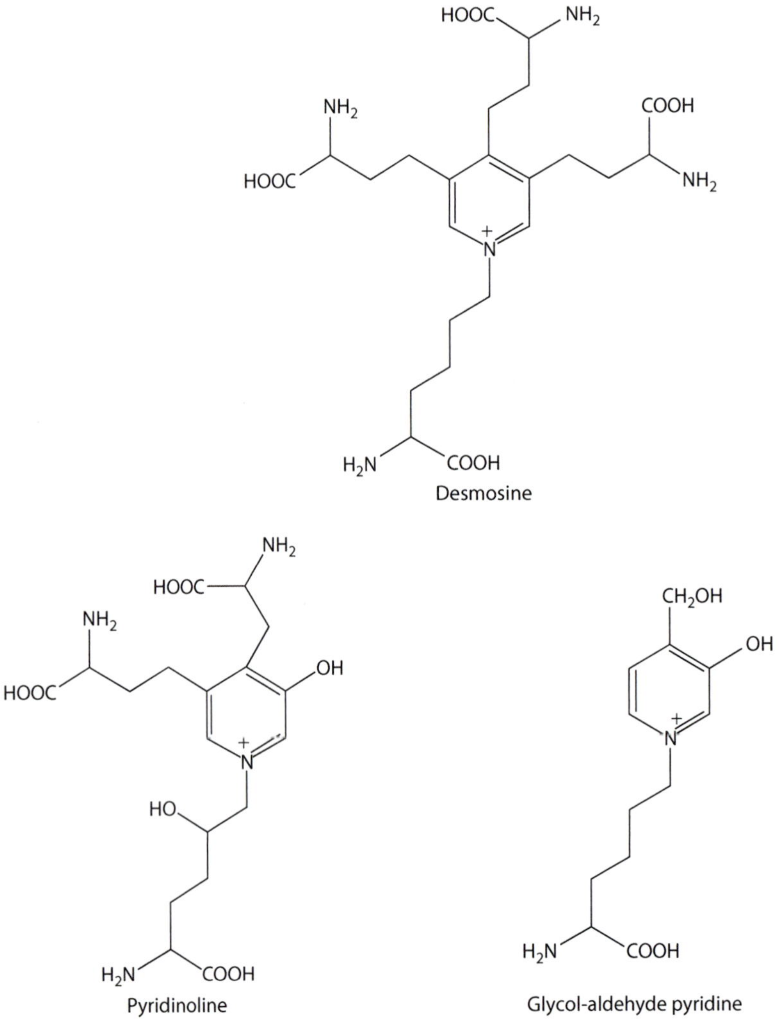

Figure 4.6 Structures of various pyridinium compounds found in the ECM of skin.

ketone groups. The most ubiquitous cellular quinone is coenzyme Q. The pterins represent a class of molecules that are typically categorized by their structural constituents, which consist of a pyrazine and pyrimidine ring, resulting in absorption in the UVA region of the spectrum and often having fluorescent properties.[8] Some molecules that belong to this group are pterin, biopterin, neopterin, and folic acid.

As a major chromophore component of the stratum corneum, *trans*-urocanic acid has received considerable attention in the literature. It is derived from the metabolism of histidine during the decomposition of filaggrin during epidermal differentiation. The absorption spectrum and chemical structure of *trans*-urocanic acid is provided in Figure 4.7.[14] The large absorption peak in the UVB region of the spectrum is thought to offer a great deal of protection for cellular amino acids and nucleic acid bases. On the other hand, *trans*-urocanic acid undergoes photoisomerization to *cis*-urocanic acid when exposed to UV irradiation, optimally at 300–310 nm. This transformation results in photosensitization and plays a major role in photoimmunosuppression.

As seen thus far, exposure to solar irradiation results in many detrimental effects to the health status of skin. However, there are instances when positive consequences are obtained from the Sun's solar UV rays. One of the last molecules provided in the list of Table 4.1 is 7-dehydrocholesterol (provitamin D_3), which is a precursor of vitamin D_3. Absorption of UVB radiation by 7-dehydrocholesterol takes place in the dermal and epidermal layers of the skin, dependent on the degree of skin pigmentation. This results in the formation of previtamin D_3, which undergoes thermal isomerization to vitamin D_3;[15,16] see Figure 4.8 for illustration. It was well established in the early part of the twentieth century that lack of exposure to sunlight may lead to the childhood disease known as rickets (osteomalacia in adults), which affects skeletal formation. In the absence of vitamin D_3, adequate levels of calcium are not present in the blood stream due to poor intestinal absorption, which causes hormonal release of calcium from the bones, ultimately leading to skeletal deformity. In order to circumvent vitamin D_3 deficiencies, many societies fortify milk with this vitamin.

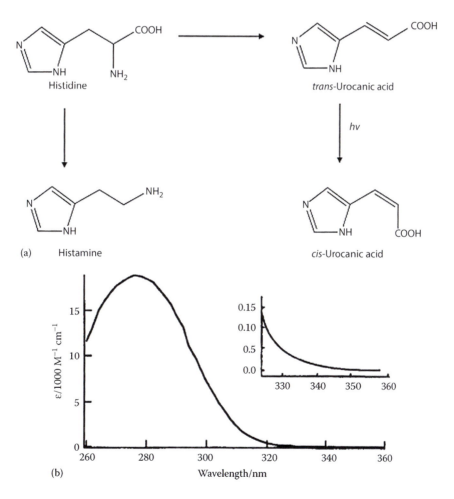

Figure 4.7 (a) Chemical structures of histidine derivatives and (b) absorption spectrum of *trans*-urocanic acid. (Reprinted with permission from Hanson, K.M. and Simon, J.D., Epidermal trans-urocanic acid and the UV-A-induced photoaging of the skin. *Proc Natl Acad Sci USA*, 95, 10576–10578. Copyright 1998 National Academy of Sciences, U.S.A.)

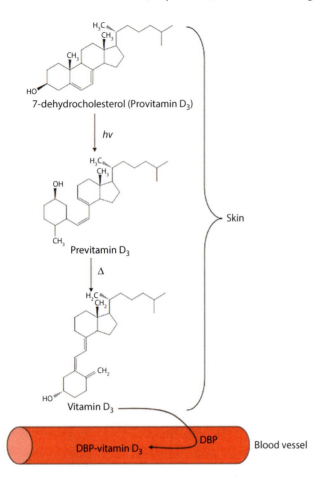

Figure 4.8 Conversion of 7-dehydrocholesterol to vitamin D_3 and its subsequent binding with vitamin D binding protein (DBP). (Adapted from Holick, M.F. et al., *Science*, 210, 203–205, 1980.)

EFFECTS OF UV LIGHT ON SKIN

In order for solar irradiation to induce a response in a plant or organism, it is necessary for some type of photochemical reaction to take place. We saw in the preceding section that skin contains many chromophores, which absorb light in the UVB, UVA, and visible regions of the electromagnetic spectrum. Typically, UVB light is thought to be most damaging to the nucleic acids followed by the proteins and various other chromophores. The mechanism of damage induced by UVA irradiation is associated with free radical reactions, which results from photosensitization of a chromophore and ultimately leads to the production of ROS or other radical species that wreak havoc on the structural components of the skin. By a similar mechanism, UVA is also responsible for damage to nucleic acids. In any event, the dose of light is of utmost importance[17] and will be governed by latitude, altitude, time of day, season, and atmospheric conditions.[1]

UVB-induced DNA damage

The genetic information in living organisms is encoded in the DNA present in the nuclei of the body's cells. DNA is composed of sequences of nucleotides of purine and pyrimidine bases (adenine, guanine, cytosine, and thymine), which form long-chain biopolymers arranged in various sequences in order to provide genetic distinctness. Through a process known as transcription, the sequence of bases in DNA are transcribed to RNA (ribonucleic acid) and ultimately expressed as proteins by way of translation. During cell division, DNA molecules must remain intact since an accurate replicate must be passed on to daughter cells. In general, DNA damage to the cellular constituents of an organism is undesirable as it could ultimately lead to mutagenesis (e.g., from DNA lesions) and ultimately carcinogenesis. Eukaryotic cells are equipped with repair mechanisms for damaged DNA in which the lesion (damaged base) is removed (e.g., by nucleotide excision repair), then replaced with new base-pairs by DNA polymerase. Unfortunately, the fidelity of this process can be compromised if these systems become overwhelmed or malfunction at times of high demand, leading to permanent mutations in DNA.[18]

It is well established that DNA damage occurs when cells are exposed to UV radiation. This damage occurs through a process of absorption by the chromophoric bases that constitute the backbone of DNA. Since maximum absorption of DNA occurs in the UVB region (*ca.* 260 nm), it stands to reason that the shorter wavelength light (290–320 nm) that reaches the terrestrial surface is the most deleterious to the structure and integrity of DNA. As a result of UVB absorption, DNA cross-links are formed between adjacent thymine residues in DNA. The two most common and lethal photoproducts are cyclobutane thymine dimers and pyrimidine (6–4) pyrimidone photoadducts. Figure 4.9 illustrates the structural modifications induced in DNA by UVB radiation.

Photosensitization reactions resulting from UVA radiation

As only 5% of incident UV radiation that strikes the Earth's surface is UVB, there is tremendous interest in elucidating the effects on skin of UVA, which constitutes the other 95%. (UVC is absorbed largely by the atmosphere; its presence at terrestrial level is negligible.) Unlike UVB, fewer photons of UVA are absorbed by DNA and, thus, the DNA photoproducts shown in Figure 4.9 are not formed to an appreciable extent as a result of exposure to UVA radiation. UVA induces a response from endogenous photosensitizers in skin, such as porphyrins and flavins, leading to several different pathways, ultimately resulting in oxidative damage to skin. Figure 4.10 provides a schematic of the general fate of a sensitizer exposed to UVA radiation, causing it to become excited to a triplet electronic energy state. It is thereby allowed to react with other molecules, resulting in the formation of ROS and other free radical species. First, absorption by UV radiation causes the sensitizer (S) to undergo excitation to a singlet state ($^1S^*$), which is followed by intersystem crossing, resulting in a triplet state. At this point, the triplet sensitizer ($^3S^*$) can follow

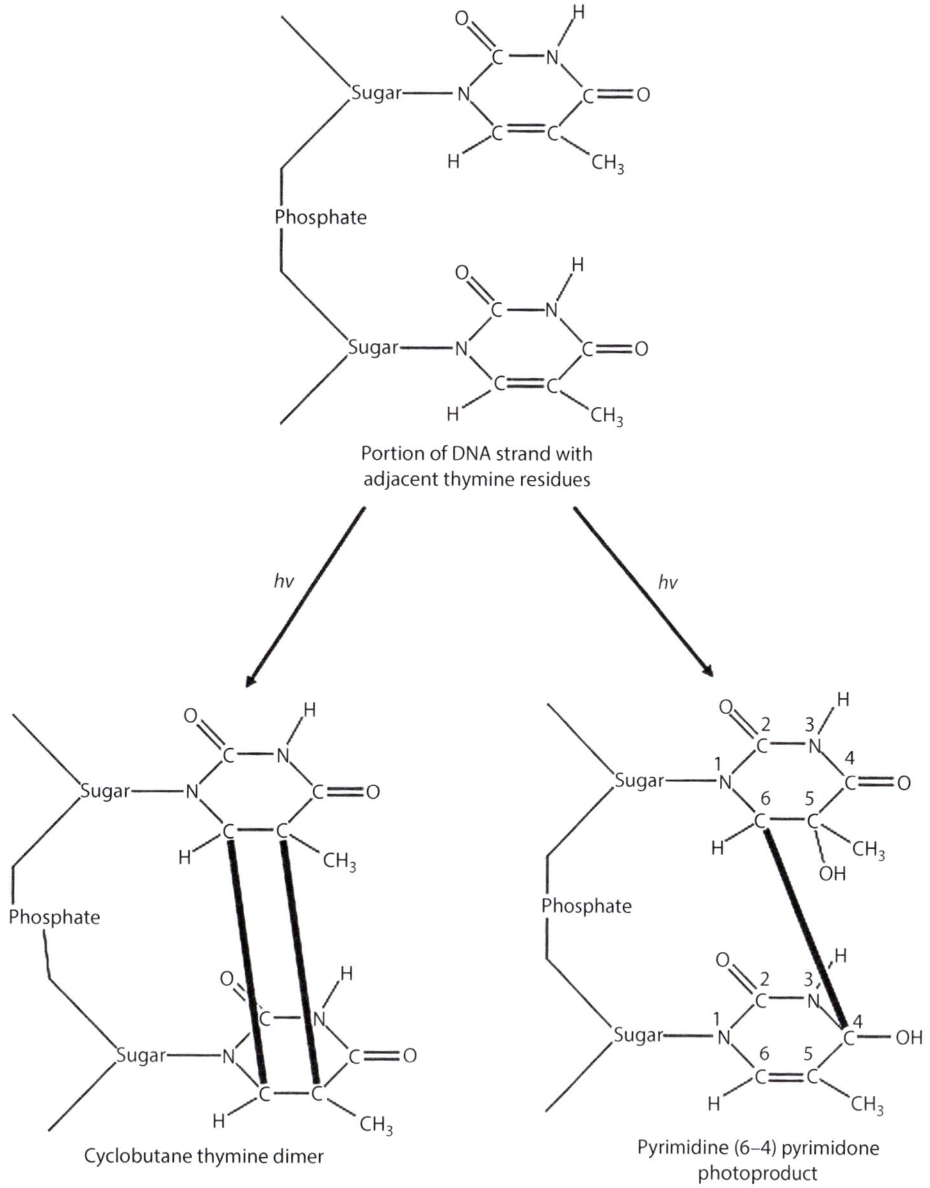

Figure 4.9 UVB-induced damage to DNA resulting in the formation of pyrimidine dimer photoproducts.

one of two distinct pathways—one in which its reaction with another molecule results in hydrogen or electron abstraction (Type I) or another in which the $^3S^*$ reacts with molecular oxygen (Type II). In the Type I mechanism, abstraction of a proton typically occurs in the presence of an unsaturated lipid. The Type II mechanism can be further classified into two pathways, one in which the $^3S^*$ reacts with molecular oxygen to form singlet oxygen ($^1O_2$) [Major Type II] or another where the $^3S^*$ reacts with O_2 to form the superoxide anion ($^1O_2^{-\bullet}$) [Minor Type II]. In the Major Type II pathway, subsequent interaction of $^1O_2$ with other endogenous species can cause further free radical reactions. The Minor Type II pathway, on the other hand, involves the dismutation of $^1O_2^{-\bullet}$ to H_2O_2, which can lead to the Fenton reaction in the presence of iron ions, ultimately yielding the extremely reactive hydroxyl radical (HO·).

In general, UVA-dependent formation of ROS and other free radicals results in damage to connective tissue, more specifically the ECM proteins of the dermis, which ultimately leads to photoaging of the skin. In addition, photosensitization reactions, caused by UVA absorption, can lead to photoaging, photoimmunosuppression, photocarcinogenesis, and other ailments of the skin.

UVA-induced DNA damage

Findings in recent years have shed light on the mode of action of UVA radiation in terms of DNA damage.[19] In the Major Type II pathway, subsequent interaction of $^1O_2$ with nucleotide bases results in chemical modification.

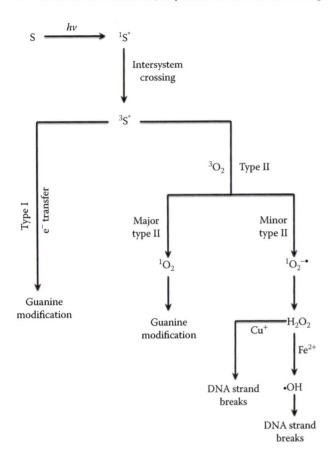

Figure 4.10 Photosensitization of a chromophore leading to three possible different pathways. (Adapted from Kawanishi, S. and Hiraku, Y., Sequence-specific DNA damage induced by UVA radiation in the presence of endogenous and exogenous photosensitizers, in Thiele, J. and Elsner, P. [Eds.], *Oxidants and Antioxidants in Cutaneous Biology. Current Problems in Dermatology*, Karger, Basel, Switzerland, 74–82, 2001.)

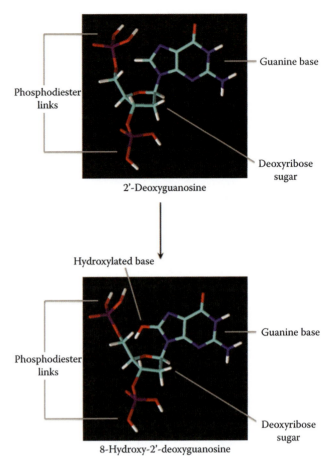

Figure 4.11 UVA-induced damage to DNA resulting in the hydroxylation of the guanine base.

As the ionization (or oxidation) potential for guanine is the lowest of the nucleotides, it is generally accepted that this base is the most frequent victim of such an electron transfer reaction.[20] Both of the Type II reactions can ultimately lead to chemical modifications to the DNA bases; however, the Minor Type II may also result in strand breaks. Figure 4.11 contains a scheme illustrating the free radical-induced formation of 8-hydroxy-2′-deoxyguanosine (8-OHdG) from guanosine. While UVA is typically associated with the formation of 8-OHdG and UVB with cyclobutane thymine dimers, studies suggest that UVA radiation may produce greater quantities of cyclobutane dimers than 8-OHdG.[21] Regardless, 8-OHdG can further undergo oxidation and reduction reactions.

Overall, both UVA and UVB contribute to the deleterious effects of solar radiation on skin.[20,22] There are numerous cellular signaling pathways as well as the induction of transcription factors that are activated by solar exposure. Due to the comprehensive nature of this subject, these topics will be discussed in a subsequent section.

IMMEDIATE MANIFESTATIONS OF UV-INDUCED DAMAGE IN SKIN

There are several well documented effects that occur immediately after exposure to UV radiation, usually on a timescale of the order of minutes to days. These include an increase in epidermal thickness, deleterious effects to immune system function, increase in vitamin D synthesis, suntan (increased pigmentation), and sunburn (erythema).[23] Photoimmunosuppression is discussed in a subsequent section and a description of vitamin D synthesis is provided in the subsection "Chromophores in the Skin" earlier in this chapter. Thus, we will briefly review erythema, solar radiation-induced pigmentation of skin, and epidermal thickening. A more comprehensive assessment of this topic may be found in the noted references.[23–25]

Exposure to solar irradiation results in an increase of melanin production and an increase in the thickness of the epidermis. Both of these effects are thought to be defense mechanisms against subsequent sun exposure. The action spectrum for sun tanning shows that UVB is primarily responsible for the induced effect; however, UVA and visible light also contribute to tanning.[23] Erythema, on the other hand, is primarily caused by UVB radiation as indicated by the action spectrum shown in Figure 4.12. Erythema is characterized by reddening, swelling, and

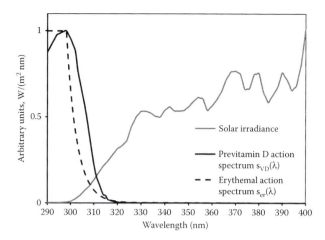

Figure 4.12 Solar spectrum of radiation reaching the Earth's surface plotted with the human erythema and previtamin D action spectra. (Reproduced from Kockott, D. et al., *PLoS ONE*, 11, e0145509, under the terms of the Creative Commons Attribution License, Copyright 2016.)

Table 4.2 Histological features of aging human skin.

Epidermis	Dermis	Appendages
Flattened dermal-epidermal junction	Atrophy	Depigmented hair
Variable thickness	Fewer fibroblasts	Loss of hair
Variable cell size and shape	Fewer mast cells	Conversion of terminal to vellus hair
Occasional nuclear atypia	Fewer blood cells	Abnormal nailplates
Fewer melanocytes	Shortened capillary loops	Fewer glands
Fewer Langerhans cells	Abnormal nerve endings	

Source: Yaar, M. and Gilchrest, B.A., Aging of skin, in *Fitzpatrick's Dermatology in General Medicine. 2*, Freedberg, I.M. et al. (Eds.), McGraw-Hill, New York, 1697–1706, 1999.

pain in the skin. The reddening results from vasodilation, while swelling is caused by vasopermeability.[23] In addition, sunburned skin often has an elevated temperature due to increased blood flow to the region.

The pigmentary change that occurs in skin immediately after solar exposure—usually several minutes later—is known as *immediate pigment darkening*. This is followed by a more extended period known as *persistent pigment darkening*. In either case, pigmentation is produced as a result of solar-induced reactions involving pre-existing melanin. Delayed tanning occurs in the aftermath in which new melanin is produced by melanocytes. Biochemically, the synthesis of melanin is upregulated by an increase in tyrosinase activity along with other factors resulting from keratinocyte activity (Appendix 2). For a more thorough treatment of this topic the reader is referred to the review by Polefka and coworkers.[1]

PHOTOAGING OF SKIN

Apart from the other aspects of photodamage, photoaging of skin refers to biochemical changes in skin as a result of chronic UV exposure that manifest in visible features such as wrinkling and pigmentary changes. The term photoaging most commonly brings to mind the notion of connective tissue damage in the dermis, which results in the development of deep furrows in the skin, and regions of hyperpigmentation, also referred to as age spots. We shall see that there is a complex series of biochemical events that lead to these symptoms and that this is still a very active field of research, not only for prevention of photoaging, but also to gain a more fundamental understanding of many of the underlying molecular pathways involved.[26–29]

Clinical and histological characteristics of photodamaged skin

The skin's capacity to perform many of its biological functions decreases with age. For example, barrier function, DNA repair mechanisms, sensory perception, thermal regulation, and sebum production all decrease as a function of age.[30] Normal aging of skin is often referred to as intrinsic aging, as it is a natural process, while photoaged skin is usually described as extrinsic aging, indicating the influence of external factors. Skin photoaging results in damage to the skin from the cumulative effects of the sun as well as the natural aging process of the skin. The ensuing damage results in visible signs that are often undesirable to the bearer.

Before continuing the discussion of photoaging, we should first discuss some of the effects associated with normal skin aging. Table 4.2 provides a list of some of the histological features associated with aged skin.

In photoaged skin, coarseness as well as fine and deep rhytides (wrinkles) are especially evident on regions of the body that are most exposed to the sun, such as the face, hands, and back of the neck. As an example, cutis rhomboidalis nuchae is a condition in which deep rhomboidal-shaped furrows develop on the back of the neck.

In addition, photoaged skin loses its elasticity and becomes less taut, thereby increasing its laxity. Pigmentary changes and disorders are also associated with photoaging and have collectively come to be known as age spots. For example, lentigines are macules that are brownish in color and are similar in shape and appearance to freckles. Telangiectasia and purpura are vascular disorders that occur in the skin as a result of photoaging. In the case of telangiectasia, vascular dilation results in the visible appearance of vessels. Purpura, on the other hand, is the result of internal bleeding in the skin and manifests as purple or red marks visible at the skin's surface.

Biochemical alterations in photodamaged skin

Photodamaged skin appears leathery, is less resilient, and loses many of its mechanical properties. These symptoms are a result of UV damage to the ECM proteins and fibroblast cells of the dermis. In general, collagen fibers provide

Table 4.3 MMPs involved in ECM degradation.

MMP	(kDa)	Subclass	Substrate
MMP-1	52, 57	Interstitial collagenases	Collagen I, collagen III
MMP-2	72	Gelatinases	Gelatin, collagen I, collagen IV, fibronectin, vitronectin, elastin
MMP-3	52, 58	Stromelysins	Laminin, fibronin, non-helical collagen
MMP-9	92	Gelatinases	Gelatin, collagen IV, collagen V

Source: Mauch, C. et al., Regulation of connective tissue turnover by matrix metalloproteinases, in *The Biology of the Skin*, Freinkel, R.K. and Woodley, D.T. (Eds.), The Parthenon Publishing Group, New York, 353–364, 2001.

skin with its mechanical tensile strength, while elastin bestows skin with its elastic properties. Irradiation with UV light damages existing macromolecules by upregulating the synthesis of matrix metalloproteinases (MMPs), which are the enzymes responsible for ECM degradation. In addition, damage to fibroblasts results in decreased ability to properly synthesize ECM proteins including collagen, elastin, and glycosaminoglycans.

MMPs are proteolytic enzymes and their expression leads to degradation of connective tissue. UV-induced upregulation of MMPs is induced by cellular signaling—discussed in the next section of this chapter.

Primarily, there are four MMPs responsible for ECM degradation, which are given in Table 4.3. The various types of MMPs have an assortment of substrates upon which they act. For example, MMP-1 serves as the catalyst for the reaction in which collagen fibers (collagen I and collagen III) are broken down by cleavage of the triple helix, allowing the remaining fragments to denature.[31] The denatured collagens can be further degraded by the gelatinases, MMP-2 and MMP-9, which are also responsible for degradation reactions of collagens located at the epidermal-dermal junction and the breakdown of gelatin.[31] MMP-3 belongs to the stromelysin subclass and is responsible for the degradation of several ECM proteins. Further, photoaging, like intrinsic aging of the skin, also results in diminished capacity to conduct collagen synthesis.

In addition to the degradation of ECM proteins, UV irradiation also causes the synthesis of dysfunctional elastic fibers, often referred to as elastotic material. This material is primarily composed of elastin; however, it also contains fibrillin, versican (a proteoglycan), and hyaluronic acid.[32] Unlike elastin, which provides skin with its elastic nature, the elastotic material leads to disorganization of the ECM.

UV-INDUCED SIGNALING CASCADES

Cellular signaling pathways are vital processes in molecular biology by which cells communicate with each other. Normally, a signal (a peptide) is secreted by one cell and then received by other cells, often via a receptor located at the plasma membrane. The receptor then activates intracellular pathways (cytosolic) that eventually make their way to the nucleus, where they activate transcription factors. As a result, upregulation of specific genes leads to RNA transcription and eventually to protein synthesis (translation). In the absence of UV radiation, such pathways are normally followed in order to regulate the proliferation, differentiation, and apoptosis of cells.[33]

It is well documented that UV light plays a key role in the induction of signaling pathways in skin. This results in ligand-independent activation of cell surface receptors, such as growth factor and cytokine receptors. Again, the activation of these receptors results in signal transduction cascades, which ultimately lead to the activation of a transcription factor. Thus, the upregulation or downregulation of a particular gene is affected by external stress factors, such as UV irradiation, which activate intracellular pathways normally induced by intercellular messengers. Although the mechanism is not fully understood, there is strong evidence that receptors are activated by ROS—probably formed as a result of UV-induced photosensitization reactions.[34]

While UV-induced cellular signaling pathways may lead to a variety of outcomes, some of the best understood pathways are those ultimately leading to skin photoaging.[34–36] Other studies, strictly concerned with molecular signaling induced as a result of UV exposure, elucidate similar or related mechanisms that may be involved in photoaging or even interconnected with photoimmunosuppression or photocarcinogenesis.[37–40] As shown in Figure 4.13, UV exposure results in the activation of cell surface receptors located at the plasma membrane: transforming growth factor-beta (TGF-beta), growth factor receptors, and cytokine receptors. As already noted, evidence indicates that the receptors are activated by UV-induced ROS.[34] In turn, the receptors trigger signal transduction pathways in the cytoplasm. The mitogen-activated protein kinases (MAPKs) regulate cell proliferation, differentiation, apoptosis, and mitosis. They consist of extracellular signal related kinase (ERK), c-Jun N-terminal kinase (JNK), and p38 MAPK. In relation to photoaging, the MAPKs activate (in the nucleus) the transcription factor activator protein-1 (AP-1). Upon activation, AP-1 upregulates the expression of MMPs that are able to degrade the ECM and downregulates the synthesis of type I procollagen, which is the precursor for collagen I.

Another signal transduction pathway is the phosphatidylinositol 3-kinase/AKT, whose upregulation inhibits keratinocyte apotosis.[34] (Apoptosis is an important mechanism for overall tissue survival and prevention of carcinomas.) In addition, the TGF-beta signaling pathway is impaired by UV irradiation. This has negative consequences, because TGF-beta is a growth factor that plays an integral role in differentiation and apoptosis. Further, the transcription factor nuclear factor-kappa beta (NF-kappa beta) is activated as a result of UV exposure. Capable of causing the expression of numerous genes, NF-kappa beta

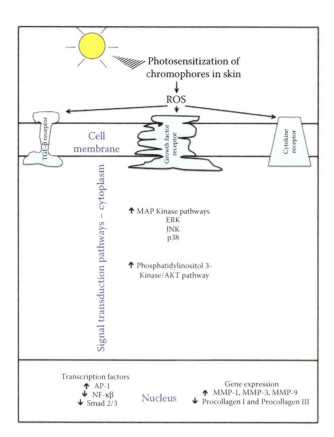

Figure 4.13 UV-induced signaling cascades in skin. (Adapted from Xu, Y. and Fisher, G.J., *J. Dermatol. Sci. Suppl.*, 1, S1–S8, 2005.)

has been associated with many diseases including inflammatory diseases and cancer.

To reemphasize, cell surface receptor activation results in signal transduction, starting at the interior of the cell membrane down through the cytoplasm until the nucleus is reached. Upon activation, transcription factors (e.g., AP-1, NF-kappa beta, or Smad2/3) can upregulate gene expression (e.g., MMP-1, MMP-3, and MMP-9) or downregulate gene expression (e.g., procollagen I and procollagen III). The upregulation of MMPs leads to increased translation, or synthesis, of these enzymes, which are responsible for the degradation of ECM proteins in the dermis. Likewise, downregulation of the procollagens (precursors to collagen) results in less connective tissue in the dermis.

The field of cellular signaling is still an active area of research that may be considered to be in its infancy. This leaves the researcher many opportunities, especially in the area of UV-induced receptor activation, to fulfill a more complete understanding of the role of ROS in receptor activation, and possible routes to inhibit UV-induced receptor activation. The pathways are much more complex than what is shown here. In fact, the pathways shown in Figure 4.13 are provided in reference to photoaging, although some may also apply to photoimmunosuppression or photocarcinogenesis. Thus, it is recommended that the reader refer to some of the accounts in the literature, which provide comprehensive reviews on this subject.[34–40]

PHOTOIMMUNOSUPPRESSION

The skin is a unique organ with an arsenal of cells capable of launching an immunological response when attacked by a foreign pathogen. However, UV radiation can have deleterious effects on this natural defense mechanism. We know this today because of the pioneering efforts of many dedicated researchers who forty years ago embarked on a journey into the unknown world of photoimmunology. Their quest to understand the effects of solar radiation on the immune system laid a solid foundation of knowledge. Yet, there remain many unanswered questions, especially concerning the molecular mechanisms responsible for UV-induced immunosuppression. The paragraphs that follow review the basic knowledge currently available in the field of photoimmunology and establish some points of reference for the mechanisms responsible for UV-induced immunosuppression.[41–49]

The origin of photoimmunology is most often credited to Michael Fisher and Margaret Kripke for their revolutionary work on mice models in the 1970s.[50] Researchers in Kripke's laboratory demonstrated that UVB irradiation suppressed immune system function, which is now known to play an integral role in the development of skin cancer. In their experiments, Fisher and Kripke exposed mice to UVB radiation, causing them to develop tumors. Next, they transplanted the tumors from these mice into non-immune suppressed mice (i.e., not exposed to UVB radiation or any other agent that could cause immunosuppression) and mice that were immune suppressed (given immunosuppressive drugs or subjected to subcarcinogenic doses of UV—both capable of suppressing the immune system). Their revolutionary discovery was that the tumors could not survive in the non-immune suppressed mice but were able to flourish in immune suppressed mice. In addition, their studies demonstrated that UV-induced tumors in skin are highly antigenic (stimulate the production of antibodies), as opposed to other tumors, and are rejected by transplant recipients if their immune system is not compromised. These studies provided a definitive link between photocarcinogenesis and immunity, resulting in the birth of a new field of photobiology, photoimmunology.

Numerous molecular and cellular events occur in skin because of exposure to UV irradiation. The onset of immunosuppression occurs because of the absorption of light by a chromophore present in the skin. The most studied and well-characterized photochemical events involved with UV-induced immunosuppression are based on absorption of light by *trans*-urocanic acid in the stratum corneum and DNA found in the epidermis (most likely in the basal layer). We still do not clearly understand many of the ensuing molecular events, that is, after chromophore absorption.

Some of the other pivotal molecular mechanisms involved with UV-induced immunosuppression involve cytokines, prostaglandins, and transcription factors. Cytokines, largely secreted by keratinocytes in response to UV irradiation, play a major role in the activation/recruitment of immune cells. At this point in time, the onset of immunosuppression by UV light is best characterized by four

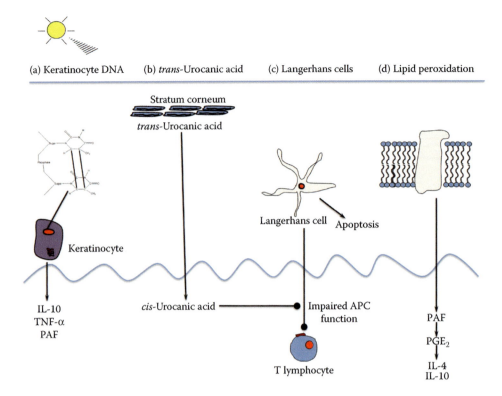

Figure 4.14 Mechanisms of UV-induced immunosuppression. (a) UV-induced DNA damage in keratinocytes resulting in the formation of cyclobutane pyrimidine dimers, or possibly another damaged form of DNA, results in keratinocyte secretion of cytokines (IL-10 and tumor necrosis factor (TNF)-alpha) and PAF. (b) *trans*-Urocanic acid in the stratum corneum can undergo conversion to the *cis* isomeric form followed by migration to lower tissues where it interferes, by a yet unknown mechanism, with the antigen presentation by Langerhans cells to T lymphocytes. (c) Langerhans cells may undergo apoptosis or suffer impaired antigen presentation capabilities. (d) UV irradiation results in free radical species, which can cause lipid peroxidation. Such events eventually lead to generation of PAF and PGE2, which result in further downstream events that produce IL-4 and IL-10. (Adapted from Leitenberger, J. et al., *Semin. Immunopathol.*, 29, 65–70, 2007.)

independent, but possibly interrelated processes involving photoreceptors in skin (DNA and *trans*-urocanic acid), lipid peroxidation, and dysfunctional or apoptotic Langerhans cells (Figure 4.14).[51] Keratinocyte DNA can undergo cross-linking as a result of UV exposure to form cyclobutane pyrimidine dimers. There is significant evidence that DNA damage causes the release of cytokines. The cytokine, interleukin-10 (IL-10), is the most notorious, likely due to its immunosuppressive behavior. The conversion of *trans*-urocanic acid to *cis*-urocanic acid and its subsequent migration from the stratum corneum to deeper tissues is also accepted as one of the critical events necessary for UV-induced immunosuppression to take place. Although the mode of action of *trans*-urocanic acid is still not completely understood, it does play a role by impeding the migration and antigen presentation of Langerhans cells to T lymphocytes. In addition to impaired antigen presenting cell function, Langerhans cells may undergo apoptosis upon UV exposure.

Lipid peroxidation also plays an important role in the induction of UV-induced immunosuppression. ROS are formed as a result of UV irradiation exposure and can have profound effects on skin health and the skin immune system. An event provoked by lipid peroxidation is the expression of platelet activating factor (PAF), which is secreted by keratinocytes as a result of oxidative stress and binds to cell membrane receptors in mast cells, monocytes, and other keratinocytes. Such an undertaking activates prostaglandin synthesis, leading further to the secretion of IL-4 and IL-10.[51] More than ten years ago, it was shown that a series of cytokines (prostaglandin E2 (PGE2), IL-4, and IL-10—in the respective order) are released due to lipid peroxidation and are in part responsible for the ensuing immunosuppression.[52]

Four decades have passed since the genesis of the field of photoimmunology. Early on, it was recognized that photocarcinogenesis and photoimmunology are intimately interrelated. Since those early days, a considerable amount of research has elucidated many of the mechanisms that occur during UV-induced immunosuppression. Initial events include the absorption of light by chromophores—termed photoreceptors—such as DNA and *trans*-urocanic acid. Likewise, damage to cell membrane components, resulting in lipid peroxidation, may be a concurrent or disparate pathway. Regardless, both routes are believed to lead to the release of cytokines, first and foremost by keratinocytes and also by other resident skin cells (e.g., Langerhans cells) as well as migrating immune cells. The signaling molecules, which carry out the most prominent role in UV-induced immunosuppression, are IL-10, TNF-alpha, PAF, and PGE2. Cytokines interact with T cells and determine whether an immune response will be cell mediated or humoral.

Another critical event, which is impaired during UV exposure, is the ability of Langerhans cells to migrate from the skin to the draining lymph nodes where they normally carry out antigen presentation. Numerous studies have shown that the antigen presenting function of Langerhans cells is diminished by UV irradiation in part due to apoptosis and also due to impairment of cell function. Since the 1970s, it has been known that T regulatory cells (formerly known as T suppressor cells) are chief participants in the cellular mechanisms responsible for UV-induced immunosuppression. As a rule, UV-induced immunosuppression can be divided into two classifications depending on whether it is local or systemic. The study of UV-induced immunosuppression is almost universally carried out utilizing murine models. Strong evidence indicates that the mouse models are accurate and predictive of events that occur in humans as a result of UV exposure.[45] In conclusion, photoimmunology remains a field with abundant possibilities for new and exciting discoveries that can benefit humankind.[53]

PHOTOCARCINOGENESIS

Carcinomas result from the over-proliferation of mutant cells (neoplasm), which can be benign (remaining at the original site) or malignant—in the latter case, they can spread to distant sites of the body (Figure 4.15)[54]. At the molecular level, carcinogenesis begins with the genes where there are defects in the DNA, which may be caused by exposure to chemical carcinogens, physical mutagens (irradiation), or in some cases, viruses. The DNA mutations are normally repaired by cellular repair mechanisms, such as nucleotide excision repair.[55] However, throughout the lifetime of an organism, mutations accumulate, eventually leading to cellular and tissue deformity.

There are three different types of skin cancer: *basal cell carcinoma*, *squamous cell carcinoma*, and *malignant melanoma*. The latter of this group is the most dangerous

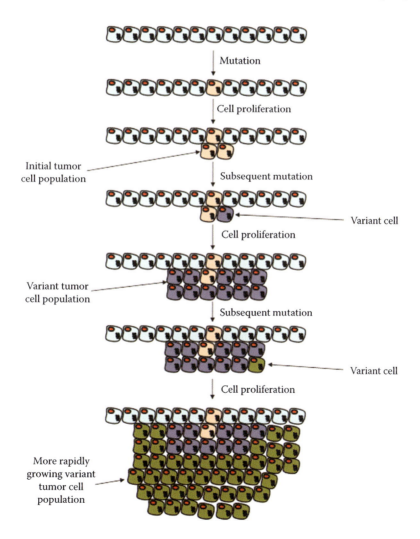

Figure 4.15 Tumor development in tissues. (Adapted from Cooper, G.M. and Hausman, R.E., *The Cell: A Molecular Approach*, 5th ed., Sinauer Associates, Sunderland, MA, 2009.)

and least frequently found type of skin cancer, substantiating only 5% of diagnosed skin cancer cases.[56] It can be found anywhere there is pigmentation; it is essentially cancer of the melanocytes, and it is able to metastasize to nearby blood vessels and lymph nodes.[56] As may be inferred from the names, basal cell carcinoma and squamous cell carcinoma arise from keratinocytes of the basal layer and the stratum spinosum, respectively. These two types of skin cancer are much more common than malignant melanoma, but much less threatening as they are less likely to metastasize before detection.

There are two types of genes particularly important in the development of genetic mutations: proto-oncogenes and tumor suppressor genes. The latter gene classification refers to genes that encode proteins that are designed to regulate cell growth, thereby preventing uncontrolled proliferation of damaged cells. In some cases, this involves controlled cell death, also known as apoptosis. The most noted example of a tumor suppressor gene is the p53 gene.[57,58] This particular gene, which is found to be mutated in 50% of cancer tumors, encodes a protein that is a transcription factor that regulates expression of proteins that prevent cell growth and division.[59] Expression of the p53 gene halts cell division long enough so that repair processes can correct the DNA mutation. When the cell repair machinery is overwhelmed or unable to correct the mutation, the p53 protein acts as a transcription factor for other proteins that induce apoptosis. Proto-oncogenes, on the other hand, are the genes responsible for promoting cell growth and mitosis.

An example of a common proto-oncogene is the *ras* gene that encodes for the ras protein, a G-coupled protein that partakes in cell signaling by relaying signals from the growth factor receptor (at the plasma membrane) to kinases (cytosol), which eventually pass the signal to a transcription factor (nucleus) that promotes cell growth. When the *ras* gene is mutated (now an oncogene), the resulting ras protein becomes excessively active. In other words, it is able to signal downstream kinases without itself receiving a signal from the growth factor receptor. Thus, gene transcription relevant to growth is more active, leading to excessive cell division and proliferation.

With specific reference to skin, Figure 4.16 provides a brief summary of the evolution of the three different

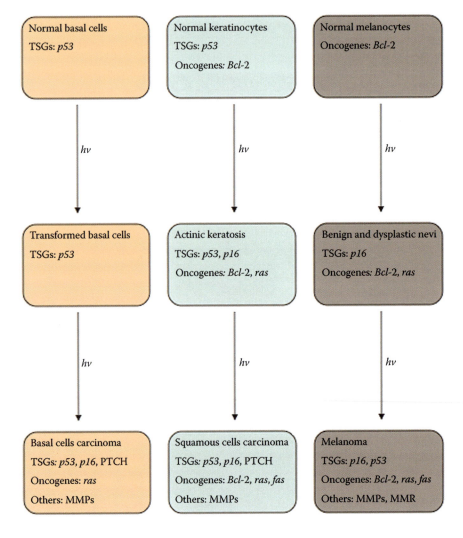

Figure 4.16 A model of carcinogenesis in skin as a result of UV-induced damage. Key tumor suppressor genes (TSGs) and oncogenes involved in these processes are listed. (Adapted from Hussein, M.R., *J. Cutan. Pathol.*, 32, 191–205, 2005.)

types of cancer along with the respective tumor suppressor genes and oncogenes involved at the various stages of tumorigenesis.[60] In all three types of cancer, the *p53* gene suffers mutation at some point during cancer development. Thus, we can assume that the ability of cells to undergo apoptosis is greatly inhibited. In addition, another tumor suppressor gene, *p16*, is present at various stages in all three types of cancer. The oncogenes, Bcl-2 and *ras*, appear to be the most prevalent mitogenic species in the skin cancers; however, in basal cell carcinoma the *ras* oncogene is not found at the early stages of tumorigenesis, but rather only at the final stage of cancer development. In addition to the tumor suppressor genes already mentioned, the patched gene (PTCH) also plays an important role in the development of the non-melanoma cancers. Also found in the carcinomas and melanomas are the MMPs, which play important roles in the growth and development of tumors. Most significantly, the MMPs degrade the ECM, creating space where tumor growth can take place.

There is a definitive connection between free radical damage and various diseases and aging.[61] Skin carcinomas are no exception to this rule. Most of this discussion thus far, in regard to photocarcinogenesis, has focused on tumor suppressor genes and oncogenes. While these molecules certainly are key effectors in these processes, we must certainly not negate the origin of such carcinomas. The previous section discussed signaling pathways in relation to photoaging. Similar pathways are consequential in skin carcinogenesis.[57,58,62] Likewise, the root of carcinomas has everything to do with the condition of the cell's DNA. As already discussed, DNA can be directly mutated by UVB radiation, resulting in DNA cross-links, or indirectly by UVA radiation through sensitization reactions and the formation of ROS. Data obtained for an action spectrum of UV-induced cancer (Figure 4.17) illustrate the contribution of both UVB and UVA radiation to the formation of skin carcinomas.[63] In closing, there is a dose-dependent response in non-melanoma skin cancers, which is correlated to cumulative exposure. Malignant melanoma, on the other hand, usually results from intensive, acute sunburn episodes that occur in childhood.

EFFECTS OF VISIBLE AND INFRARED LIGHT ON SKIN

Historically, most of the damaging effects of solar radiation on skin were believed to be a result of electromagnetic radiation in the UVB and UVA region of the spectrum. Visible and infrared light were thought to be innocuous. It was not until recent years that researchers began to gain a better understanding of these light bands on the health state of skin. Visible light was shown to induce erythema, produce pigmentation, cause thermal damage, and produce free radicals in skin.[3,4,64] Further evidence suggests the likelihood that visible light activates sensitizers (endogenous and exogenous chromophores) in skin, resulting in ROS formation and DNA damage.[3] Likewise, infrared radiation was shown to induce the production of free radicals in human skin.[65,66] Infrared-induced radicals in skin can be detected by electron spin resonance or (indirectly)

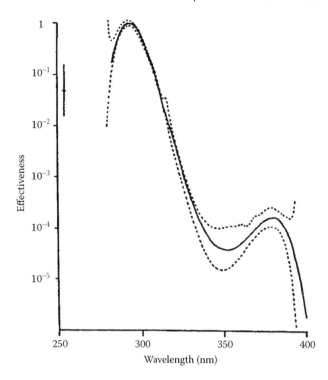

Figure 4.17 Action spectrum for UV-induced cancer in the hairless mouse. The dashed lines were obtained from experiment, while the solid represents an average of the experimental curve. (Reprinted from *Cancer Res.*, 53, 53–60, de Grujil, F.R. et al., Wavelength dependence of skin cancer induction by UV irradiation of albino hairless mice, Copyright 1993, with permission from AACR.)

by probing the behavior of the endogenous antioxidants, such as beta-carotene and lycopene, with Raman spectroscopy when they become radicalized.[66,67] While the signaling pathways have yet to be elucidated, infrared and visible light were also shown to activate the matrix-degrading enzymes, MMPs, which result in the structural breakdown of collagen in the skin.[68–70] Approaches to ameliorate the effects of visible light on skin were shown to provide minimal protection,[69] while the use of sunscreens by another research laboratory did show some promise for protection against infrared radiation, most likely attributable to the high degree of light scattering that occurs when these formulations are utilized.[71] It was also shown that treatment with topical beta-carotene provided protection against infrared radiation.[67] The idea that visible and infrared light cause damage to skin is a progressive concept still in its infancy.[72,73] Future work in this area should shed more light on just how detrimental it is to skin as compared to UV light.

EFFECT OF AIR POLLUTION ON THE SKIN

With increasing population levels and a greater awareness of the effects of burning of fossil fuels for energy and transportation, the effects of air pollution on the skin has become an important area of research in the dermatological and cosmetic science community.[74] It is well established that exposure to air pollutants causes a variety of adverse effects in skin including inflammatory and allergic skin conditions, such as acne, atopic dermatitis, eczema, lentigines, psoriasis, and urticaria.[75–79]

Extrinsic skin aging—as opposed to the natural intrinsic aging process—also results from exposure to air pollution.[80–82] Most of our understanding of extrinsic aging in relation to pollution only extends to its clinical manifestations. For example, a positive correlation was found between the development of pigment spots and pronounced wrinkles.[81] At present, there does not appear to be a good understanding of the changes in skin elastic tissue as a result of exposure to air pollution. Further research is still needed to compare extrinsic aging caused by UV and air pollution exposure.

The most serious ailment possibly caused by air pollutants is skin cancer, although there are a very limited number of studies that have sought to establish a causal relationship between pollution and the disease.[83] In recent years, two large-scale clinical studies carried out in major polluted urban centers (Mexico City and Shanghai) demonstrated the effects of air pollution on the barrier function of skin and the modification of the regulation of several important biochemical markers—squalene, vitamin E, and lactic acid—that are indicators of cutaneous oxidative status.[84–86]

The principal components of air pollution are oxides (nitrogen oxides and sulfur oxides), O_3, PM, polycyclic aromatic hydrocarbons, tobacco smoke, and VOCs. In the following sections, we outline the composition of these various air pollutants and how they adversely influence skin health. Finally, in the last section we examine general strategies that are being employed to combat the adverse effects of pollution on the skin.

Oxides

Nitrogen oxides and sulfur oxides are produced in nature and by human combustion processes. There is serious concern due to their presence in the environment, which greatly affects the quality of ambient air, and also their involvement in the formation of acid rain and smog. In nature, these gases can be produced by volcanic eruptions and lightning strikes. However, the greatest concern stems from their production as a result of fossil fuel burning by electrical power plants and their production by combustion engines in automobiles. The nitrogen oxides, nitric oxide (NO) and nitrogen dioxide (NO_2), are two gases of particular concern, which are formed when nitrogen reacts with oxygen. It should be noted that NO_2 is very poisonous. Likewise, sulfur dioxide (SO_2) is used as an indicator of the total sulfur oxides in the air. In addition, the formation of carbon monoxide in the environment is also troubling as it interacts with hemoglobin, and competes with its interaction with oxygen, hence interfering with oxidative metabolism.

Surprisingly, not many studies have focused on the specific effects of oxides on the skin. A recent study by Krutmann and co-workers demonstrated that exposure to NO_2 correlated with the development of lentigines on the cheeks in both Asian and Caucasian (German) populations.[77] In other studies, researchers investigated the effects of traffic pollution, again a rich source of oxides, on the incidence of eczema, showing a positive correlation between the two.[87] Despite the lack of studies attributing skin damage from fossil fuel production to specific oxides, it is well established that the various forms of pollutants from industrial and motorized vehicle sources have a significant negative impact on the health state of the skin.[74]

Ozone

O_3 is a very reactive form of oxygen that can produce ROS (see Chapter 2). Most of the O_3 that is present in the Earth's atmosphere can be found in the stratosphere. At this level—ca. 10–50 km above the Earth's surface—it provides a paramount service for the inhabitants of Earth by filtering UVC and UVB light via a photochemical reaction mechanism known as the Chapman cycle. O_3 present in the stratosphere forms what we know as the O_3 layer.

Tropospheric O_3—ca. 0–10 km above the Earth's surface—results from photochemical reactions involving air pollutants, such as nitrogen oxides, carbon monoxide, and VOCs. O_3 is a key component of smog and has been known for a long time to negatively impact respiratory health.[88–90]

It is well known that exposure to O_3 causes oxidative stress in the skin resulting in damage to proteins and lipids.[91–93] It has also been demonstrated to deplete the levels of endogenous antioxidants in skin.[93,94] While O_3 exposure appears to affect the stratum corneum more than other layers of skin—leading to disruption of its barrier function—there is also evidence that it is involved in cutaneous inflammation and might play a role in carcinogenesis.[94] Interestingly, there is some evidence that treatment with antioxidants, specifically beta-carotene, may be able to mediate O_3-induced oxidative stress.[95]

In more recent years, it has been shown that exposure of skin to O_3 can have a dual nature. As we already know, chronic O_3 exposure can lead to a number of deleterious events in skin. On the other hand, acute treatment with O_3 has been shown to provide therapeutic benefits, especially in the cleansing of wounds as a disinfectant and increasing the degree of oxygenation in the wound area.[96] In certain circumstances, traditional medicines are ineffective at treating infected wounds—for example, due to antimicrobial resistance to antibiotics. In those cases, ozonated ointments could be very useful as wound dressing agents.[97]

Particulate matter

PM is a mixture of solid particles and liquid droplets in the atmosphere that are contaminants. It may consist of aerosols, ash, dirt, dust, fumes, pollen, smoke, and soot. Some particulates are visible to the naked eye, while others are much smaller in size and require microscopy to view and identify them. PM_{10} describes PM with a diameter of 10 μm or smaller that can be inhaled. On the other hand, $PM_{2.5}$ refers to inhalable PM with a diameter less than 2.5 μm. As a point of reference, imagine a hair fiber, which depending on its racial origin can have a diameter ranging from 50 to 120 μm. Typically, Caucasian hair has an average diameter of 70 μm.

PM may be produced directly from various sources, such as factory exhaust, construction sites (dust), and fires. However, most PM is produced via the burning of fossil fuels (energy plants, automobiles, airplanes, etc.), resulting in the production of nitrogen and sulfur oxides. Ultimately, these gaseous pollutants undergo reactions that produce PM.

It is well known that PM has detrimental effects on human health. The World Health Organization estimates that PM air pollution is linked with 800,000 premature deaths each year.[98] Cardiovascular and respiratory diseases are the illness most associated with particular matter. It should be noted that PM produces the gravest health effects as compared to other air pollutants.

In recent years, significant attention has been given by a number of research groups investigating the effects of PM on the health state of skin.[99,100] Evidence indicates that PM plays a major role in the development of inflammatory skin diseases, such as acne, atopic dermatitis, and psoriasis as well as skin aging in the form of pigmentation spots.[81,101] In addition, trans-epidermal water loss and increased permeability of the skin—allowing for the entry of foreign substances—are manifestations resulting from exposure of the skin to PM.[102] Furthermore, fine PM is able to penetrate into the skin, bringing with it toxic compounds that affect the homeostasis of skin cells.[103] The most threatening skin disease correlated with PM exposure is malignant melanoma.[101]

Inflammatory processes in PM-exposed skin are purported to result from the creation of ROS that lead to the expression of inflammatory cytokines. Several notable ROS found in skin exposed to PM are $^1O_2$, superoxide anion ($^1O_2^{-\bullet}$), and hydroxyl radial (HO$^\bullet$).[99,100] Some of the pro-inflammatory cytokines expressed by keratinocytes are TNF-alpha, IL-1 alpha, and IL-8.[100] See Figure 4.18 for an illustration of the cascade of events related to ROS produced by PM. As noted in the figure, eventually this process leads to upregulation of MMPs that degrade proteins of the ECM of the dermis. Furthermore, ROS can produce damaging effects to the DNA of skin cells, causing a cascade of reactions that results in a loss of tissue viability.

Polycyclic aromatic hydrocarbons

Polycylic aromatic hydrocarbons, often referred to as PAHs, represent a group of several hundred molecules that are produced during combustion in nature (e.g., forest fires) or during combustive processes in man-made sources (e.g., automobile emissions, energy plants, cigarette smoke, etc.).[104] They are also present naturally in coal, crude oil, and gasoline, and are also found in charred foods. Their toxicity in organisms stems from the ability to impair the function of cell membranes and associated proteins. In addition, they are mutagenic and carcinogenic to organisms. Structurally, polycyclic aromatic hydrocarbons are composed of two or more aromatic rings fused together in a variety of structural motifs (Figure 4.19).

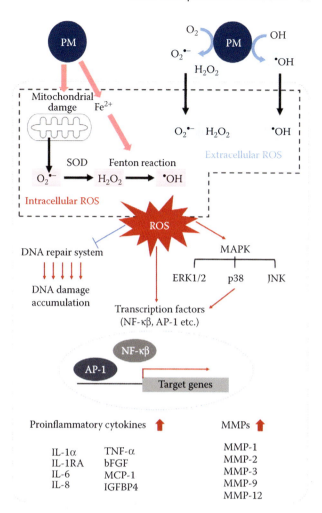

Figure 4.18 Reactive oxygen species generation by PM and subsequent cellular signaling pathways leading to the upregulation of pre-inflammatory cytokines and MMPs. (Reprinted from *Life Sci.*, 152, Kim, K.E. et al., Air pollution and skin diseases: Adverse effects of airborne PM on various skin diseases, 126–134, Copyright 2016, with permission from Elsevier.)

Researchers have been interested in understanding the penetration of polycyclic aromatic hydrocarbons in the skin for quite some time. One study appeared in the late 1980s examining the skin surface levels of polycyclic aromatic hydrocarbons of roofing workers exposed to tar.[105] To better understand the trans-dermal absorption characteristics of polycyclic aromatic hydrocarbons, investigators at the University of Nijmegen in the Netherlands applied a coal-tar ointment to various anatomical sites of the body and monitored the amount of 1-hydroxypyrene in urine as well as the disappearance of polycyclic aromatic hydrocarbons from the surface of skin as indicators of the systemic levels of the pollutants.[106] Essentially, these findings demonstrated the following order of absorption: shoulder > forehead, forearm, groin > ankle, hand. Although, it should be noted that the differences between the different anatomical sites were marginal. Other studies demonstrated the carcinogenic properties of polycyclic aromatic hydrocarbons in relation to the skin.[107] A comparison was

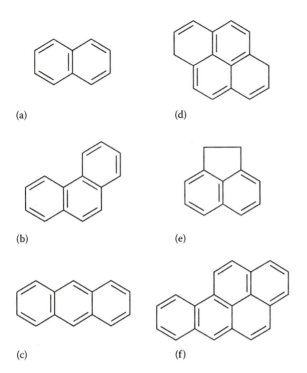

Figure 4.19 Molecular structures of common polycyclic aromatic hydrocarbons resulting from combustible processes that contaminate the atmosphere: (a) napthalene, (b) phenanthrene, (c) anthracene, (d) pyrene, (e) acenaphthene, and (f) benzo[a]pyrene.

made between two types of polycylic aromatic hydrocarbons (benzo[a]pyrene and dibenzo[def, p]chrysene) and pollutant matter (coal tar, diesel particulate, and cigarette smoke condensate). Dibenzo[def, p]chrysene was found to be the most potent agent, followed by benzo[a]pyrene.

Tobacco smoke

Despite its adverse effects on human health, tobacco use in industrialized and developing countries still persists. In addition to other ailments, it is responsible for many grave conditions including cancer, cardiovascular disease, and chronic obstructive pulmonary disease.[108] Cigarette smoke contains more than 5,000 chemicals, which includes numerous toxic and carcinogenic compounds.[109]

Tobacco smoke is an aerosol consisting of solid (tar) and gas phases. The solid phase consists of PM with a large quantity of stable free radicals that have very long lifetimes, such as the semiquinone radical system. These radicals oxidize O_2, resulting in its conversion to $^1O_2^{-\bullet}$ (detected in tar), and further to H_2O_2, which in the presence of Fe^{2+} (tar contains high levels of Fe^{2+}) leads to the formation $HO^{\bullet}$ via the Fenton reaction.[110]

The gas phase of tobacco smoke contains many volatile organic carbons as well as numerous quantities of free radical species. NO is one of the gas phase species that has received considerable attention.[110] While it plays an integral role in human health at low concentrations (as a signaling molecule), it becomes toxic at high concentrations, reacting with $^1O_2^{-\bullet}$, forming peroxynitrite ($O = NNO^-$), which is extremely damaging to biomolecules.

A number of studies have demonstrated the adverse effects of tobacco smoke on the health state of skin. It is associated with accelerated aging of the skin, resulting in premature wrinkling, especially in the facial region.[111–113] In addition, smoking has been correlated with androgenetic alopecia.[100] In an attempt to better understand the mechanism of tobacco smoke-induced aging, the role of tobacco smoke at inducing lipid peroxidation in skin has been the subject of several research investigations.[114,115] In addition to its role in environmental aging, tobacco smoke use has also been associated with higher incidences of acne, psoriasis, and squamous cell carcinoma.[75]

Volatile organic compounds

Volatile organic compounds (VOCs) are generally defined as molecules that are emitted as gases from solids or liquids due to the compound's low vapor pressure. VOCs are produced from a variety of common household substances including paints, aerosol sprays, cleansers and disinfectants, and solvents. According to a study conducted by the Environmental Protection Agency in the United States, the level of VOCs in indoor environments can be two to five times higher than outside.[116] While by definition VOCs can be a number of different molecules—even natural compounds, such as odors, that become volatized—the regulatory definition is restricted to compounds that have adverse effects on the environment. Some of the most common and dangerous VOCs, especially for long-term exposure, consist of benzene; carbon tetrachloride; 1,4-dichlorobenzene; methylene chloride; perchloroethylene; tetrachloroethylene; toluene; 1,1,1-trichloroethane; styrene; and xylene.

Exposure of skin to VOCs may result in adverse effects to the skin. Studies have shown that VOCs absorbed on the skin's surface can enter the bloodstream and become systemic.[117] In addition to immediate symptoms, such as headache as well as ocular and nasal irritation, exposure to common VOCs can cause skin irritation.[118] Surprisingly, not much is known about the long-term effects of VOCs derived from pollution on skin health.[119]

In vitro studies with keratinocytes revealed that exposure to VOCs (hexane, toluene, acetaldehyde, formaldehyde and acetone) is damaging to proteasome, an important cellular entity involved in the cell cycle, apoptosis, transcription, DNA repair, protein quality control, and antigen presentation.[120]

In a completely different context, there has been a significant amount of research focusing on VOCs that emanate from human skin—some stemming from the use of personal care products and others due to metabolic emissions.[121]

Protection strategies against air pollution

Most strategies for combating the effects of air pollutants on the skin focus on active ingredient treatments or exclusion technology, which provides a protective barrier over the skin. From the active ingredient standpoint, extracts containing antioxidants are used to counteract or prevent damage caused by ROS produced by pollutant matter. Forming a protective barrier on the surface of skin is yet another approach to combat air pollutants, which can be achieved with film-forming polymers.

BLUE LIGHT AND ITS EFFECT ON THE SKIN

Over the last several years there has been growing concern about the effect of blue light on the skin. This has mostly been fueled by increasing amounts of exposure to this type of light by artificial light sources (e.g., compact fluorescent lamps) and electronic devices that use light emitting diodes (LEDs), such as television screens, computer monitors, tablets, and smart phones.

For many years, most home lighting systems were based on incandescent light in which a metal filament is energized, resulting in a glowing effect or illumination of the metal. However, in the last decade there have been radical changes in indoor lighting as well as the widespread use of electronic devices that emit blue light. Most technologists agree that our exposure to blue light will continue to increase over time in tandem with the increasing use of these lighting sources and devices.

Blue light (400–500 nm) represents a portion of the visible electromagnetic spectrum that is adjacent to the UVA region in terms of emitted wavelength or energy of the light waves. It actually corresponds to the spectral distribution of both violet (400–450 nm) and blue (450–495 nm) light. Although many artificial light sources appear white, they give off an intense emission in the blue light region, which is stronger than that present in natural sunlight.

There has been growing concern due to the damaging effects of blue light on eye physiology, which leads to degradation of retinal photoreceptors and could be implicated in macular degeneration.[122,123] Ironically, blue light has been used to treat sleep disorders, in which it functions to reset circadian rhythms.[124] It is also beneficial for the treatment of infants with neonatal jaundice, where bilirubin accumulates in the blood and tissues (eyes, skin, etc.), resulting in an overall yellow appearance. Since blue light can penetrate fairly deep into the skin, it is used as a form of photodynamic therapy to dissolve bilirubin so that it can be excreted from the body.[125]

Acne vulgaris is a common disease, which is reported to affect approximately 80% of the population.[126] The bacteria, *Propionibacterium acnes*, is implicated in the development of acne, and is the primary target of most medical treatments, which usually consist of antibiotics or immunotherapy. Blue light therapy has been found to be efficacious in the treatment of certain infectious diseases, especially in the case of acne.[127–129] While the exact mechanism of how blue light functions to combat acne has not been elucidated, it is well known that blue light has broad spectrum antimicrobial activity against gram-positive and gram-negative bacteria. In contrast to UV light therapy, it does not require the use of exogenous photosensitizers and, overall, is considered less damaging to mammalian cells.[130]

Notwithstanding the beneficial effects of blue light on the skin, there is considerable concern in the skin research community in regard to its deleterious effects. A recent study highlights the depletion of carotenoids in skin by blue light, which is believed to be facilitated by the generation of ROS.[131] Mechanistically, it has been shown that exposure to visible light leads to the excitation of cellular photosensitizers, ultimately leading to ROS production, specifically $HO^\bullet$, $^1O_2^{-\bullet}$, and $^1O_2$.[132] In pigmented cells, melanin and lipofuscin have been identified as photosensitizers; however, in non-pigmented cells the photosensitizers remain unknown, although it appears that flavin-containing oxidases, the cytochrome system, heme-containing proteins, and tryptophan-rich proteins are likely candidates.[132]

While not specifically focused on blue light, a number of studies have shown that visible light can promote melanogenesis and erythema in skin and lead to the production of ROS.[73,133,134] On the other hand, a clinical study at the Radboud University Nijmegen Medical Centre in Nijmegen, Netherlands demonstrated that short-term blue light use in skin therapy does not cause DNA damage or premature photoaging.[135] Regardless, there is still a great deal of interest in this subject, which has even led to the launch of commercial products designed to protect the skin from blue light emitted from smart phones, tablets, and laptops.

CONCLUDING REMARKS

Exposure to solar radiation can be detrimental to the health state of the skin. It leads to photoaging, photoimmunosuppression, and photocarcinogenesis. At the same time, there are positive outcomes to solar exposure, such as vitamin D synthesis, which facilitates the absorption of calcium. Historically, most of the concern about solar radiation exposure centered around UVB radiation and its immediate and long-term effects on various structures of the skin. In more recent years, a wealth of research demonstrated that exposure to UVA radiation is also of paramount importance and is responsible for many photosensitization reactions that ultimately lead to free radical-induced DNA lesions. Today, researchers are unveiling the mechanisms and possible roles played by visible and infrared radiation in the generation of ROS in skin. Advances in our understanding of solar radiation exposure have changed our approach to solar protection. Nowadays, most commercial sunscreen formulations contain antioxidants, in addition to traditional solar filters, to combat ROS generated during solar exposure. In addition, there has been growing concern about exposure to air pollutants and the role of ROS in damaging the skin. Many advances have been made in this area in the past decade. Another area of growing interest is the effect of artificial blue light on the skin. This field is still in its infancy and researchers are still determining to what extent it affects public health.

REFERENCES

1. Polefka TG et al. *J Cosmet Dermatol*. 2012;11:134–143.
2. Anderson RR, Parrish JA. *J Invest Dermatol*. 1981;77:13–19.
3. Mahmoud BH et al. *Photochem Photobiol*. 2008;84:450–462.
4. Mahmoud BH et al. *J Invest Dermatol*. 2010;130:2092–2097.
5. Kohen E et al. *Photobiology*. San Diego, CA: Academic Press; 1995.
6. Young AR. *Phys Med Biol*. 1997;42:789–902.
7. Wondrak GT et al. *Photochem Photobiol Sci*. 2006;5:215–237.
8. Wondrak GT et al. *J Biol Chem*. 2004;279:30009–30020.
9. Sober HA (Ed.). *Handbook of Biochemistry*. Cleveland, OH: CRC Press; 1968.
10. Yin D. *Free Radic Biol Med*. 1996;21:871–888.
11. Terman A, Brunk UT. *Inf J Biochem Cell Biol*. 2004;36:1400–1404.
12. Schmid F. *Encyclopedia of Molecular Biology*. New York: John Wiley & Sons; 1999.
13. Boyer RF. *Modern Experimental Biochemistry*. Redwood City, CA: Benjamin/Cummings; 1993.
14. Hanson KM, Simon JD. *Proc Natl Acad Sci USA*. 1998;95:10576–10578.
15. Holick MF et al. *Science*. 1980;210:203–205.
16. Holick MF. *J Cell Biochem*. 2003;88:296–307.
17. Diffey B. *Phys Med Biol*. 1980;25:405–426.
18. Marrot L, Meunier J-R. *J Am Acad Dermatol*. 2008;58:S139–S148.
19. Schuch A et al. *Free Rad Biol Med*. 2017;107:110–124.
20. Cadet J et al. Effects of UV and visible radiations on cellular DNA. In: Thiele J, Elsner P (Eds.). *Oxidants and Antioxidants in Cutaneous Biology. Current Problems in Dermatology*. Basel, Switzerland: Karger; 2001, pp. 74–82.
21. Mouret S et al. *Org Biomol Chem*. 2010;8:1706–1711.
22. Kawanishi S, Hiraku Y. Sequence-specific DNA damage induced by UVA radiation in the presence of endogenous and exogenous photosensitizers. In: Thiele J, Elsner P (Eds.). *Oxidants and Antioxidants in Cutaneous Biology. Current Problems in Dermatology*. Basel, Switzerland: Karger; 2001, pp. 74–82.
23. Soter NA. Sunburn and suntan: Immediate manifestations of photodamage. In: Gilchrest BA (Ed.). *Photodamage*. Cambridge, MA: Blackwell Science; 1996, pp. 12–25.
24. Moyal D, Fourtanier A. Acute and chronic effects of UV on skin: What are they and how to study them? In: Rigel DS, Weiss RA, Lim HW, Dover JS (Eds.). *Photoaging. Basic and Clinical Dermatology, 28*. New York: Marcel Dekker; 2004, pp. 15–32.
25. Kockott D et al. *PLoS ONE*. 2016;11(1):e0145509.
26. Yaar M, Gilchrest BA. *Br J Dermatol*. 2007;157:874–887.
27. Rabe JH et al. *J Am Acad Dermatol*. 2006;55:1–19.
28. Wölfle U et al. *Skin Pharmacol Physiol*. 2014;27:316–332.
29. Birch-Machin M, Bowman A. *Br J Dermatol*. 2016;175(Suppl. S2):26–29.
30. Yaar M, Gilchrest BA. Aging of skin. In: Freedberg IM, Eisen AZ, Wolff K, Austen KF, Goldsmith LA, Katz SI et al. (Eds.). *Fitzpatrick's Dermatology in General Medicine, 2*. New York: McGraw-Hill; 1999, pp. 1697–1706.
31. Mauch C et al. Regulation of connective tissue turnover by matrix metalloproteinases. In: Freinkel RK, Woodley DT (Eds.). *The Biology of the Skin*. New York: The Parthenon Publishing Group; 2001, pp. 353–364.
32. Jenkins G. *Mech Age Dev*. 2002;123:801–810.
33. Petrazzuoli M, Goldsmith LA. Molecular mechanisms of cellular signaling. In: Freedberg IM, Eisen AZ, Wolff K, Austen KF, Goldsmith LA, Katz SI et al. (Eds.). *Fitzpatrick's Dermatology in General Medicine, 1*. 5th ed. New York: McGraw-Hill; 1999, pp. 114–131.
34. Xu Y, Fisher GJ. *J Dermatol Sci Suppl*. 2005;1:S1–S8.
35. Rittié L, Fisher G. *Ageing Res Rev*. 2002;1:705–720.
36. Wenk J et al. UV-induced oxidative stress and photoaging. In: Thiele J, Elsner P (Eds.). *Oxidants and Antioxidants in Cutaneous Biology, 29*. Basel, Switzerland: Karger; 2001, pp. 83–94.
37. Peus D, Pittelkow MR. Reactive oxygen species as mediators of UVB-induced mitogen-activated protein kinase activation in keratinocytes. In: Thiele J, Elsner P (Eds.). *Oxidants and Antioxidants in Cutaneous Biology, 29*. Basel, Switzerland: Karger; 2001, pp. 114–127.
38. Klotz L-O et al. UVA and singlet oxygen as inducers of cutaneous signaling events. In: Thiele J, Elsner P (Eds.). *Oxidants and Antioxidants in Cutaneous Biology, 29*. Basel, Switzerland: Karger; 2001, pp. 95–113.
39. Bender K et al. *J Photochem Photobiol B: Biol*. 1997;37:1–17.
40. Bode AM, Dong Z. Mitogen-activated protein kinase activation in UV-induced signal transduction. *Sci STKE*. 2003;2003(167):RE2.
41. Amerio P et al. *Anti-Inflamm Anti-Allergy Agents Med Chem*. 2009;8:3–13.
42. Aubin F. *Eur J Dermatol*. 2003;13:515–523.
43. Beissert S, Schwarz T. *J Invest Derm Symp Proc*. 1999;4:61–64.
44. de Gruijl FR. *Photochem Photobiol*. 2008;84:2–9.
45. McMullen RL. UV-induced immunosuppression of skin. In: Dayan N, Wertz PW (Eds.). *Innate Immune System of Skin and Oral Mucosa: Properties and Impact in Pharmaceutics, Cosmetics, and Personal Care Products*. Hoboken, NJ: John Wiley & Sons; 2011.
46. Norval M et al. *Photochem Photobiol*. 2008;84:19–28.

47. Schwarz T. *Keio J Med.* 2005;54:165–171.
48. Schwarz T. *Photochem Photobiol.* 2008;84:10–18.
49. Ullrich SE. *Mol Carcinog.* 2007;46:629–633.
50. Fisher MS, Kripke ML. *Proc Natl Acad Sci USA.* 1977;74:1688–1692.
51. Leitenberger J, Jacobe HT, Cruz Jr. PD. Photoimmunology—illuminating the immune system through photobiology. *Semin Immunopathol.* 2007;29:65–70.
52. Shreedhar V et al. *J Immunol.* 1998;160:3783–3789.
53. Ullrich SE et al. *Exp Dermatol.* 2002;11(Suppl. 1):1–4.
54. Cooper GM, Hausman RE. *The Cell: A Molecular Approach.* 5th ed. Sunderland, MA: Sinauer Associates; 2009.
55. Rass K, Reichrath J. UV damage and DNA repair in malignant melanoma and nonmelanoma skin cancer. In: Reichrath J (Ed.). *Sunlight, Vitamin D and Skin Cancer.* New York: Landes Bioscience and Springer Science + Business Media; 2008.
56. Marieb EN, Hoehn K. *Human Anatomy & Physiology,* 9th ed. Menlo Park, CA: Benjamin Cummings; 2012.
57. Gruber F et al. *Coll Antropol.* 2007;31(Suppl. 1):101–106.
58. Melnikova VO, Ananthaswamy HN. *Mutat Res.* 2005;571:91–106.
59. Reece J et al. *Campbell Biology,* 6th ed. San Francisco, CA: Benjamin Cummings; 2010.
60. Hussein MR. *J Cutan Pathol.* 2005;32:191–205.
61. Halliwell B, Gutteridge JMC. *Free Radicals in Biology and Medicine,* 5th ed. Oxford, UK: University Press; 2015.
62. Katiyar S. *Toxicol Appl Pharmacol.* 2007;224:220–227.
63. de Gruijl FR et al. *Cancer Res.* 1993;53:53–60.
64. Zastrow L et al. *Skin Pharmacol Physiol.* 2008;22:31–44.
65. Darvin M et al. *J Invest Dermatol.* 2010;130:629–631.
66. Darvin M et al. *J Biophotonics.* 2011;4:21–29.
67. Darvin M et al. *Exp Dermatol.* 2011;20:125–129.
68. Buechner N et al. *Exp Gerontol.* 2008;43:633–637.
69. Liebel F et al. *J Invest Dermatol.* 2012;132:1901–1907.
70. Schroeder P et al. *J Invest Dermatol.* 2008;128:2491–2497.
71. Meinke M et al. *Photochem Photobiol.* 2011;87:452–456.
72. Zastrow L, Lademann J. *Anticancer Res.* 2016;36:1389–1394.
73. Sklar L et al. *Photochem Photobiol Sci.* 2013;12:54–64.
74. Krutmann J et al. *J Dermatol Sci.* 2014;76:163–168.
75. Drakaki E, Dessinioti C, Antoniou C. Air pollution and the skin. *Front Environ Sci.* 2014;2(Article 11):1–6.
76. Ahn K. *J Allergy Clin Immunol.* 2014;134:993–999.
77. Hüls A et al. *J Invest Dermatol.* 2016;136:1053–1156.
78. Kim Y et al. *PLoS One.* 2017;12(4):e0175229.
79. Kousha T, Valacchi G. *J Toxicol Environ Health A.* 2015;78:524–533.
80. Lanuti E, Kirsner R. *J Invest Dermatol.* 2010;130:2696.
81. Vierkötter A et al. *J Invest Dermatol.* 2010;130:2719–2726.
82. Vierkötter A, Krutmann J. *Dermatoendocrinol.* 2012;4:227–231.
83. Baudouin C et al. *Cell Biol Toxicol.* 2002;18:341–348.
84. Pham D et al. *Int J Cosmet Sci.* 2015;37:357–365.
85. Lefebvre M et al. *Int J Cosmet Sci.* 2015;37:329–338.
86. Lefebvre M et al. *Int J Cosmet Sci.* 2016;38:217–223.
87. Lee Y et al. *J Invest Dermatol.* 2008;128:2412–20.
88. Lippmann M. *JAPCA.* 1989;39:672–695.
89. Chen T et al. *Am J Med Sci.* 2007;333:244–248.
90. Jerrett M et al. *N Engl J Med.* 2009;360:1085–1095.
91. Thiele J et al. *FEBS Lett.* 1998;422:403–406.
92. Cotovio J et al. *Toxicol In Vitro.* 2001;15:357–362.
93. Valacchi G et al. *FEBS Lett.* 2000;466:165–168.
94. Thiele J et al. *Biol Chem.* 1997;378:1299–1305.
95. Valacchi G et al. *Toxicol Ind Health.* 2009;25:241–247.
96. Valacchi G et al. *Br J Dermatol.* 2005;153:1096–1100.
97. Travagli V et al. *Mediators Inflamm.* 2010:610418.
98. Anderson J et al. *J Med Toxicol.* 2012;8:166–175.
99. Magnani N et al. *Toxicol Sci.* 2016;149:227–236.
100. Kim K et al. *Life Sci.* 2016;152:126–134.
101. Kim H et al. *Toxicol Lett.* 2017;273:26–35.
102. Pan T et al. *J Dermatol Sci.* 2015;78:51–60.
103. Mancebo S, Wang S. *J Eur Acad Dermatol Venereol.* 2015;29:2326–2332.
104. Abdel-Shafy H, Mansour MSM. *Egypt J Pet.* 2016;25:107–123.
105. Wolff M et al. *Arch Environ Health.* 1989;44:157–163.
106. VanRooij J et al. *J Toxicol Environ Health.* 1993;38:355–368.
107. Siddens L et al. *Toxicol Appl Pharmacol.* 2012;264:377–386.
108. U.S. Department of Health and Human Services. *The Health Consequences of Smoking: 50 Years of Progress. A Report of the Surgeon General.* Atlanta, GA: U.S. Department of Health and Human Services, Centers for Disease Control and Prevention, National Center for Chronic Disease Prevention and Health Promotion, Office on Smoking and Health; 2014.
109. Talhout R et al. *Int J Environ Res Public Health.* 2011;8:613–628.
110. Valavanidis A et al. *Int J Environ Res Public Health.* 2009;6:445–462.
111. Kadunce D et al. *Ann Intern Med.* 1991;114:840–844.
112. Ernster V et al. *Am J Public Health.* 1995;85:78–82.
113. Koh J et al. *Int J Dermatol.* 2002;41:21–27.
114. Egawa M et al. *Int J Cosmet Sci.* 1999;21:83–98.
115. Pelle E et al. *Skin Pharmacol Appl Skin Physiol.* 2002;15:63–68.
116. EPA. Volatile Organic Compounds' Impact on Indoor Air Quality, https://www.epa.gov/indoor-air-quality-iaq/volatile-organic-compounds-impact-indoor-air-quality, 2017.
117. Simon L, Ospina J. et al. *Chem Eng Comm.* 2017;204:698–704.

118. Norbaeck D et al. *Sci Total Environ.* 2017;592:153–160.
119. Lee H et al. *Mol Cell Toxicol.* 2016;12:337–343.
120. Dezest M et al. *Sci Rep.* 2017;7(1):10707.
121. Tang X et al. *Environ Sci Technol.* 2016;50:12686–12694.
122. Tosini G et al. *Mol Vis.* 2016;22:61–72.
123. Jaadane I et al. *Free Radic Biol Med.* 2015;84:373–384.
124. Holzman D. *Environ Health Perspect.* 2010;118:A22–A27.
125. Ennever J. *Clin Perinatol.* 1990;17:467–481.
126. Liu P et al. *Curr Drug Metabol.* 2015;16:245–254.
127. Gold M et al. *J Clin Aesthet Dermatol.* 2009;2:44–50.
128. Charakida A et al. *Am J Clin Dermatol.* 2004;5:211–216.
129. Ammad S et al. *J Cosmet Dermatol.* 2008;7:180–188.
130. Dai T et al. *Drug Resist Updat.* 2012;15:223–226.
131. Vandersee S et al. *Oxid Med Cell Longev.* 2015. doi:10.1155/2015/579675.
132. Godley B et al. *J Biol Chem.* 2005;280:21061–21066.
133. Randhawa M et al. *PLoS One.* 2015;10(6):e0130949.
134. Darvin M et al. *Skin Pharmacol Physiol.* 2010;23:40–46.
135. Kleinpenning M et al. *Photodermatol Photoimmunol Photomed.* 2010;26:16–21.

Lipid peroxidation and its measurement

> The oxidation of unsaturated fatty acids is one of the most fundamental reactions in lipid chemistry.
>
> —Edwin N. Frankel
> *Lipid Oxidation*

Lipids perform various functions in cosmetic science including their role as biological structural components of skin and hair, sebum constituents, and functional ingredients in cosmetic preparations. From a biological standpoint, the plasma membrane of keratinocytes and other cells of the viable epidermis and dermis are composed principally of phospholipids with small quantities of cholesterol, free fatty acids, and other lipids. The stratum corneum, on the other hand, mostly contains ceramides with lesser quantities of cholesterol and free fatty acids. A major consideration for all lipids related to skin and skin care technologies is their potential to become oxidized. As the outermost protective organ of the body, the skin continuously finds itself under assault from external insults. Lipids under attack by free radicals undergo oxidation reactions that alter their structure and debilitate them to the point where they can no longer perform their normal biological functions. In cell membranes, this results in loss of membrane fluidity and could disrupt membrane channels that permit the passage of ions and molecules into and out of the cell. Lipid peroxidation and its prevention are not only important in vivo, but also play an important role in the stability of cosmetic products. Cosmetic preparations may contain long-chain polyunsaturated fatty acids (PUFAs), which are ideal targets of lipid oxidation. Much of the current knowledge about lipid peroxidation comes from a tremendous amount of research conducted in the rubber and food industries. In the last couple of decades, biological lipid peroxidation has gained a more prominent position in the scientific realm due to its involvement with many pathological conditions as well as the free radical theory of aging. This chapter discusses the fundamental aspects of lipid oxidation as well as in vivo scenarios of biochemically relevant oxidation processes in skin. Further, potential lipid oxidation schemes that may be encountered in cosmetic formulations and colloidal-based systems are outlined, and techniques and assays employed to measure lipid oxidation in vitro and ex vivo are also reviewed.

LIPID PEROXIDATION
Mechanism of lipid peroxidation

With regard to the skin, lipid peroxidation may occur (or be studied) in a variety of situations: in vivo systems (epidermis or dermis), in vitro cell cultures (keratinocytes or fibroblasts), ex vivo skin biopsies, or skin care formulations. These reactions can occur as the result of (1) a free radical-mediated chain reaction, (2) non-enzymatic, non-radical photo-oxidation, or (3) enzymatic reaction.[1] In biological systems, all three possibilities can occur, while in formulation we are only likely to encounter the first and second case. Fortunately, most formulations are protected against UV irradiation by their packaging. The most familiar lipid peroxidation mechanism is the free radical-mediated chain reaction, which follows the steps: *initiation*, *propagation*, *branching*, and *termination*.[1]

The initiation step takes place due to the formation of a radical, either by heat, light, or chemistry (metals). The radical is capable of abstracting a proton from the lipid (L_1H), thus forming a lipid radical ($L_1^{\bullet}$).

Initiation

$$L_1H + R^{\bullet} \rightarrow L_1^{\bullet} + RH \quad (5.1)$$

The lipid radical may then react with molecular oxygen (O_2) to form a lipid peroxyl radical ($L_1OO^{\bullet}$), which can react with a second lipid molecule (L_2H). This second step of the free radical-mediated chain reaction is known as propagation, or, simply, chain reaction.

Propagation

$$L_1^{\bullet} + O_2 \rightarrow L_1OO^{\bullet} \quad (5.2)$$

$$L_1OO^{\bullet} + L_2H \rightarrow L_2^{\bullet} + L_1OOH \quad (5.3)$$

The second lipid molecule, now in its radical form ($L_2^{\bullet}$), can follow the same pathway as the first lipid molecule and form a lipid hydroperoxide (L_1OOH and L_2OOH). Lipid hydroperoxides often break down or react with other species, resulting in the formation of ketones, aldehydes, and other compounds that are often toxic in vivo. They may also revert back to free radical species, such as $LOO^{\bullet}$ or alkoxyl ($LO^{\bullet}$) radicals, or the extremely reactive hydroxyl radical ($HO^{\bullet}$). Often, the degradation of $LOOH$ is catalyzed by transition metals, such as iron.

Termination

$$L_2^{\bullet} + AOH \rightarrow L_2H + A^{\bullet} \quad (5.4)$$

Reaction of $LOO^{\bullet}$, or any other radical species, with an antioxidant neutralizes the radical and creates a radical from the antioxidant, which normally is stable and persistent. Alternatively, free radicals may react with each other to render dimers and other products that do not contain an unpaired electron and are not highly reactive.

Lipid peroxidation chemistry follows similar pathways regardless of the type of system encountered, be it biological, formulation, food, and so forth. The chemical and physical environment may be different and affect reactivity; however, the general process of lipid oxidation follows the pathway shown earlier.

Lipid peroxidation in vivo

Lipid peroxidation is a series of degradative events that result from free radical attack and render a lipid dysfunctional. In addition, the lipid radicals themselves, or their degradation products, may react with other important biological molecules, thereby undermining the structural or functional role played by that molecule in the cell. Such targets can range from integral proteins located in the cell membrane to DNA in the nucleus. As a consequence, DNA strand breaks or even genetic defects may occur, carbohydrates become susceptible to chain breaks, and proteins may undergo fragmentation. In DNA, the most well-noted free radical mechanism that causes damage is a result of the production of 8-hydroxyguanosine—a marker of free radical DNA damage. In proteins, $HO^{\bullet}$ can attack amino acid residues, while H_2O_2 is capable of oxidizing the sulfhydryl groups of methionine and cysteine.[2] These reactive oxygen species (ROS) and the ensuing reactions often evolve from lipid peroxidation. Figure 5.1 provides an example of lipid peroxidation, as it is proposed to occur in cellular membranes, in which a phospholipid has its polar headgroup in contact with the water phase and its hydrophobic tail at the interior of the membrane.[3] The hydrocarbon tail has two points of unsaturation, making the lipid susceptible to free radical attack and a further cascade of transformations into a lipid hydroperoxide, thereby losing its normal biological function. The scheme also demonstrates how the lipid peroxidation cascade is terminated by alpha-tocopherol, resulting in the formation of a lipid hydroperoxide, and the regeneration of alpha-tocopherol by ascorbic acid. The figure also contains a representation of the combined action of several enzymes, which are able to convert the damaged lipid (lipid hydroperoxide) back to a functioning lipid.

Iron plays an important role in lipid peroxidation. This is especially true with the well-known Haber–Weiss and Fenton reactions in which oxidized iron (Fe^{2+}) catalyzes the breakdown of H_2O_2 into the deleterious $HO^{\bullet}$. As shown in Figure 5.2, the Fenton-produced $HO^{\bullet}$ may rapidly react with lipids, causing the onset of lipid peroxidation.[4] In skin, a lipid radical may be formed as a result of the conversion of reduced iron (Fe^{3+}) to Fe^{2+}, which is able to occur due to the presence of superoxide anion ($O_2^{\bullet-}$). In turn, $O_2^{\bullet-}$ is produced due to the interaction of UV light with O_2. In addition to the generation of $HO^{\bullet}$, iron-containing compounds can also act as catalysts in the decomposition of lipid hydroperoxides, leading to the formation of $LO^{\bullet}$ and $LOO^{\bullet}$ species. These intermediates are able to undergo further reactions, ultimately generating a myriad of compounds, notably aldehydic and ketonic molecules (discussion of which follows).

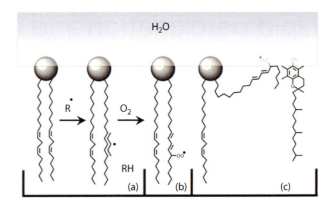
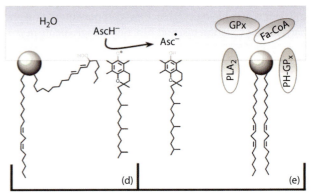

Figure 5.1 Membrane lipid peroxidation. The lipid bilayer shows a phospholipid with its polar headgroup in contact with an H_2O layer and the unsaturated alkyl chains present in the lipid phase of the membrane. (a) A radical ($R^{\bullet}$) abstracts a hydrogen atom from the unsaturated chain rendering a lipid radical. (b) The lipid radical then reacts with O_2 to produce a lipid peroxyl radical with a conjugated diene structure. (c) The lipid peroxyl radical portion of the phospholipid migrates to the lipid-H_2O interface, where it interacts with alpha-tocopherol. (d) The lipid peroxyl radical is converted to a lipid hydroperoxide leaving the alpha-tocopheroxyl radical, which can react with aqueous phase ascorbic acid. (e) The alpha-tocopheroxyl radical is regenerated by ascorbic acid to its original form, alpha-tocopherol. Various enzymes aid in the repair of the lipid hydroperoxide: phospholipase A2 (PLA2), phospholipid hydroperoxide glutathione peroxidase (PH-GPx), fatty acyl-coenzyme A (FA-CoA), and glutathione peroxidase (GPx). (Adapted from Buettner, G., *Arch. Biochem. Biophys.*, 300, 535–543, 1993. With permission.)

In the human body, lipids serve a variety of functions such as fat storage, structural components of cell membranes, and hormonal functions similar to those exhibited by the prostaglandins. Several classes of lipids include fatty acids, steroids (e.g., cholesterol), phospholipids (e.g., phosphoglycerides, sphingolipids, and glycosphingolipids), triglycerides (storage fats), waxes, and fat-soluble vitamins (e.g., vitamin E). These lipids serve various biological functions and are found throughout the body in almost all cell types. In most cases, fatty acids serve as the structural building blocks for these lipids and the original structure of the fatty acid can be seen in the skeletal structure of the lipid, most notably as the alkyl chain.

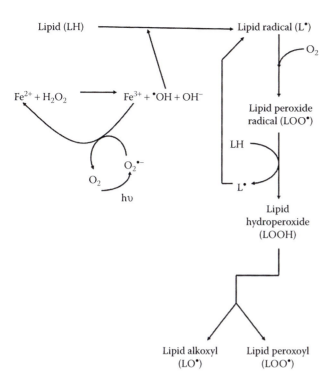

Figure 5.2 UV-induced epidermal free radicals. (Adapted from Ogura, R. and Sugiyama, M., Reactive oxidants in skin: UV-induced lipid peroxidation, in Fuchs, J. and Packer, L. [Eds.], *Oxidative Stress in Dermatology. Clinical Dermatology*, Marcel Dekker, New York, 49–66, 1993.)

In nature there are three major classes of fatty acids: saturated, monounsaturated, and polyunsaturated. Of these three classes, a PUFA is the most likely target to undergo lipid peroxidation due to multiple double bonds located on its long alkyl chain, only separated from each other by a methylene group. Figure 5.3 provides the structures for the most common PUFAs found in nature, which are particularly relevant to the current discussion. In this particular conjugated arrangement of the PUFA, the hydrogen atoms (allylic hydrogen) on the methylene group that is sandwiched between two double bonds are susceptible to removal since the C–H bond is very labile due to resonance imparted by the double bonds. Regardless, attack by a radical removes one of the hydrogen atoms on the methylene group, leaving a carbon-centered radical. Then, the lipid radical rearranges to form the more stable conjugated diene. This is followed by uptake of oxygen, resulting in the LOO• radical species, which goes on to form a LOOH. Again, formation of the LOOH hinders the molecule's ability to carry out its normal biological function.

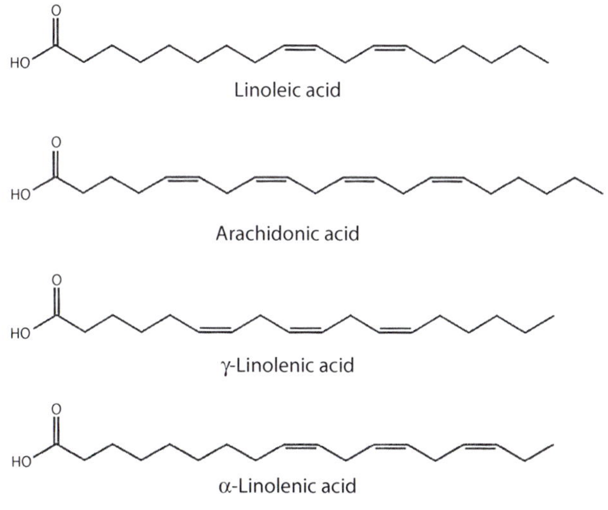

Biological lipids are synthesized by the body using fatty acid precursors, such as those shown in Figure 5.3. Therefore, the alkyl chains of some lipids contain a double bond arrangement inherent to omega-3 and omega-6 fatty acids. Thus, lipids that are composed of PUFAs are likely targets of lipid peroxidation. Linoleic, arachidonic, and gamma-linolenic acids are omega-6 fatty acids, while alpha-linolenic acid is an omega-3 fatty acid. The use of the nomenclature—omega-3 and omega-6—stems from the position of the first double bond from the end of the alkyl chain, which is either three or six carbon atoms away. These fatty acids are also referred to as essential fatty acids, since they cannot be synthesized by the human body from smaller molecules and must be obtained through the diet. Arachidonic acid is probably the most commonly found component of phospholipids that constitute cell membranes. It is also a precursor for the biosynthesis of prostaglandins (Eicosanoid family)—an important group of lipids that regulate many important biochemical processes. In humans, linoleic acid (found in many vegetable oils) can undergo bioconversion through a sequence of reactions to yield arachidonic acid. Therefore, it is also a precursor of prostaglandins. While we often think of long-chain lipids with multiple double bonds as targets of lipid peroxidation, cholesterol may also undergo oxidative decomposition by several different pathways—any one of which results in the intermediate formation of a hydroperoxide.[2]

Lipid peroxidation results in the formation of numerous by-products, some known to be biologically toxic. This is because lipid hydroperoxides are not very stable compounds and further decompose into unsaturated aldehydes, ketone compounds, and hydrocarbons. These compounds may include: *n*-alkenals; 2,4-alkadienals; alkatrienals; alpha-hydroxyalkenals; hydroperoxyalkanals; 4-hydroxyalkenals; malondialdehyde (MDA); alpha-dicarbonyls; alkanes; and alkenes.[5] In this chapter, particular interest will be paid to MDA since it is one of the most frequently probed compounds to determine the extent of lipid peroxidation. Also noteworthy is 4-hydroxy-2-*trans*-nonenal (HNE), a 4-hydroxyalkenal, which has been the subject of great interest not only as a lipid peroxidation end-product, but also a toxic aldehyde in vivo.[6] The primary products of decomposition of the omega-6 fatty acids are HNE

Figure 5.3 Structures of several PUFAs that are targets of lipid peroxidation. Linoleic, arachidonic, and gamma-linolenic acids are omega-6 fatty acids, while alpha-linolenic acid is an omega-3 fatty acid.

and hexanal, whereas omega-3 lipid peroxidation leads primarily to the formation of 4-hydroxy-2,3-*trans*-hexenal and propanal. Many of the unsaturated aldehydes that are produced from oxidation may react with the pendant amine groups of amino acids such as lysine to form Schiff bases, which ultimately lead to protein cross-linking.

Lipid peroxidation with reference to the skin

As discussed in Chapter 1, the lipid composition of the skin varies significantly throughout the strata that constitute the morphological structure of the epidermis. At the basal layer, columnar-shaped keratinocytes serve as reproductive cells of the epidermis. The lipid components in the lower layers of the epidermis are like those of most other metabolically active cells in the body, with phospholipids being the principal components followed by much lower concentrations of cholesterol, free fatty acids, triglycerides, and glucosyl ceramides.[7] In addition, lipids form membranes around many organelles of the cell. As we make our way up from the lower layers of the epidermis to the outermost stratum corneum, the lipids and their structural organization become very unique. At the stratum granulosum, we observe the secretion by keratinocytes of specialized organelles known as lamellar bodies (or lamellar granules), which extrude lipid packets at the uppermost section of the stratum granulosum into the intercellular space, ultimately forming the protective lipid barrier of the skin at the stratum corneum. These packets mostly contain ceramides, cholesterol, free fatty acids, and enzymes. As a result, the stratum corneum lipid composition drastically changes, being almost entirely composed of lipids from the lamellar bodies.[7]

Figure 5.4 contains the structures of various lipids found in the epidermis (and skin surface lipids), which could potentially undergo lipid peroxidation. Phospholipids are found in all of the viable layers of the epidermis and often contain unsaturated chains, which may be oxidized. Phosphotidylcholine, phosphatidylethanolamine, and sphingomyelin are the major phospholipids that form the keratinocyte plasma membrane and are found in the viable lamellae of skin.[8,9] Cholesterol, found in all layers of the epidermis, is also known to undergo oxidation and even form cholesterol hydroperoxide.[2] Likewise, squalene—a metabolic precursor of cholesterol—is found in the viable epidermis and stratum corneum, and is also a candidate of oxidation.[10] Linoleic, oleic, and palmitoleic acids are reported to be major components of stratum corneum lipids. Under normal physiological conditions, it is doubtful that the monounsaturated fatty acids undergo autooxidation; however, they are very likely candidates for photooxidation. The ceramides—the principal lipids of the stratum corneum—represent a unique group of sphingolipids containing a sphingosine component with a polar headgroup (less polar than phospholipids) and an aliphatic tail. In addition, ceramides contain amide-linked fatty acids, which may include normal fatty acids, alpha hydroxy acids, or omega hydroxy acids.[11] It is the amide-linked fatty acid portion of the molecule that would appear most susceptible to oxidation, specifically in the case of omega hydroxy acids. In fact, it is rather surprising that there is no available data in the literature regarding lipid peroxidation of ceramides. Unpublished studies completed by Wertz et al. demonstrated the ability of the linolenate-containing ceramides, ceramide EOS, ceramide EOP, and ceramide EOH, to undergo lipid peroxidation.[12]

A complex mixture of lipids is secreted by the sebaceous gland, which is associated with the hair follicle (pilosebaceous unit). Lipids extrude from the gland onto the mature hair shaft and are brought to the surface of the skin, where they form the acid mantle protecting the skin. The principal components of sebum lipids are squalene, wax esters, triglycerides, free fatty acids, cholesterol esters, cholesterol, and phospholipids.[13] As already mentioned, squalene, cholesterol, and phospholipids are susceptible to lipid peroxidation. Cholesterol esters were also found to undergo peroxidation reactions.[14] Triglycerides (triacylglycerols) are energy storage molecules in plants and animals and contain a glycerol backbone esterified with three fatty acid residues. As shown in Figure 5.4, the fatty acid composition may vary from chain to chain and also among different molecules. Some of the chains may be saturated and unlikely to undergo oxidation, while other unsaturated chains are susceptible to oxidation. Wax esters are esters of long-chain saturated/unsaturated fatty acids and long-chain alcohols.[15] They are found in many species in the plant and animal kingdoms, where they are secreted on the exterior surfaces to provide protection and prevent water loss. In skin, there appears to mostly be saturated or monounsaturated (only one double bond) wax esters.[16] Sterol esters (the class of compounds to which the cholesterol esters belong) are reported to follow similar chain length patterns as those found in wax esters.[16] It was reported that 50% of the fatty acids found in the various esters and triglycerides are monounsaturated and are unique to the skin.[17] It is extremely interesting to note that sebaceous lipids also contain antioxidants, such as vitamin E and coenzyme Q.[18] Such findings suggest the need to protect sebum lipids from oxidation in order to remain functional. Whether protection is destined for sebaceous lipids while in the gland, on/in the hair fiber, or at the skin surface has yet to be determined.

In general, PUFAs are considered the most common molecules that undergo in vivo lipid peroxidation. However, when considering integral skin lipids as well as skin surface lipids (sebum), we must keep in mind that these regions are frequently exposed to UV radiation. Thus, photooxidation may bring about lipid peroxidation reactions in lipids that normally would not experience autoxidation. For example, we would not expect oleic acid to undergo autoxidation at physiological temperature (37°C), unless perturbed by free radical species. However, it has been shown that such monoenes may form lipid hydroperoxides quite readily by the action of UV light.[19] Furthermore, a comprehensive study demonstrated the ease of squalene photooxidation—a chief component of

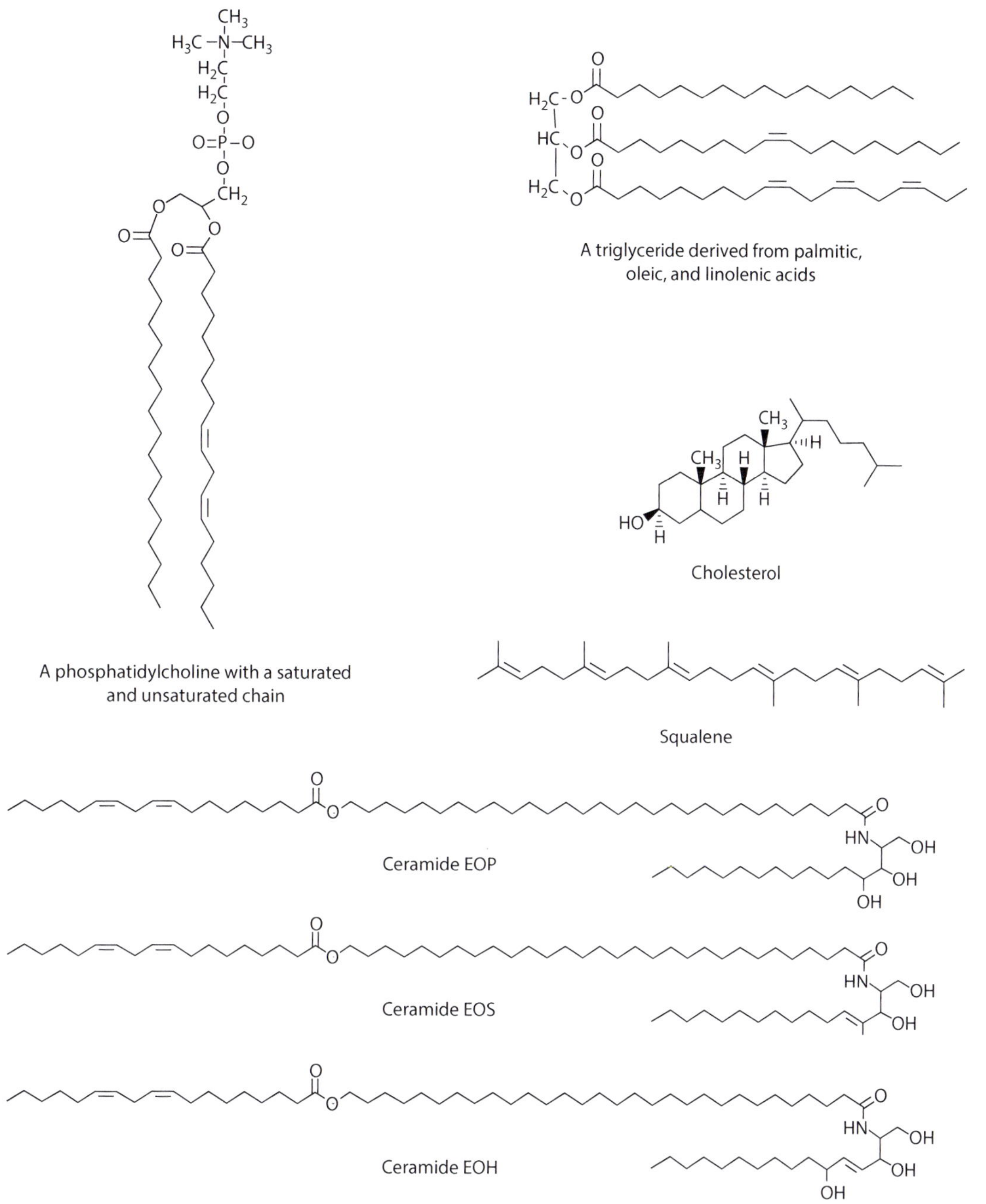

Figure 5.4 Structures of several skin lipids and skin surface lipids susceptible to lipid peroxidation. Their predominant location is provided in text; the triglyceride shown is given as an illustration of one with saturated and unsaturated chains. While this particular species may occur in nature or other parts of the body, it is not certain that it is present in skin.

skin surface lipids also present in the stratum corneum and remaining epidermis.[10] Therefore, many lipids one may expect to be stable on the skin surface or in the skin structure may undergo photooxidation, yielding similar products as autoxidation. For a complete summary of skin lipids, the reader is referred to several book chapters dedicated to this topic.[13,20]

Lipid peroxidation in cosmetic formulations

Thus far, most of this discussion has centered on lipid peroxidation relevant to in vivo circumstances or studies of ex vivo or in vitro systems. It is now worth noting some key considerations with regard to formulations. Antioxidants are frequently employed in cosmetic formulations to maintain product stability, and they are also often used as active ingredients to be delivered to the skin, where they are meant to ward off free radical species. Hence, it is often necessary to preserve lipids present in the formulation as well as to prevent an active ingredient antioxidant from becoming oxidized. Lipids serve a variety of functions in cosmetic formulations. They provide stability, especially for water-in-oil emulsions, and they can be used to manipulate viscosity and control the solubility of active ingredients. In a textural context, lipids play a very important role in skin feel. In addition, they are film formers that can be utilized as waterproofing agents in sunscreen formulations or as occlusive agents preventing transepidermal water loss (TEWL), thereby acting as moisturizers.[21] Further uses include attempts to regenerate skin barrier function by replenishing lost or damaged lipids of the stratum corneum.

Some of the most common lipid ingredients used in cosmetic formulations are petrolatum, beeswax, lanolin, jojoba oil, esters, natural glycerides, silicones, and ceramides.[21] Many of these ingredients are complex mixtures of many different lipids. For example, beeswax is composed of wax esters, free fatty acids, fatty alcohols, and hydrocarbons. Not all lipid ingredients used in cosmetics undergo lipid oxidation. Saturated ceramides, which do not contain double bonds along the aliphatic chains, are not likely to oxidize. Likewise, many of the saturated hydrocarbon ingredients, such as those found in petrolatum, will not readily oxidize under normal environmental conditions. Silicones are also very stable and do not require antioxidant preservation. On the other hand, triglycerides, jojoba oil (which contains omega fatty acids), certain esters, lecithin, and many natural oils from plant sources are susceptible to oxidation. As the use of natural ingredients becomes more prevalent in cosmetic formulations, it will become imperative to prevent oxidation in these samples, since naturals tend to contain more unsaturated lipids than synthetic compositions.[22,23]

Environmental conditions play a major role in lipid peroxidation and greatly influence kinetics. For example, in vivo we generally need not worry about temperatures exceeding 40°C. Therefore, most of the usual targets of lipid peroxidation are PUFAs, cholesterol, and so on. However, monounsaturated fatty acids such as oleic acid—a commonly used ingredient in cosmetics—may also undergo lipid peroxidation, although the reaction is catalytically slow below 60°C.[24] This may be a very important factor for long-term stability. We already discussed the importance of lipid peroxidation in the context of the omega-3 and omega-6 fatty acids. In these molecules, the double bonds are separated by two single bonds, making them unconjugated PUFAs, which follow the lipid peroxidation scheme already discussed. Conjugated PUFAs may also undergo oxidation. These fatty acids are characterized by a chemical structure in which at least two double bonds are separated by only one single bond. Linoleic acid is a typical example of a conjugated PUFA, which is found in cosmetic compositions. Often thought to be inert, saturated fatty acids may also undergo oxidation, although this requires relatively high temperatures, normally exceeding 100°C.[24] Palmitic and stearic acids are two ingredients frequently utilized in cosmetics that fall into the category of saturated fatty acids.

The role played by iron in lipid peroxidation and the possibility of the Fenton and Haber–Weiss reactions occurring in vivo, ex vivo, or in vitro in biological substrates have been mentioned. Likewise, the presence of iron in formulations may also be troublesome. To circumvent any problems that could be introduced by iron, a sequestering agent such as disodium ethylenediaminetetraacetic acid (EDTA) is normally used in the formulation.

Lipid oxidation and antioxidants in colloidal systems

Cosmetic formulations, especially skin care products, typically employ emulsion systems, be it an oil-in-water (o/w) or water-in-oil (w/o) emulsion. In the case of an o/w emulsion, oil droplets are dispersed in a continuous water phase, while the contrary is true for a w/o emulsion. Emulsifiers are typically employed to stabilize an otherwise thermodynamically unstable emulsion. Other common colloidal systems—usually formed by surface active compounds—also used in cosmetic products consist of liposomes and micelles. Emulsions, especially o/w, are very common in food chemistry. For this reason, a great deal of research has been conducted on food colloidal systems and their oxidative stability. This is in sharp contrast to the cosmetic industry, where there is little literature available in the public domain that discusses lipid oxidation in emulsion systems or other common colloidal structures found in cosmetics. One reason for greater attention in the area of food chemistry is the more frequent use of PUFAs in food emulsions. Historically, saturated or monounsaturated fatty acids were probably more commonly found in most commercial cosmetic products. However, as we enter the *green* age and find increasing levels of naturals/botanicals in cosmetic formulations, we will likely find higher concentrations of PUFAs.[22] Regardless, we will draw from much of the literature associated with food chemistry to gain a better understanding of lipid oxidation in emulsions and other colloidal structures.

The chemical and physical environment of an antioxidant will play a major role in its activity. When planning to prevent lipid oxidation in colloidal systems one must understand what type of antioxidant will perform optimally under certain conditions. It is not as simple as choosing a lipid-soluble antioxidant to protect lipid phase molecules. There is a phenomenon—which has come to be known as the *polar paradox* (also termed the *antioxidant paradox*)—that essentially states that hydrophilic (or polar) antioxidants are more efficacious in bulk oil systems than lipophilic (or nonpolar) antioxidants. It also states that lipophilic (or nonpolar) antioxidants are more effective than hydrophilic (or polar) antioxidants in systems that have a substantial aqueous phase, such as oil-in-water emulsions.[25–28] The ability of polar antioxidants to provide greater protection than lipophilic antioxidants in bulk oil systems has been attributed to the tendency to position itself at the air–oil interface where oxidation is most likely to occur due to the presence of oxygen, resulting in oxidation products. Due to its low solubility in pure oil, the hydrophilic antioxidant will migrate from the bulk oil phase to the interface where it will be found at highest concentrations.[26–28] It is also believed that reverse micelles are formed within the bulk oil phase, such as in air bubbles, which is another likely location of oxidation and a place where polar antioxidants may congregate.[28] In o/w emulsions, it is believed that nonpolar antioxidants will be present in the oil droplet and will migrate to surface of the droplet, the oil-water interface, where oxidation reactions are most likely to occur.[26–28] It is also believed that most lipid oxidation reactions take place at the oil-water interface in o/w emulsions, where hydroperoxides (from the lipids) interact with heavy metals in the aqueous phase.[29]

Electrostatic interactions are also believed to play an important role in determining antioxidant efficacy in colloidal systems. For example, it has been shown that charged antioxidants are more efficacious in liposomes than non-charged species.[27] Therefore, one should expect the pH of a formulation to influence the ability of an antioxidant to interact with other charged species and thus affect the antioxidant's efficacy. As an example of electrostatic effects, Frankel points out that the negatively charged antioxidants, ascorbic acid and trolox, are more efficacious in linoleic acid micelles stabilized with a cationic emulsifier (hexadecyltrimethyl ammonium bromide) than the same micellar system stabilized with an anionic emulsifier (sodium dodecyl sulfate). He explains that this phenomenon occurs due to repulsion between the negatively charged antioxidants and the negatively charged headgroups of sodium dodecyl sulfate.[27]

While many different behaviors have been elucidated for antioxidant-colloid systems in food chemistry, there are still numerous possibilities and avenues to be explored. This is especially true due to the vast quantity of antioxidants available to the formulator. In addition, when used in unison they often act synergistically and their physical or chemical environment may very well affect efficacy. As indicated by Frankel, there is an imperative need to examine homologous series of antioxidants in various colloidal systems to better understand their behavior.[27] Recent studies—systematically examining structure-property relationships of antioxidants—demonstrate that some molecules do not follow the guidelines normally expected by the polar paradox.[30] For more information in this area, the reader is referred either to the textbook by Frankel or one of the recent articles that addresses many contemporary issues with lipid peroxidation in colloidal systems.[27,28]

LIPID PEROXIDATION MEASUREMENT TECHNIQUES FOR IN VITRO LIPID MODEL SYSTEMS AND BIOLOGICAL SAMPLES

The quantification of lipid peroxidation is a difficult task that has challenged scientists over the last century.[31] This is mainly due to the complex nature of the lipid peroxidation process from a kinetic viewpoint but is also due to the many different products that are formed. The complexity in vivo stems from the many different events that occur on the cellular level as well as the reality that biological substrates are very complex systems that do not always have predictable behavior like model systems. In vitro, many advances in the current understanding of lipid peroxidation and its measurement have evolved from a wealth of research that was conducted in part by researchers associated with the food industry to elucidate and prevent rancidity in food products as well as research conducted in the rubber industry in the earlier part of the twentieth century.[26,32,33] In food, the decomposition of fats and oils results in degradation of many important food properties, such as taste, odor, texture, nutritional value, and shelf life. In this context, many analytical techniques have been developed to quantify lipid peroxidation and its prevention. Much of this technology was garnered and further advanced by those working at the interface of biology, biotechnology, biochemistry, and chemistry with primary interests focused on in vivo lipid peroxidation. Likewise, we may also utilize the transfer of technology not only to produce better cosmetic and pharmaceutical formulations, but also in the quest to target and deliver antioxidants to the skin where they may act as active ingredients and influence skin's biological function.

Lipid peroxidation may be measured at several different stages during the transformation and subsequent decomposition of the lipid.[34–36] First, we can monitor the loss of unsaturated fatty acid in the sample under investigation. A second and more common approach is to monitor the formation of primary lipid peroxidation products. This could be the measurement of conjugated dienes or lipid hydroperoxides in the initial stages of oxidation. A third strategy for the measurement of lipid peroxidation is to screen the formation of secondary lipid peroxidation products (e.g., MDA, HNE, etc.), such as those already mentioned and those to be discussed in further detail as this chapter progresses. In addition, electron spin resonance spectroscopy can be used in conjunction with spin traps (see Chapter 7) to monitor the free radicals produced at all of the intermediate steps. An outline of the various stages of lipid peroxidation and possible analytical techniques for quantification is provided in Figure 5.5.[35] The primary lipid peroxidation products (conjugated dienes and lipid hydroperoxides) can be quantified using UV spectroscopy, iodometric titration, the ferrous oxidation in xylenol orange (FOX) assay, and chemiluminescence. Once a LOOH is formed, there are two possible pathways that can be followed, leading to further lipid decomposition and the formation of secondary lipid peroxidation products. In the route that leads to the formation of alkoxyl radicals, further products include alkenes and various aldehydes. Review of the literature indicates that the aldehydes are probably the most frequently monitored species by those working in the field. Most likely, this is the case because aldehydes not only provide an indication of lipid peroxidation, but some (e.g., HNE) are cytotoxic to mammalian cells. Of all these tests, the thiobarbituric acid reactive substances (TBARS) assay remains one of the most commonly employed in laboratories throughout the world. In this assay, the formation of MDA can be monitored for in vitro cell cultures, ex vivo skin samples, and in vitro model systems whether they are suspensions of lipids or even more complex formulations. While the TBARS assay finds universal application, there is quite a bit of controversy as to its accuracy.

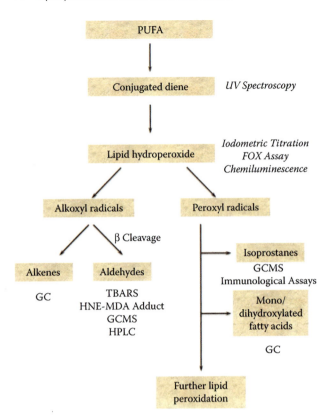

Figure 5.5 Scheme of products formed during lipid peroxidation and various procedures employed to conduct measurements. (Adapted from Moore, K. and Roberts, L.J.I., *Free Rad. Res.*, 28, 659–671, 1998.)

Several of the techniques outlined in Figure 5.5 will be discussed further as this chapter progresses. Much attention will be given to the most commonly employed techniques, namely UV spectroscopy to measure conjugated dienes, iodometric titration, TBARS assay, FOX assay, and chemiluminescence. In addition, two special interest sections are included. The first, "model lipid systems", reviews techniques available for the preparation of pure lipid systems to study lipid peroxidation that are very useful to determine the efficacy of antioxidants. A second section, titled "analysis of in vivo, ex vivo, and in vitro samples", provides general procedures for tissue homogenization and subsequent fractionation of cellular and molecular components. The second section is very relevant to studies of skin cell cultures and ex vivo skin sections, in which case it is necessary to isolate molecules of interest from a complex biological matrix.

Diene conjugation

Lipid peroxidation of unsaturated lipids and fatty acids results in the formation of conjugated diene structures. Normally, unsaturated fatty acids and lipids contain unconjugated dienes, where each double bond is separated by two single bonds. However, during the lipid peroxidation process these fatty acids and lipids undergo conversion where double bonds become separated by only one single bond, which is referred to as a conjugated diene. As shown in Figure 5.6, conversion of an unconjugated diene to a conjugated diene is the result of hydrogen atom abstraction and subsequent free radical formation. It is important to note that in the process of lipid peroxidation, conjugated dienes are intermediate products, which are eventually converted to lipid hydroperoxides.

Conjugated dienes absorb in the UVC region of the electromagnetic spectrum, making their detection facile in model lipid systems. This phenomenon was discovered in 1931, when it was found that lipids stored over a period of time developed an increase in absorption in the region 230–235 nm. Since the 1960s, this procedure has been used universally in the food industry to monitor the lipid quality of food products.[1] Figure 5.7 contains a UV absorption spectrum of ethyl linoleate demonstrating the utility of UV-visible spectrophotometry in monitoring lipid peroxidation. An intense band occurs at 200–210 nm due to absorption by non-conjugated dienes. As a result of conjugated diene formation, a shoulder develops at 200–235 nm where peak intensity measurements are made to quantify lipid peroxidation.

The sensitivity of this technique can be greatly enhanced by performing second-derivative spectrophotometry or using high-performance liquid chromatography (HPLC) to separate the various forms of conjugated dienes.[2] Results are generally best obtained from pure lipid samples, and it is advised to use extreme caution when analyzing samples obtained from biological sources and fluids as these contain many chromophores that interfere with conjugated diene absorption.[37] In conclusion, while this method has been and may be used for the study of lipid peroxidation in biological systems, its best use is probably to monitor lipid peroxidation of lipid-containing formulations or model lipid systems, such as micelles, lamellar structures, and liposomes.

Thiobarbituric acid reactive substances assay

MDA—also referred to as malondialdehyde or malonaldehyde—and other related aldehydes are formed in foods, cosmetics, in vitro cultures, and in vivo as a result of lipid peroxidation.[38] Often, these compounds are utilized as probes to determine the extent of oxidative deterioration in a substrate. As noted in previous sections of the text, lipid hydroperoxides are formed during the process of lipid peroxidation. As shown in Figure 5.8, lipid hydroperoxides can be further decomposed through a sequence of steps to MDA. Only PUFAs containing three or more double bonds are able to decompose to lipid hydroperoxides and further to MDA. The three most notable examples are linoleic, linolenic, and arachidonic acids (Figure 5.3).

The formation of MDA is often utilized as an indicator of lipid peroxidation, and one of the tests most commonly used to quantify MDA formation is the TBARS assay. In order to detect MDA, TBARS is added to the sample, allowing the reaction shown in Figure 5.9 to proceed. The resulting MDA-TBARS complex is red in color

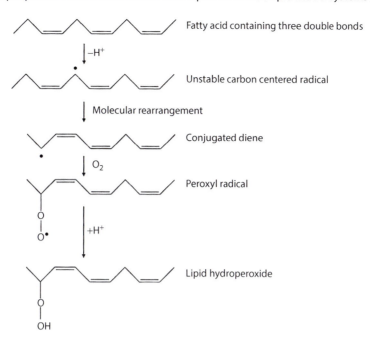

Figure 5.6 Formation of lipid hydroperoxide. (Adapted from Gutteridge, J.M.C., *Clin. Chem.*, 41, 1819–1828, 1995.)

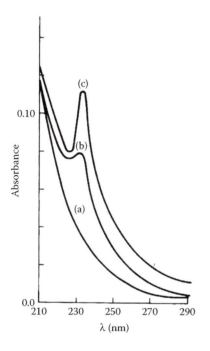

Figure 5.7 Formation of conjugated dienes in ethyl linoleate. (a) Purified ethyl linoleate, (b) after oxidation with air for 8 hours at 30°C, and (c) after exposure to nitrogen dioxide to accelerate lipid peroxidation. (Courtesy of William Pryor; From Halliwell, B. and Gutteridge, J., *Free Radicals in Biology and Medicine*, 5th ed., Oxford University Press, Oxford, UK, 2015, by permission of Oxford University Press.)

(λ_{max} = 532–535 nm) and its formation can be followed using spectrophotometry. The assay must be conducted at low pH and slightly elevated temperature. While this assay can be carried out on biological samples, it works best with model lipid systems such as microsomes or liposomes. It has also been universally used to determine the oxidation of various food products and is an official method of the American Oil Chemists' Society (AOCS).

Provided below are some of the caveats of the TBARS assay as well as some recommendations to improve the sensitivity of the method. In general, most of these items apply to complex biological systems in which many other substances may interfere with the spectroscopic determination of MDA.

Caveats of the thiobarbituric acid reactive substances assay[39–41]

1. MDA can only be formed from fatty acids that contain a series of three conjugated double bonds in the aliphatic portion of the molecule, such as linolenic acid or arachidonic acid.
2. TBA may react with substances other than MDA, such as other aldehydes, carbohydrates, amino acids, and bile pigments. Other aldehydes are often produced at much greater concentrations than MDA.
3. In vivo, MDA may form Schiff bases or react with lysine and arginine, which results in cross-linking reactions, ultimately generating advanced glycation products.
4. In the case of many lipids, MDA is not formed as a result of oxidation.
5. Normally, lipid hydroperoxides are formed during the oxidation process. MDA, on the other hand, is not formed until the TBARS assay is executed. This has the advantage that it amplifies the amount of MDA present; however, it does not represent the true amount of MDA present in the sample where oxidation has occurred.
6. Only trace amounts of MDA are produced from the physiologically most abundant polyunsaturated fatty acid (linolenic acid).

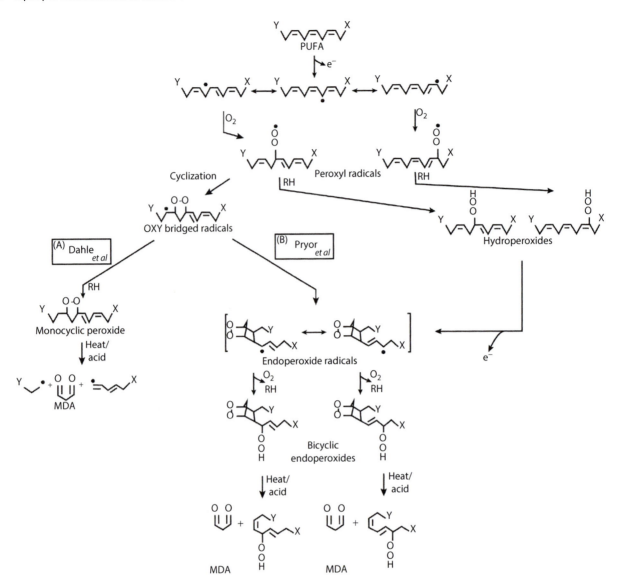

Figure 5.8 Possible mechanisms for the formation of MDA from PUFAs. (Reprinted from *Free Rad. Biol. Med.*, 9, Janero, D.R., Malondialdehyde and thiobarbituric acid-reactivity as diagnostic indices of lipid peroxidation and peroxidative tissue injury, 515–540, copyright 1990, with permission from Elsevier.)

Methods to improve the thiobarbituric acid reactive substances assay[41]

1. Utilize spectrofluorescence to detect the MDA-TBA complex (λ_{ex} = 532 nm, λ_{em} = 553 nm).
2. Use inline high-performance liquid chromatography (HPLC) separation to purify the MDA-TBA complex prior to obtaining the spectrophotometric measurement.
3. HPLC may also be used in combination with spectrofluorescence.

Due to the practical, but controversial, nature of MDA-related assays, a tremendous amount of research has been conducted to develop a better understanding in this area.[6,42–48] More recent developments have focused on refining methods with more modern chromatographic techniques.[49,50] There are also several guidelines provided in the literature in regard to handling biological samples when conducting the TBARS assay.[51–56] Like most fields of molecular biology, studies concentrating on lipid peroxidation in skin utilize the TBARS assay as a guideline. Table 5.1 contains a list of references where the TBARS assay has been used to measure lipid peroxidation in skin systems.

Ferrous oxidation in xylenol orange assay

Lipid hydroperoxides, which are produced as a result of lipid peroxidation, are capable of oxidizing ferrous iron (Fe^{2+}) to the ferric ion (Fe^{3+}). The FOX assay, originally developed by Simon P. Wolff, is an acronym for ferrous oxidation in xylenol orange.[87] It is based on the reaction of Fe^{3+} with a molecular probe, xylenol orange [o-cresolsulfonephthalein-3′,3′-bis(methylimino)diacetic acid, sodium salt], resulting in the formation of a colored

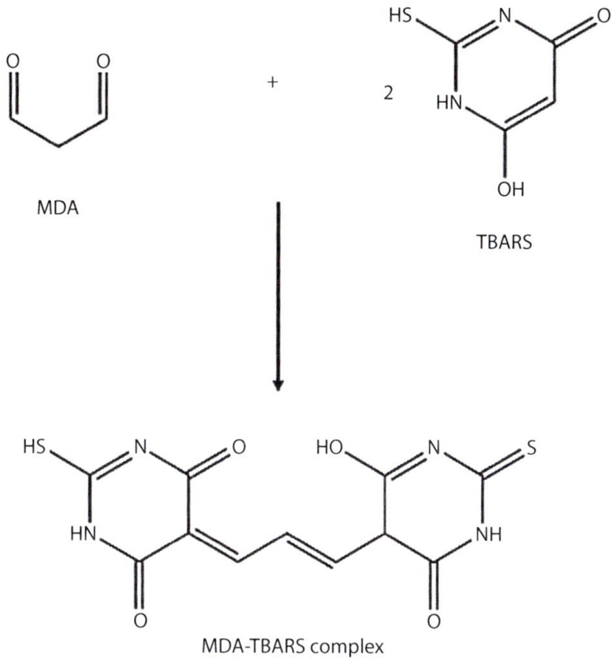

Figure 5.9 Reaction of MDA and TBARS to produce the MDA-TBARS complex, which has a λ_{max} = 532–535 nm.

In fact, two versions of the FOX assay were described in the literature to measure both water-soluble hydroperoxides and lipid-soluble hydroperoxides.[88]

The FOX assay for water-soluble hydroperoxides was designed to measure the concentration of H_2O_2 and other hydroperoxides, such as butyl and cumyl hydroperoxides.[87] In order to increase the sensitivity of the FOX assay for water-soluble hydroperoxides, the hydroperoxide signal can be amplified by the addition of sorbitol, which is included as an ingredient of the assay that reacts with alkoxyl radical (RO•) produced in Reaction 5.5. Through a reaction consisting of several steps, one of sorbitol's many hydroxyl groups is transformed into a peroxyl radical, which disassociates, ultimately yielding the ketone form of sorbitol and hydroperoxyl radical (HOO•). Formation of HOO• allows the following reaction to proceed:

$$Fe^{2+} + HOO^{\bullet} \rightarrow Fe^{3+} + H_2O_2 \quad (5.7)$$

Thus, addition of sorbitol to the assay reaction medium results in an artificially high reading of the hydroperoxides present in a sample.

The water-soluble FOX assay is carried out with the following reagents: xylenol orange, ammonium ferrous sulfate,

Table 5.1 Analysis of TBARS in skin utilizing various substrates.

Substrate	References
Skin biopsies or tissue models	Tomaino et al.,[57] Katiyar et al.,[58] Nakayama et al.,[59] McArdle et al.,[60] McArdle et al.[61]
Murine models	Thiele et al.,[62] Evelson et al.,[63] Khettab et al.,[64] Kobayashi et al.,[65] Wei et al.,[66] Şener et al.,[67] Toklu et al.,[68] Pugliese et al.[69]
Keratinocyte cultures	Afaq et al.,[70] Djavaheri-Mergny et al.,[71] Mora-Ranjeva et al.,[72] Quiec et al.,[73] Tebbe et al.,[74] Zhu et al.[75]
Fibroblast cultures	Han et al.,[76] Morlière et al.,[77] Morlière et al.,[78] Moysan et al.[79]
Melanocytes	Kvam and Dahle[80]
Model lipid systems	Trommer and Neubert,[81] Trommer et al.,[82] Sapino et al.,[83] Lasch et al.,[84] Lee and Choi,[85] Calabrese et al.[86]

(blue-purple) complex with an absorption maximum at 560 nm (ε_{560} = 1.5 × 10^4 M^{-1} cm^{-1}). As already stated, Fe^{2+} can react with a hydroperoxide to produce Fe^{3+}, hydroperoxyl radical, and hydroxy anion (HO$^-$):

$$Fe^{2+} + ROOH \rightarrow Fe^{3+} + RO^{\bullet} + HO^{-} \quad (5.5)$$

The Fe^{3+} that is produced as a result of this reaction can react with xylenol orange to form a complex detectable by UV-visible spectrophotometry:

Fe^{3+} + Xylenol orange → Fe-xylenol orange complex (5.6)

This technique was designed to offer a more selective technique to detect *authentic* lipid hydroperoxides.[87] This statement refers to TBARS assays and the like, which have been criticized for non-specificity toward the detection of lipid hydroperoxides as well as other inherent problems.

sorbitol, and H_2SO_4. Acid is added to prevent oxidation of Fe^{2+} at physiological pH. An aqueous sample, suspected to contain hydroperoxides, is added to the reagent system and incubated for 30 minutes after vortexing. The absorbance of the resulting mixture is read at 560 nm. A calibration curve is obtained using various concentrations of H_2O_2.

Lipid-soluble hydroperoxides are monitored using a different version of the FOX assay.[88] It was designed to measure hydroperoxides in liposomes and low-density lipoproteins. In this version of the assay, sorbitol is not used to amplify the quantity of hydroperoxide present.

There are not very many examples of the utilization of the FOX assay in cosmetic science. Regardless, it has been applied to model lipid systems to monitor UV-induced degradation of PUFAs relevant to skin care.[89] It may, however, be applied to many other applications where the intent is to measure lipid hydroperoxide concentration.

Measurement of cytotoxic aldehydes—4-hydroxy-2-*trans*-nonenal

As already noted, lipid peroxidation of omega-6 PUFAs such as linoleic and arachidonic acid results in the generation of numerous metabolites that may cause further oxidative reactions or other toxic compounds that can, in turn, cause membrane and cellular damage. Certain aldehydes formed as a result of PUFA oxidation are usually classified as 2-alkenals, 4-hydroxy-2-alkenals, and ketoaldehydes.[90] In particular, lipid peroxidation of linoleic and arachidonic acid is known to generate the cytotoxic compound HNE, which is highly reactive and is readily able to attack biological molecules, such as DNA, proteins, and lipids. This compound, shown in Figure 5.10, has an extremely reactive double bond due to resonance with the neighboring carbonyl group. It can be classified as an electrophilic molecule with an alpha, beta-unsaturated carbonyl group that is capable of undergoing Michael Addition reactions. HNE was discovered by the late Hermann Esterbauer[6,91] and is considered to play such an important biological role that the 4-HydrOxynonenal Club (www.hne-club.org) was established to focus study and attention on this topic—and an entire issue of *Molecular Aspects of Medicine* was likewise dedicated to the subject.[92] Due to its discovery as a metabolite of biologically important lipids (PUFAs) and its cytotoxic properties, much interest in the free radical community has focused on the mechanistic study of HNE formation and quantitative measurements of it in vitro. As skin cells (e.g., keratinocytes and fibroblasts) contain PUFAs and are capable of such biological degradation reactions, detection of HNE for skin in in vitro systems is extremely relevant.

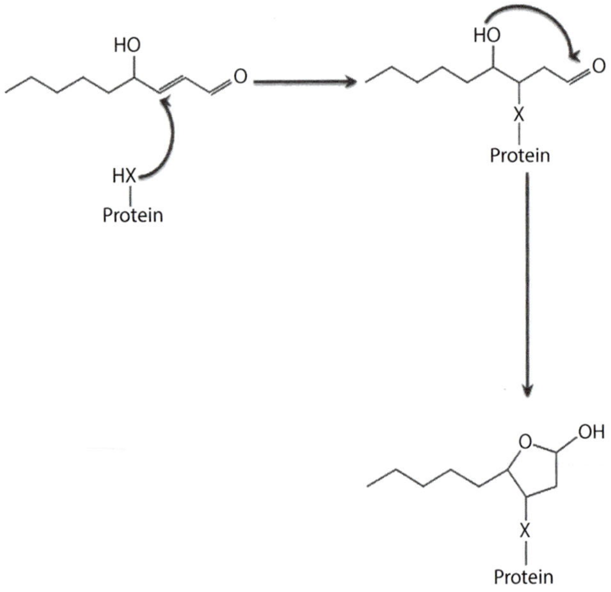

It should be noted, however, that free hydroxyalkenals are extremely volatile and unstable.[93] For this reason, the presence of HNE in vitro should be detected qualitatively, not quantitatively. A typical technique for HNE detection is to employ thin-layer chromatography (TLC) in conjunction with HPLC. In this methodology, the sample is treated with dinitrophenylhydrazine (DNPH), which reacts with aldehydes in the sample. By reacting with DNPH, the aldehyde-DNPH derivatives are more stable and less volatile than free aldehydes.[46] After the reaction with DNPH takes place, the sample is placed on a TLC plate where the different DNPH derivatives will migrate based on polarity. The separated constituents can be gathered and analyzed by HPLC. In addition to using HPLC and TLC, HNE and other aldehydes can be measured directly by HPLC or gas chromatography–mass spectrometry (GC-MS) if they are in the free form.

One of the most damaging aspects of HNE is its ability to react with nucleic acids of DNA or RNA and amino acids of proteins, causing the biomolecule to lose its intended function. In particular, much attention has been given to the reaction of HNE with proteins.[90,94,95] A scheme for the reaction of HNE with a protein adduct is shown in Figure 5.10 and proceeds by Michael Addition. In addition to the measurements described earlier, one may also find some interesting work dealing with the detection of HNE adducts with proteins.[96,97]

Considering how important HNE is considered in redox biology, it is rather surprising that very little data seems to be available concerning HNE and skin.[98–102] There was, however, a useful study of antioxidant protection of a skin tissue culture model with a botanical extract where the authors demonstrated the utility of HNE as a biomarker of oxidative stress.[57]

Quantification of F_2-isoprostanes

Arachidonic acid is an omega-6 fatty acid that is incorporated into the structure of many phospholipids in eukaryotic cells. In normal metabolic circumstances it is converted to prostaglandins by the enzyme cyclooxygenase (COX). However, during lipid peroxidation arachidonic acid may be converted by a free radical mechanism (COX is not involved) to prostaglandin-like compounds, which belong to the family of isoprostanes and are toxic. Figure 5.11 shows a common F_2-isoprostane that is often used as a probe of isoprostane formation. The F_2-isoprostanes have become accepted as key biomarkers

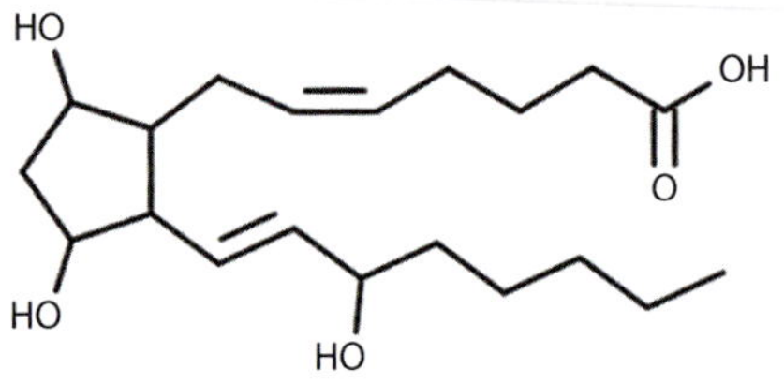

Figure 5.10 Reaction scheme of HNE with proteins, which proceeds by a Michael-type addition. X represents the sulfhydryl group of cysteine, imidazole group of histidine, or ε-amino group of lysine. (Adapted from Uchida, K., *Prog. Lipid Res.*, 42, 318–343, 2003.)

Figure 5.11 Molecular structure of 8-iso-prostaglandin F2alpha (8-iso-PGF2alpha), a common isoprostane.

of oxidative stress in vivo and are usually present in tissues or fluids suffering from oxidative damage at elevated concentrations.[103–108]

There are several methods to quantify F_2-isoprostanes in body tissues and fluids. A great deal of work has been conducted using GC-MS and liquid chromatography–mass spectrometry (LC-MS).[103,104] A very detailed description is provided by Morrow's group, who developed this technology beginning in the early 1990s.[103] While these techniques are very specific, the limited availability of instrumentation in many research laboratories prevents their application as routine analysis. Immunological methods are also used to assess F_2-isoprostane concentration, with the most common being the enzyme immunoassay (EIA). This test is widely employed due to its low cost and ease of use. One problem associated with EIA is that only one class of F_2-isoprostane is detected, while all classes may be detected with GC-MS and LC-MS. A brief description of the EIA method is provided in the paragraph below, while the reader is referred to Milne et al. for a complete description of GC-MS and LC-MS.[103]

EIAs are often designed to be competitive assays in which an antibody to a specific isoprostane (the antigen) is attached to a well plate. There are two antigens: (1) the tracer, which is added and contains the isoprostane of interest with a covalently attached probe that allows for fluorescence or UV-visible measurements, and (2) the isoprostane present in the sample to be analyzed. The tracer and the sample to be analyzed are added to the well plate so that they may compete for binding with the antibody. When absorbance or fluorescence measurements are obtained, they are due to the tracer. Therefore, the concentration of isoprostane present in the sample is inversely proportional to the amount of antibody-bound tracer.

Most of the research dealing with the detection and study of isoprostanes has been conducted with plasma, urine, and other bodily tissues. Isoprostanes have also been detected in skin cells and skin tissue, and it has been shown that photoirradiation produces them in a dose-dependent manner.[109] In fact, high levels of 8-isoprostane were detected in skin afflicted by basal cell carcinoma as well as healthy UVA-irradiated skin.[110] It was even found that the isoprostane levels were higher in chronic wounds (versus acute), presumably due to the persistent state of oxidative stress.[111]

Model lipid systems

When testing for antioxidant efficacy, often model lipid systems are used rather than biological substrates. This allows for facile categorization of specific lipid peroxidation without interference from numerous biological factors. Pure or mixed lipid systems may be employed and they may form a variety of colloidal structures or organized assemblies, such as micelles, lamellar phases, emulsions, or liposomes. For example, a simple o/w system can be created by dispersing linolenic acid in water using a laboratory flask shaker.[81] More complex systems, such as liposomes or multi-lamellar vesicles, require a little extra preparation, employing several distinct types of lipids: for example, cholesterol, linolenic acid, and dipalmitoylphosphatidylcholine (DPPC)—a phospholipid.[81] Comprehensive studies were conducted with a range of phospholipids, free fatty acids, and cholesterol in attempt to mimic viable skin lipids and the effects of UV irradiation and transition metal ions on lipid peroxidation.[82] In many cases, lipid peroxidation is induced by adding a chemical initiator or transition metal salts. Regardless of the initiation procedure, one of the assays described in the previous section may then be employed to measure lipid peroxidation—it can be as simple as adding TBA to the model lipid system followed by spectrophotometric measurements. Table 5.2 provides a list of studies published in cosmetic science literature that utilized model lipid systems to investigate lipid peroxidation.

Analysis of in vivo, ex vivo, and in vitro samples

Often, experiments involving free radical- and lipid peroxidation-related research are carried out on many different subjects. The closest method of analysis to the final application—at least for topical application of antioxidants—would be in vivo testing on humans. Unfortunately, these tests are normally limited to the analysis of skin surface lipids or punch biopsies. Murine models are typically employed in rigorous academic research, whether it be to study free radical biology or test the efficacy of antioxidants. The hairless mouse (SKH-1) is the most frequently utilized rodent due to its reputation as a standard in skin research and its commonality with human skin. Researchers also employ the Wistar rat and guinea pig, but with much less frequency. Lipid peroxidation experiments are also performed on skin cell cultures (keratinocytes, fibroblasts, and, sometimes, melanocytes) or tissue models of skin. Skin tissue may be harvested in the laboratory (requires a clean room) or can be purchased from a suitable supplier (e.g., EpiSkin).

In experiments involving surgically removed skin from mice, typically the mice are sacrificed at the end of the study and the portion of skin that has undergone treatment and UVR exposure is removed with a scalpel. Most often, treatment is administered in the dorsal region of the mouse. For punch biopsies of humans, the subjects are not sacrificed. Once the skin is removed, subcutaneous fat is removed and the skin is placed on ice, or frozen, until it is time to undergo further processing. If desired (which often is the case), the epidermis and dermis are separated by first heating at slightly elevated temperature for a short duration of time (e.g., 60°C for 30–60 seconds) and then making an incision with a scalpel between these two layers of skin to facilitate their separation. The section of skin to be analyzed, typically the epidermis, is then homogenized. This is accomplished by placing the tissue in a buffer solution and sonicating it for short period of time (on the order of a few minutes), resulting in a suspension of the biological sample. The homogenate may then be centrifuged and the supernatant may be subjected to further analysis involving lipid peroxidation detection. A crucial step prior to

Table 5.2 Studies conducted on model lipid systems to determine antioxidant efficacy.

Author	Summary	Parent method
Carini et al.[112]	Fatty acid solutions and micellar systems. FT-IR, NMR, and UV-visible spectrometry	
Jeon et al.[113]	Lipid peroxidation system containing linolenic acid. Measure optical density at 500 nm	Igarashi et al.[126]
Kroyer[114]	Effect of O_3 on a model lipid system	Nicolaides[127]
Courbebaisse et al.[115]	Induction of lipid peroxidation in liposomes	Babizhayev et al.[128]
Kim et al.[116,117]	Lipid peroxidation system containing ethyl linoleate. TBARS assay	Ohkawa et al.[55]
Hong et al.[118]	Lipid peroxidation system containing ethyl linoleate. TBARS assay	Ohkawa et al.[55]
Kuno et al.[119]	Lipid peroxidation of linoleic acid induced by HO•. TBARS assay	Tamura and Yamagami[47]
Lee et al.[120]	Lipid peroxidation system induced by Fenton's reagent. TBARS assay	Ohkawa et al.[55]
Sasaki et al.[121]	Linoleic acid (0.1%) suspended in sodium dodecyl sulfate solution (0.8%) Peroxidation was induced by UV lamps and measured by the TBARS assay	
Bonina et al.[122]	DPPC/linoleic acid unilamellar vesicles. Peroxidation induced by 2,2′-azobis(2- amidinopropane) hydrochloride	
Lee et al.[85]	Lipid system containing ethyl linoleate; peroxidation induced by Fenton's reagent	
Motoyoshi et al.[123]	Investigated fat- and water-soluble lipid peroxidation systems. Fat-soluble: L-alpha-glycerophosphorylcholine and squalene. Water-soluble: Liposomes of L-alpha-glycerophosphorylcholine. Peroxidation induced by chemical initiators	
Kim et al.[124]	In vitro analysis of primrose oil (73% linoleic acid and 9.7% alpha-linolenic acid)	Peers and Swoboda[129]
Carini et al.[89]	Photooxidation of PUFAs (linoleic, linolenic, and arachidonic acids) in sodium dodecyl sulfate micelles	
Bonina et al.[125]	Unilamellar vesicles of DPPC/linoleic acid	

sonication or homogenization is the addition of butylated hydroxytoluene (BHT) to the sample to prevent any further oxidation reactions from occurring. Likewise, skin cell cultures may also be homogenized and the supernatant analyzed by assay. An alternate approach to homogenizing skin tissue is to extract the epidermis with a mixture of ethanol, sodium dodecyl sulfate, BHT, and chloroform. The chloroform phase may then be collected and be analyzed by an appropriate assay.[62] Another approach to study lipid peroxidation is to collect surface lipids (sebum) from the skin and measure the lipid peroxidation status using the assays described in the earlier sections. Lipids present on the surface of the skin may be collected by using a cotton swab followed by Soxhlet extraction of the swab with an organic solvent, or mixture of solvents.

More details on the preparation of tissue samples and cell cultures may be found in a textbook by Graham and Rickwood.[130] For further information on laboratory preparatory techniques involving free radical research, the reader is referred to the work of Rice-Evans and coworkers.[93]

IN VITRO LIPID PEROXIDATION ASSAYS FOR MEASURING FAT/OIL STABILITY
Tests to measure oxidation of fats/oils
Peroxide value determination by iodometric titration

The peroxide value (PV) is often used as an indicator of the concentration of peroxides (ROOR) and hydrogen peroxides (ROOH) that are present in a given sample. It is typically determined by performing iodometric titration; however, there are a number of different methods that may be used to measure peroxides.[1] In the iodometric titration technique, the peroxides oxidize iodide (I^-) to iodine (I_2), which can be measured by standard titration techniques. This is an official method of the American Oil Chemists Society (AOCS) and is frequently utilized to monitor lipid peroxidation in food and cosmetic samples.[131–133] The iodometric titration is typically carried out by reacting potassium iodide (the source of I^-) with the sample to be analyzed, which often is a lipid oil system that is suspected of containing ROOR and/or ROOH. By performing the titration, one may quantify the amount of peroxides present in the sample and also investigate the possible prevention of oxidation by antioxidants.

The initial reaction takes place in a solvent system containing acetic acid and chloroform. Potassium iodide is then added to the reaction vessel, followed by addition of the sample to be investigated. As already mentioned, the potassium iodide is able to react with ROOH (or ROOR), resulting in liberated I_2. The balanced equation for the reaction of iodide with ROOH is:

$$ROOH + 2H^+ + 2I^- \rightarrow I_2 + ROH + H_2O \qquad (5.8)$$

After production of I_2, the titration is carried out in which sodium thiosulfate ($S_2O_3^{2-}$) acts as the titrant and, normally, starch is utilized as the end-point indicator. The reaction between the thiosulfate and I_2 results in the production of I^-, which can further complex with added starch, resulting in a dark blue color, indicating that the reaction shown below (Reaction 5.9) has been completed.

$$I_2 + 2S_2O_3^{2-} \rightarrow S_4O_6^{2-} + 2I^- \quad (5.9)$$

The results are typically expressed as milliequivalents of active (peroxide) oxygen per mass of sample using the formula:

$$PV = \frac{V \cdot T}{m} \cdot 1000 \quad (5.10)$$

where:

V and T are the volume and normality of the $S_2O_3^{2-}$ solution, respectively

m is the mass (in kg) of the investigated sample

The iodometric titration technique has several limitations; the two most notable sources of error are:[134]

1. Absorption of I_2 at unsaturated bonds.
2. If O_2 is present in the solution, it can react with potassium iodide and release I_2.

It is also noteworthy that during lipid peroxidation, peroxides are intermediate products that are eventually converted to carbonyl and hydroxyl compounds. Therefore, measurement with this technique is limited to the early stages of lipid peroxidation.

Even with these limitations, iodometric titration is still considered the standard procedure to monitor peroxide oxygen. It is employed universally in the analysis of lipid peroxidation in the food industry, and also finds common usage in the analysis of cosmetic formulations. It is especially useful for measuring lipid peroxidation in bulk samples of lipids and may also be utilized to analyze peroxidation in biological samples if proper solvent extraction procedures are employed.[34] In addition to iodometric titration, several other volumetric techniques are commonly used to determine lipid peroxidation, especially in the food industry. They are used for the determination of free fatty acids, carbonyl oxidation products, and epoxides.[135] While these methods are very simple to employ and have been around for many years, they have been replaced with instrumental techniques because they require large quantities of solvent.[135]

Kreis test

Named after Hans Kreis, this test was designed more than a century ago, in 1899, to measure oxidation in fats and oils, and is based on the detection of the oxidative end-product epihydrinaldehyde, a derivative of MDA.[136] This assay consists of adding phloroglucinol to a lipid sample and monitoring its reaction with epihydrinaldehyde, which produces a complex that absorbs at 540 nm. The original assay underwent some modifications during its first fifty years of existence; however, it has existed in its current form since the 1950s.[1] The procedure that is typically employed consisted of dissolving a fat sample (3 g) in benzene with the resulting solution then shaken in concentrated HCl for 1 minute. A small amount (few drops) of phloroglucinol is then added to the reaction mixture and absorbance readings are obtained.[137]

p-Anisidine value

As already stated, peroxides are usually the first intermediate products of lipid peroxidation, followed by further decomposition to aldehydes and ketones. The p-anisidine value (AV) test measures the amount of aldehydes, predominantly 2-alkenals and 2,4-dienals, that react with the probe, p-anisidine. This assay, developed almost 40 years ago, is still in common use today.[138,139] It is a modification of an earlier developed test to determine benzidine value, in which case benzidine was replaced by p-anisidine due to its carcinogenecity.[140,141] It should be noted, however, that the toxicological profile of p-anisidine is such that it should not be allowed to come in contact with skin.[141,142] The test for AV measures the amount of secondary lipid oxidation products present in the sample due to the reactivity of p-anisidine with compounds containing carbonyl groups. Figure 5.12 illustrates possible reaction routes that may be followed by p-anisidine and several forms of aldehydes.

In addition to its frequent present-day use,[143,144] there are several official methods of analysis that describe this technique.[42,145] The procedure consists of dissolving the

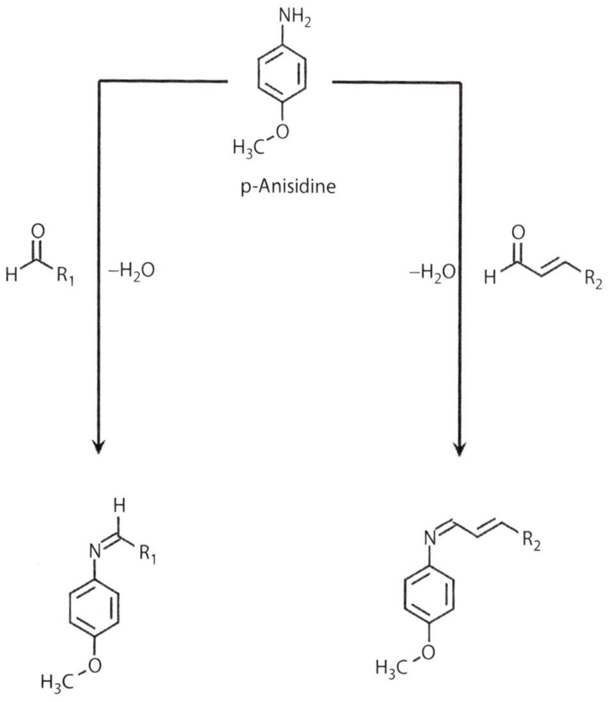

Figure 5.12 Possible reactions of p-anisidine with compounds containing carbonyl groups. (Adapted from Pokorný, J. et al., Ultraviolet-visible spectrophotometry in the analysis of lipid oxidation, in *Analysis of Lipid Oxidation*, Kamal-Eldin, A., Pokorný, J. [Eds.], AOCS Press, Champaign, IL, 2005.)

sample (fat or oil) in isooctane and glacial acetic acid, followed by addition of p-anisidine and measurement of the optical absorbance at 350 nm. Using Equation 5.11 the AV may be determined.

$$AV = \frac{25(1.2 A_b - A_s)}{m} \quad (5.11)$$

where:
- A_b is the absorbance of the fat solution
- A_s is the absorbance of the fat solution after reaction with p-anisidine
- The mass of the original fat or oil sample is denoted by m.

As with all tests for lipid oxidation, there are some considerations that need to be kept in mind. First, the products produced from the reaction of p-anisidine with carbonyl compounds are yellowish in color. When conducting investigations of pure oils this facet may be troublesome due to the inherent color of the oil. In cosmetic products, this will also be the case. Further, H_2O is formed as a result of reactions between p-anisidine and aldehydes. As a result, one must take special care to ensure that no H_2O is present in all reagents used in this method. Normally, a Karl Fisher determination is completed to ensure that H_2O levels of 0.1% or less are present in each reagent.[143]

TOTOX value

Under most circumstances, the peroxide and AVs are considered to be equally important. The PV is indicative of primary (intermediate) lipid peroxidation products. In the food industry, oils and fats are commonly studied using some method to determine the PV. Since many oils and fats are heated to high temperatures, the intermediate peroxides formed during lipid oxidation may further decompose to secondary lipid oxidation products, such as the aldehydic compounds measured by the AV test. Therefore, in order to take into account both primary and secondary lipid oxidation products, food scientists developed the TOTal OXidation value, which is calculated using results from tests to determine peroxide and AV according to the formula:

$$TOTOX = 2PV + AV \quad (5.12)$$

While this equation is very empirical in nature, it is used frequently for the evaluation of refined oils in the food industry.[141] In the determination of the TOTOX value, the PV is multiplied by a factor of two due to the importance of PV on oil stability. It should be noted, however, that it is not recommended to use this equation when PV exceeds 5 mEq/kg.[141]

2,4-Dinitrophenylhydrazine

The formation of secondary lipid oxidation products, such as ketones and aldehydes, can be monitored by following their reaction with 2,4-dinitrophenylhydrazine to form 2,4-dinitrophenylhydrazones (Figure 5.13). This test for lipid oxidation decomposition products, like many of the assays for bulk lipids, has been in use for more than 100 years.[40,141,146,147] The formation of 2,4-dinitrophenylhydrazones is normally followed with UV-visible spectrophotometry.[148]

Accelerated stability tests

Weight gain

Probably one of the oldest tests for measuring lipid oxidation, the Weight Gain test consists of measuring the change in mass of the sample as it becomes oxidized.[149,150] In most experimental circumstances, the sample (an oil or fat) is heated and mass measurements are obtained with a laboratory scale at prescribed time intervals. Hypothetically, the lipids in the sample react with and incorporate O_2 into their structure. Thus, the addition of O_2 to lipid structures results in an increase in the mass of the sample.

This method has been criticized for its lack of sensitivity and its poor correlation with shelf-life predictions.[25,149] Furthermore, the formation of volatile oxidation products may also negatively interfere with estimations of oxidation, as this would cause weight loss rather than weight gain. It is advised to utilize the official method by the

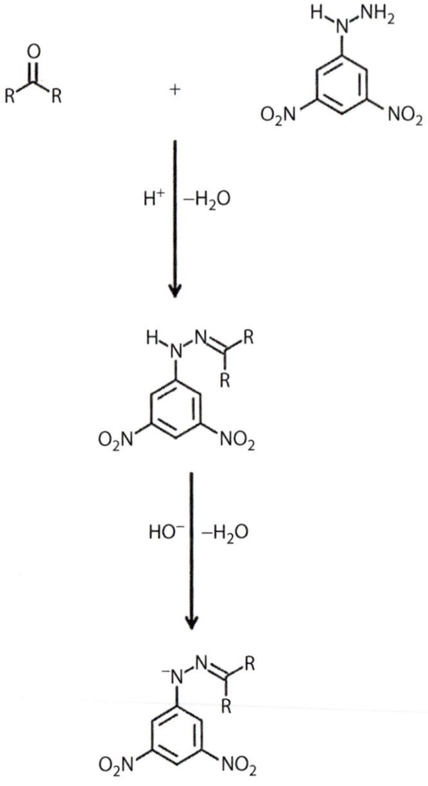

Figure 5.13 Reaction of carbonyls with 2,4-dinitrophenylhydrazine to produce hydrozones. (Adapted from Shahidi, F. and Wanasundara, U. N., Methods for measuring oxidative rancidity in fats and oils, in *Food Lipids: Chemistry, Nutrition, and Biotechnology*, Akoh, C.C. and Min, D.B. [Eds.], Marcel Dekker, New York, 465–487, 2002.)

AOCS, Oven Storage Test for Accelerated Aging of Oils, which recommends an oven temperature of 60°C.[151]

Schaal oven test

One of the most practical tests for lipid oxidation consists of placing a sample in an oven and monitoring oxidation at regular time intervals. Traditionally, rancidity used to be measured by sensory tests at intermittent stages of the Schaal Oven Test; however, more quantitative data can be obtained by measuring PV or another suitable indicator of lipid oxidation status. Several different temperatures have been described in the literature for use in this test, ranging from 50°C to 70°C.[149,152,153] There is, however, an oven stability test described in the Official Methods and Recommended Practices of the AOCS, which specifies a guideline temperature of 60°C.[151] It is imperative not to exceed temperatures of 80°C because doing so will change the oxidation mechanism and will not allow the test to be an extrapolation of ambient temperature conditions for extended shelf life.[151]

As will be discussed in the measurement of the Oil Stability Index (OSI), there is an initial Induction Period, which is a slow oxidation process. This step is followed by a rapid increase in the rate of oxidation. The Induction Period can be determined by measuring PV and plotting it as a function of time. A precaution that must be taken when performing the Schaal Oven Test is to ensure proper cleanliness of any glassware containers used to store the samples. Ions capable of catalyzing lipid oxidation and oxidized lipids from previous tests may cause autoxidation of the sample.[153] Overall, the Schaal Oven Test is considered to be one of the standard accelerated stability tests for oils with the least amount of inherent problems.[154]

Active oxygen method

Historically referred to as the Swift Stability Test, the Active Oxygen Method (AOM) is widely employed throughout the oil and fat industry to measure the stability of fat/oil samples. In this test, the sample is kept at constant elevated temperature (90°C–100°C) in a tube by passing air through hot oil. PVs are then measured at selected time intervals to obtain a plot of oil stability.[148] From the graph, the induction period may be determined. Similar to the PV determination assay (described previously), there are some intrinsic problems with the AOM. Most notably, AOM measures peroxides, which are intermediate products of lipid peroxidation that eventually break down to smaller, more stable compounds.[148]

Oil stability index

As already stated, the onset of lipid oxidation is a slow process until a certain point is reached and rapid oxidation takes place. The time period from the beginning of the experiment until the rapid oxidation point is reached is known as the Induction Period. The duration of the Induction Period depends on various factors of the fat/oil under investigation such as degree of saturation in the alkyl chains and the presence of antioxidants or pro-oxidants (e.g., transition metals) in the sample.[155] In this method, purified air is passed through a thermostated sample cell, which contains the fat/oil under investigation, and further to a sample of deionized water. The conductivity of water is measured as a function of time to obtain a plot that contains a fingerprint of the lipid oxidation state of the sample. As the lipid sample becomes oxidized, it first develops secondary, nonvolatile oxidation products that are then further degraded to volatile tertiary oxidation products (short-chain organic acids), which are carried by the purified air from the sample cell to the deionized H_2O container. As a result, the conductivity of H_2O increases with increasing concentration of the short-chain fatty acids. Typically, a second derivative plot is constructed from the raw data in order to resolve the point where the maximum change in the rate of oxidation occurs.[155] The time that elapses from the outset of the experiment until the peak maximum in the second derivative curve is reached is the aforementioned Induction Period and reported as the OSI. The resulting OSI value is reported in units of time and the temperature that the test was conducted.

The OSI is an official method of the AOCS.[155] It was proposed by AOCS for this test to serve as an automated replacement for the AOM already discussed. This test is often referred to in the literature as the Rancimat Assay due to the commercialization of an instrument by the same name. This technique is universally accepted and has been thoroughly reviewed, and it is considered to be superior to the AOM, not only for its automation and continuous collection of data, but also due to its low variability among different laboratories.[49]

Summary of standard methods to measure the stability/oxidation of fats and oils

Throughout this chapter we have referenced a variety of methods, notably those adapted by the AOCS and the International Union of Pure and Applied Chemistry (IUPAC). These organizations set standards for the oil and fat industry. Most of their methods involve the determination of a chemical attribute related to the development of rancidity in a food product. In most cases, they describe analytical procedures to characterize bulk oil samples as opposed to multiphase systems, such as emulsions and liposomes, or aqueous systems. Therefore, special care must be taken by those working in the area of cosmetics where multiphase systems are commonly found. Thus, many of these tests may not be directly applicable to the systems we wish to study and some modifications may be required.

Often, the methods developed by AOCS and IUPAC are adopted by what is considered to be a higher authority, AOAC International, formerly Association of Official Analytical Chemists. AOAC International is considered to be one of the highest authorities for approved methods due to international adoption of its methods by various regulatory and government agencies.[156] Tables 5.3 and 5.4 contain methods discussed earlier as well as some additional techniques to measure the stability or oxidation of fats and oils that are official methods of the AOCS and IUPAC.

Table 5.3 Selected AOCS official methods and recommended practices for the evaluation of fat/oil stability and oxidation with possible application to cosmetic products.

Method title	Method number
PV acetic acid–chloroform method[a]	Cd 8-53
PV acetic acid–isooctane method	Cd 8b-90
Fat stability, AOM	Cd 12-57
Oil stability index (OSI)[a]	Cd 12b-92
p-Anisidine value[a]	Cd 18-90
2-Thiobarbituric acid value direct method[a]	Cd 19-90
Recommended practices for assessing oil quality and stability	Cg 3-91
Volatile organic compounds (VOC) in fats and oils by gas chromatography	Cg 4-94
Oven storage test for accelerated aging of oils[a]	Cg 5-97
Accelerated light exposure of edible vegetable oils	Cg 6-01
Techniques for assessing the effects of antioxidants in oils and fats	Cg 7-05

Source: Firestone, D. (Ed.), *Official Methods and Recommended Practices of the American Oil Chemist's Society*, 5th ed., AOCS, Champaign, IL, 1998.

[a] Discussed in the previous sections.

Table 5.4 Selected techniques described in IUPAC *Standard Methods for the Analysis of Oils, Fats and Derivatives*.

Method title	Method number
Determination of PV[a]	2.501
Determination of the *oxidized acids* (insolubilization method)	2.502
Determination of the p-anisidine value (p-A.V.)[a]	2.504
Evidence of purity and deterioration from ultraviolet spectrophotometry	2.505
Determination of stability (the modified *swift test*)	2.506

Source: Dieffenbacher, A. and Pocklington, W. D. (Eds.), *IUPAC Standard Methods for the Analysis of Oils, Fats and Derivatives*, 7th ed., Blackwell Scientific Publications, Oxford, UK, 1992.

[a] Discussed in the previous sections.

It should be noted that the AOM is still listed as an official method by AOCS; however, it is primarily provided for historical reference. The AOCS recommends that the OSI method be used in place of the AOM. You will, of course, see it described in many of the texts concerned with the measurement of lipid oxidation in fats and oils.

Several techniques set forth by IUPAC in *Standard Methods for the Analysis of Oils, Fats and Derivatives* are listed in Table 5.4. These methods come from a section in the text specifically devoted to the determination of the quality and stability of oils and fats. Many of the procedures outlined in the manual are similar to those published by AOCS. The PV and AV determinations have already been discussed. The Determination of *Oxidized Acids* method is based on the insolubility of oxidized fats in hexane and their solubility in ethanol. Method 2.505, Evidence of the Purity and Deterioration from Ultraviolet Spectrophotometry, could be classified with the methods discussed in the Diene Conjugation section of this chapter. The Determination of Stability test is conducted by passing air through a sample and measuring the PV (according to Method 2.501) at regular time intervals. The test is finished when a PV of 100 is reached and the data are reported as the time required to reach this value.

CONCLUDING REMARKS

Lipid peroxidation is a significant concern for scientists involved in cosmetic technology. First and foremost, free radical damage, commonly encountered due to exposure to UV radiation, causes lipid peroxidation to structural components of skin. Ultimately, repeated oxidative injury can lead to a pathological state and even carcinoma. Finding strategies to ward off such adversities requires sound knowledge of the measurement techniques presented in this chapter. Many of these assays are expected to provide guidance in the choice of antioxidants utilized to minimize lipid peroxidation. Second, formulation stability depends on the redox state of the cosmetic preparation. Work in the food industry has shed light on antioxidant concepts when preventing lipid peroxidation in colloidal systems. Knowing the target of lipid peroxidation in the formula (for example, is it at the interface of the continuous phase and the emulsion or the air-solution interface?) allows us to more judicially choose an antioxidant with structural properties that will allow it to migrate to the region of interest. Several lipid peroxidation assays are already used extensively in the personal care industry (e.g., the TBARS assay). In addition, model lipid peroxidation systems are also employed in the cosmetic industry to determine antioxidant efficacy. Moreover, we also present information related to a battery of stability tests for lipids—commonly employed in the food industry—with hope that researchers in cosmetic science will adopt them and help advance the current state of the art.

REFERENCES

1. Antolovich M et al. *Analyst.* 2002;127:183–198.
2. Halliwell B, Gutteridge J. *Free Radicals in Biology and Medicine*, 5th ed. Oxford, UK: Oxford University Press; 2015.
3. Buettner G. *Arch Biochem Biophys.* 1993;300: 535–543.
4. Ogura R, Sugiyama M. Reactive oxidants in skin: UV-induced lipid peroxidation. In: Fuchs J, Packer L (Eds.). *Oxidative Stress in Dermatology. Clinical Dermatology*. New York: Marcel Dekker; 1993, pp. 49–66.

5. de Zwart LL et al. *Free Rad Biol Med.* 1999;26:202–226.
6. Esterbauer H et al. *Free Rad Biol Med.* 1991;11:81–128.
7. Yardley HJ. *Int J Cosmet Sci.* 1987;9:13–19.
8. Mier PD, Cotton DWK. *The Molecular Biology of the Skin.* Oxford, UK: Blackwell; 1976.
9. Wertz PW. *Adv Drug Deliv Rev.* 1996;18:283–294.
10. Ekanayake Mudiyanselage S et al. *J Invest Dermatol.* 2003;120:915–922.
11. Harding C et al. Ceramides and the skin. In: Baran R, Maibach HI (Eds.). *Textbook of Dermatology.* London, UK: Taylor & Francis Group; 2005.
12. Wertz PW. Personal communication, 2010.
13. Möller H. The chemistry of natural and synthetic skin barrier lipids. In: Förster T (Ed.). *Cosmetic Lipids and the Skin Barrier. Cosmetic Science and Technology, 24.* New York: Marcel Dekker; 2002, pp. 1–35.
14. Leitinger N. *Mol Apects Med.* 2003;24:239–250.
15. Nelson DL, Cox MM. *Lehninger: Principles of Biochemistry.* New York: W.H. Freeman and Company; 2008.
16. Nicolaides N et al. *Lipids.* 1972;7:506–517.
17. Downing DT et al. *Int J Cosmet Sci.* 1986;8:115–123.
18. Passi S et al. *Free Rad Res.* 2002;36:471–477.
19. Kieber RJ et al. *Limnol Oceanogr.* 1997;42:1454–1462.
20. Michniak BB, Wertz PW. Ceramides and lipids. In: Paye M, Barel AO, Maibach HI (Eds.). *Handbook of Cosmetic Science and Technology*, 2nd ed. New York: Taylor & Francis Group; 2006, pp. 281–288.
21. Lanzendörfer G. Lipidic ingredients in skin care formulations. In: Förster T (Ed.). *Cosmetic Lipids and the Skin Barrier. Cosmetic Science and Technology Series, 24.* New York: Marcel Dekker; 2002, pp. 255–297.
22. Gorcea M. Personal communication. 2010.
23. Draelos ZD, Thaman LA. *Cosmetic Formulation of Skin Care Products.* Jungermann E (Ed.). New York: Taylor & Francis Group; 2006.
24. Swern D. Primary products of olefinic autoxidations. In: Lundberg WO (Ed.). *Autoxidation and Antioxidants, 1.* New York: John Wiley & Sons; 1961, pp. 1–54.
25. Porter WL et al. *J Agric Food Chem.* 1989;37:615–624.
26. Frankel EN. *Lipid Oxidation*, 2nd ed. Edgewater, UK: The Oily Press; 2005.
27. Frankel EN. *Antioxidants in Food and Biology: Facts and Fiction.* Bridgewater, UK: The Oily Press; 2007.
28. Decker EA et al. *J Agric Food Chem.* 2005;53:4303–4310.
29. McClements DJ, Decker EA. *J Food Sci.* 2000;65:1270–1282.
30. Laguerre M et al. *J Agric Food Chem.* 2009;57:11335–11342.
31. Kamal-Eldin A, Pokorný J. *Analysis of Lipid Oxidation.* Champaign, IL: AOCS Press; 2005.
32. Lundberg WO. *Autoxidation and Antioxidants.* New York: John Wiley & Sons; 1961.
33. Akoh CC, Min DB. *Food Lipids: Chemistry, Nutrition, and Biotechnology*, 2nd ed. New York: Marcel Dekker; 2002.
34. Gutteridge JMC, Halliwell B. *Trends Biochem Sci.* 1990;15:129–135.
35. Moore K, Roberts LJI. *Free Rad Res.* 1998;28:659–671.
36. Gutteridge JMC. *Clin Chem.* 1995;41:1819–1828.
37. Halliwell B, Chirico S. *Am J Clin Nutr.* 1993;57(suppl):715S–725S.
38. Janero DR. *Free Rad Biol Med.* 1990;9:515–540.
39. Laguerre M et al. *Prog Lipid Res.* 2007;46:244–282.
40. Wheatley RA. *Trends Anal Chem.* 2000;19:617–628.
41. Södergren E. *Lipid Peroxidation In Vivo: Evaluation and Application of Methods for Measurement.* Uppsala, Sweden: Uppsala University; 2000.
42. Bird RP, Draper HH. *Methods Enzymol.* 1984;105:299–305.
43. Buege JA, Aust SD. *Methods Enzymol.* 1978;52:302–310.
44. Dahle LK et al. *Arch Biochem Biophys.* 1962;98:253–261.
45. Draper HH, Hadley M. *Methods Enzymol.* 1990;186:421–431.
46. Esterbauer H, Cheeseman KH. *Methods Enzymol.* 1990;186:407–421.
47. Tamura H, Yamagami A. *J Agric Food Chem.* 1994;42:1612–1615.
48. Wright JR et al. *Arch Biochem Biophys.* 1981;206:296–304.
49. Lefèvre G et al. *Ann Biol Clin (Paris).* 1998;56:305–319.
50. Liu J et al. *Anal Biochem.* 1997;245:161–166.
51. Botsoglou NA et al. *J Agric Food Chem.* 1994;42:1931–1937.
52. Fukunaga K et al. *J Chromatogr.* 1993;621:77–81.
53. Fernández J et al. *Food Chem.* 1997;59:345–353.
54. Lykkesfeldt J. *Clin Chem.* 2001;47:1725–1727.
55. Ohkawa H. *Anal Biochem.* 1979;95:351–358.
56. Slater TF, Sawyer BC. *Biochem J.* 1971;123:805–814.
57. Tomaino A et al. *Toxicol In Vitro.* 2006;20:1395–1402.
58. Katiyar SK et al. *Carcinogenesis.* 2001;22:287–294.
59. Nakayama S et al. *J Invest Dermatol.* 2003;121:406–411.
60. McArdle F et al. *Free Rad Biol Med.* 2002;33:1355–1362.
61. McArdle F et al. *Am J Clin Nutr.* 2004;80:1270–1275.
62. Thiele JJ et al. *FEBS Lett.* 1997;401:167–170.
63. Evelson P et al. *J Photochem Photobiol B.* 1997;38:215–219.
64. Khettab N et al. *Biochimie.* 1988;70:1709–1713.
65. Kobayashi S et al. *Photochem Photobiol.* 1996;63:106–110.
66. Wei H et al. *Cancer Lett.* 2002;185:21–29.
67. Şener G et al. *Burns.* 2005;31:587–596.
68. Toklu HZ et al. *Burns.* 2007;33:908–916.
69. Pugliese PT, Lampley CB. *J Appl Cosmetol.* 1985;3:129–138.
70. Afaq F et al. *J Invest Dermatol.* 2007;127:222–232.
71. Djavaheri-Mergny M et al. *FEBS Lett.* 1996;384:92–96.
72. Mora-Ranjeva MP et al. *Chem Phys Lipids.* 2006;141:216–224.
73. Quiec D et al. *J Invest Dermatol.* 1995;104:964–969.
74. Tebbe B et al. *J Invest Dermatol.* 1997;108:302–306.
75. Zhu Q et al. *Toxicology.* 2005;209:55–67.

76. Han Y et al. *Pharmacol Res.* 2004;49:265–274.
77. Morlière P et al. *Biochim Biophys Acta.* 1991;1084:261–268.
78. Morlière P et al. *Free Rad Biol Med.* 1995;19:365–371.
79. Moysan A et al. *J Invest Dermatol.* 1993;100:692–698.
80. Kvam E, Dahle J. *J Invest Dermatol.* 2003;121:564–569.
81. Trommer H, Neubert RHH. *J Pharm Pharmaceut Sci.* 2005;8:494–506.
82. Trommer H et al. *Eur J Pharm Biopharm.* 2001;51:207–214.
83. Sapino S et al. *J Cosmet Sci.* 2005;56:227–251.
84. Lasch J et al. *Biochim Biophys Acta.* 1997;1349:171–181.
85. Lee KK, Choi JD. *J Cosmet Sci.* 1998;49:351–359.
86. Calabrese V et al. *J Appl Cosmetol.* 1995;13:27–34.
87. Jiang Z-Y et al. *Lipids.* 1991;26:853–856.
88. Jiang Z-Y et al. *Anal Biochem.* 1992;202:384–389.
89. Carini M et al. New bioanalytical markers of the oxidative stress status of human keratinocytes following UVB exposure. Proceedings of the 20th IFSCC International Congress; 1998; Cannes, France.
90. Uchida K. *Prog Lipid Res.* 2003;42:318–343.
91. Benedetti A et al. *Biochim Biophys Acta.* 1980;620:281–296.
92. Poli G, Schaur J. *Mol Apects Med.* 2003;24(4–5):147–313.
93. Rice-Evans CA et al. *Techniques in Free Radical Research: Laboratory Techniques in Biochemistry and Molecular Biology.* Burdon RH, van Knippenberg PH (Eds.). Amsterdam, the Netherlands: Elsevier; 1991.
94. Forman HJ et al. *Arch Biochem Biophys.* 2008;477:183–195.
95. Schaur RJ. *Mol Aspects Med.* 2003;24:149–159.
96. Carini M et al. *Mass Spectrom Rev.* 2004;23:281–305.
97. Uchida K, Stadtman ER. *Methods Enzymol.* 1994;233:371–385.
98. Aldini G et al. *J Mass Spec.* 2003;38:1160–1168.
99. Yang YS et al. *J Biol Chem.* 2003;278:41380–41388.
100. Zhaorigetu S et al. *J Photochem Photobiol B: Biol.* 2003;71:11–17.
101. Tanaka N et al. *Arch Dermatol Res.* 2001;293:363–367.
102. Poot M et al. *Eur J Biochem.* 1987;162:287–291.
103. Milne G et al. *Methods Enzymol.* 2007;433:113–126.
104. Berdeaux O et al. *Pathol Biol.* 2005;53:356–363.
105. Montuschi P et al. *Curr Med Chem.* 2007;14:703–707.
106. Roberts LJ, Morrow JD. *Biochim Biophys Acta.* 1997;1345:121–135.
107. Roberts LJ, Morrow JD. *Free Rad Biol Med.* 2000;28:505–513.
108. Morrow JD, Roberts LJ. *Prog Lipid Res.* 1997;36:1–21.
109. Schneider LA et al. *Br J Dermatol.* 2006;154:1147–1154.
110. Belli R et al. *Int J Immunopathol Pharmacol.* 2005;18:497–502.
111. Yeoh-Ellerton S, Stacey MC. *J Invest Dermatol.* 2003;121:918–925.
112. Carini M et al. Protective effect of procyanidines from vitis vinifera seeds on UV-induced photodamage: In vitro and in vivo studies. *Proceedings of the 19th IFSCC International Congress*; 1996; Sydney, Australia.
113. Jeon C-O et al. Anti-melanogenesis effect of 2,5 dimethy-4-hydroxy-3 [2H]-furanone. *Proceedings of the 19th IFSCC International Congress*; 1996; Sydney, Australia.
114. Kroyer G, Evaluation of antioxidative cosmetic additives for the protection of human skin lipids against air polluting substances. *Proceedings of the 19th IFSCC International Congress*; 1996; Sydney, Australia.
115. Courbebaisse Y et al. Pseudopeptides: New compounds with a broad-spectrum activity against oxidative stress. A study of their "universal" protective effect and their ability to repair cell membrane damage. *Proceedings of the 19th IFSCC International Congress*; 1996; Sydney, Australia.
116. Kim JH et al. Biological screening of 100 plant extracts for cosmetic use. (1) Antioxidative activity and free radical scavenging activity. *Proceedings of the 19th IFSCC International Congress*; 1996; Sydney, Australia.
117. Kim BJ et al. New anti-aging and anti-wrinkle cosmetic ingredient: Inner nutshell of *Castanea mollisima BL* chestnut. *20th IFSCC International Congress*; 1998; Cannes, France.
118. Hong IT et al. Antioxidative and anti-inflammatory activities of *Phaseolus aureus*. *Proceedings of the 19th IFSCC International Congress*; 1996; Sydney, Australia.
119. Kuno N et al. New anti-aging cosmetic ingredients—lignan glycosides in germinated sesame seeds. *Proceedings of the 20th IFSCC International Congress*; 1998; Cannes, France.
120. Lee K et al. Efficacy of biological activities of a new anti-aging agent obtained from *areca catechu*. *Proceedings of the 20th IFSCC International Congress*; 1998; Cannes, France.
121. Sasaki S et al. Enhancement of human fibroblast growth and other dermatological effects induced by cell extract from heat-shocked blue green alga (Cyanobacterium). *Proceedings of the 22nd IFSCC International Congress*; 2002; Edinburgh, UK.
122. Bonina F et al. *J Cosmet Sci.* 2002;53:321–335.
123. Motoyoshi K et al. *IFSCC Mag.* 2000;3(3):31–38.
124. Kim YD et al. *IFSCC Mag.* 2001;4(4):269–276.
125. Bonina F et al. *Int J Cosmet Sci.* 1998;20:331–342.
126. Igarashi K et al. *Agric Biol Chem.* 1990;54:1053–1055.
127. Nicolaides N. *Science.* 1974;186:19–26.
128. Babizhayev MA. *Biochim Biophys Acta.* 1989;1004:363–371.
129. Peers KE, Swoboda PAT. *J Sci Food Agric.* 1979;30:876–880.
130. Graham JM, Rickwood D (Eds.). *Subcellular Fractionation: A Practical Approach.* Oxford, UK: IRL Press; 1997.

131. Firestone D. Cd 8-53: Peroxide value acetic acid–chloroform method. *Official Methods and Recommended Practices of the American Oil Chemist's Society*, 5th ed. Champaign, IL: AOCS; 1998.
132. Paquot C, Hautfenne A. *Standard Methods for the Analysis of Oils, Fats and Derivatives*, 7th ed. Oxford, UK: Blackwell Scientific; 1987, pp. 199–200.
133. Lea CH. *J Sci Food Agric*. 1952;3:586–594.
134. Gray JI. *J Amer Oil Chem Soc*. 1978;55:539–546.
135. Pokorný J. Volumetric analysis of oxidized lipids. In: Kamal-Eldin A, Pokorný J (Eds.). *Analysis of Lipid Oxidation*. Champaign, IL: AOCS Press; 2005.
136. Kreis H. *Chemiker-Ztg*. 1899;23:802–803.
137. Ostendorf JP. *J Soc Cosmet Chem*. 1965;16:203–220.
138. Holm U, Ekborn K. p-Anisidine as a reagent of secondary oxidation products in oils and fats. *Proceedings of the International Society for Fat Research Congress*, Gothenburg, Sweden, 1972.
139. List GR et al. *J Amer Oil Chem Soc*. 1974;51:17–21.
140. Holm U et al. *J Amer Oil Chem Soc*. 1957;34:606–609.
141. Pokorný J et al. Ultraviolet-visible spectrophotometry in the analysis of lipid oxidation. In: Kamal-Eldin A, Pokorný J (Eds.). *Analysis of Lipid Oxidation*. Champaign, IL: AOCS Press; 2005.
142. Firestone D. Cd 18-90: P-Anisidine Value. *Official Methods and Recommended Practices of the American Oil Chemist's Society*, 5th ed. Champaign, IL: AOCS; 1998.
143. Ali M et al. *Pak J Nutr*. 2008;7:717–720.
144. Carelli A et al. *Grasas Aceites*. 2005;56:303–310.
145. Dieffenbacher A, Pocklington WD. Determination of the p-Anisidine Value (p-A.V.): Method 2.504. IUPAC. *Standard Methods for the Analysis of Oils, Fats and Derivatives*, 7th ed. Oxford, UK: Blackwell Scientific Publications; 1992.
146. Henick AS et al. *J Amer Oil Chem Soc*. 1954;31:88–91.
147. Esterbauer H, Zollern H. et al. *Free Rad Biol Med*. 1989;7:197–203.
148. Shahidi F, Wanasundara UN. Methods for measuring oxidative rancidity in fats and oils. In: Akoh CC, Min DB (Eds.). *Food Lipids: Chemistry, Nutrition, and Biotechnology*. New York: Marcel Dekker; 2002, pp. 465–487.
149. Verleyen T et al. Accelerated stability tests. In: Pokorný J, Kamal-Eldin A (Eds.). *Analysis of Lipid Oxidation*. Champaign, IL: AOCS Press; 2005.
150. Mikula M, Khayat A. *J Amer Oil Chem Soc*. 1985;62:1694–1698.
151. Firestone D. Cg 5-97: Oven storage test for accelerated aging in oils. *Official Methods and Recommended Practices of the American Oil Chemist's Society*, 5th ed. Champaign, IL: AOCS; 1998.
152. Mehlenbacher VC. *Analysis of Fats and Oils*. Champaign, IL: Garrard Press; 1960.
153. Rossell JB. Classical analysis of oils and fats. In: Hamilton RJ, Rossell JB (Eds.). *Analysis of Oils and Fats*. London, UK: Elsevier Applied Science; 1986.
154. Frankel EN et al. *Trends Food Sci Tech*. 1993;4:220–225.
155. Firestone D. Cd 12b-92: Oil stability index (OSI). *Official Methods and Recommended Practices of the American Oil Chemist's Society*, 5th ed. Champaign, IL: AOCS; 1998.
156. Baur FJ. Analytical methods for oils and fats. In: Lawson H (Ed.). *Food Oils and Fats: Technology, Utilization, and Nutrition*. New York: Chapman & Hall; 1995.

Antioxidant assays 6

A fool with a tool is still a fool.

—Albert M. Kligman

In nature, there are a plethora of different antioxidants in plants and other biological species. Extracts from these species are often used in cosmetic preparations. To determine the antioxidant potential of such extracts and other antioxidants in cosmetics, foods, and biological systems, antioxidant assays are commonly employed to determine the reaction efficiency between a selected antioxidant and a chemical probe. As a result of such high demand, a number of assays to measure antioxidant efficacy have become available in the last twenty years. These assays differ from the lipid peroxidation assays discussed in Chapter 5 insofar as antioxidant assays measure reaction kinetics and do not investigate degradation products of lipids. In general, the assays are easy to employ and provide useful information about antioxidant systems, especially when comparing a series of antioxidants. There are, of course, criticisms of the assays. For example, it can be argued that the reaction kinetics observed with an assay probe will be intrinsically different than the actual in vivo situation. Moreover, molecular mobility will not be the same in vivo as in a solution containing only a few reagents. A similar argument could be proposed for complex formulations, such as those found in cosmetics. Regardless, these tools (the assays) provide insight concerning the feasibility of antioxidant species with prospective use in skin care applications.

2,2-DIPHENYL-1-PICRYLHYDRAZYL RADICAL ASSAY

The 2,2-diphenyl-1-picrylhydrazyl (DPPH) assay is an in vitro test that is used in many areas of antioxidant research. The assay is based on the depletion of the 2,2-diphenyl-1-picrylhydrazyl radical (DPPH·) by a free radical scavenger. Normally, it is monitored using either electron spin resonance (ESR) or UV-visible spectrophotometry. This persistent free radical, whose structure is shown in Figure 6.1, is converted to a hydrazine as a result of the reaction with a free radical scavenger. As seen in the figure, A-H represents an antioxidant, which is able to donate a proton. In general, the DPPH assay is simple to employ and is very reproducible.[1,2] One reason for its widespread use is the inherent stability of DPPH· as it is a persistent free radical. This eliminates the need for the experimenter to generate free radicals in situ since DPPH· can be purchased in its radical form.[1]

Another reason for the widespread use of the DPPH assay is its facile implementation. The assay only requires the presence of the free radical species, DPPH·, and the antioxidant whose efficacy is to be determined. Typically, DPPH· is dissolved in ethanol or methanol and to this an alcoholic antioxidant solution is added. As mentioned previously, the assay may be carried out using either ESR or UV-visible spectrophotometry. An ESR spectrum for DPPH· is shown in Figure 6.2, and its depletion by reaction with a free radical scavenger (antioxidant) can be monitored as seen in the spectra of lower intensities (see Chapter 7 for more about ESR).[3] The most common method, however, of monitoring DPPH· depletion by a free radical scavenger is by UV-visible spectrophotometry, in which one may take advantage of the property of DPPH· to absorb visible light (ca. 515 nm).

The reduction of DPPH·, by either another radical or an antioxidant, results in a non-absorbing species

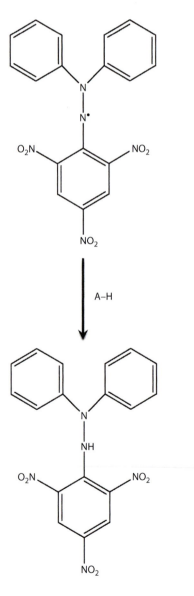

Figure 6.1 Conversion of DPPH· to DPPHH in the DPPH assay. A-H is a proton-donating antioxidant.

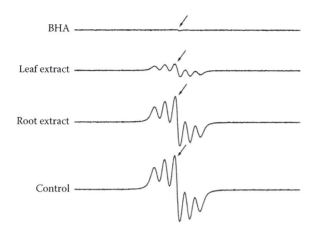

Figure 6.2 ESR spectra of DPPH· (control) and DPPH· treated with various antioxidants. (From Kušar, A. et al., *Hum. Exper. Toxic.*, 25, 599–604, 2006. Reprinted by permission of Sage.)

(Figure 6.3).[4] Therefore, a decrease in visible absorption corresponds to depletion of DPPH· and formation of products by one of the two pathways shown here:

$$DPPH^\bullet + AH \rightarrow DPPH\text{-}H + A^\bullet \quad (6.1)$$

$$DPPH^\bullet + R^\bullet \rightarrow DPPH\text{-}R \quad (6.2)$$

In Equations 6.1 and 6.2, AH and R· represent an antioxidant and a free radical, respectively. The amount of DPPH remaining can be calculated using an equation similar to that provided here:

$$\%DPPH^\bullet_{REM} = \frac{[DPPH^\bullet]_O - [DPPH^\bullet]_T}{[DPPH^\bullet]_O} \times 100 \quad (6.3)$$

In which case $\%DPPH^\bullet_{REM}$, $[DPPH^\bullet]_T$, and $[DPPH^\bullet]_O$ are indicative of the amount of DPPH· remaining, the concentration of DPPH· at a particular time during the experiment, and the initial concentration of DPPH·, respectively. Thus, the reaction kinetics may be followed and one can plot $\%DPPH^\bullet_{REM}$ as a function of reaction time as shown in Figure 6.4. Typically, numerous plots are obtained for different initial concentrations of the antioxidant under study. From these plots (Figure 6.4), the $\%DPPH^\bullet_{REM}$ can be determined when a steady state concentration is reached. That is, the value of $\%DPPH^\bullet_{REM}$ when the plot of $\%DPPH^\bullet_{REM}$ versus time reaches a plateau. As exemplified in Figure 6.5, the value of $\%DPPH^\bullet_{REM}$ at the steady state, for various concentrations of antioxidant, may then be plotted as a function of antioxidant concentration, often expressed as the ratio of antioxidant to DPPH· concentration. From this final graph, we can then express the efficacy of the antioxidant by a value referred to as EC_{50}, which is the efficient concentration of antioxidant when the residual $\%DPPH^\bullet_{REM}$ is 50%. The EC_{50} value can then be used to compare the efficacy of various antioxidants. Often, the EC_{50} value is expressed as its inverse form, $1/EC_{50}$, which is referred to as the antiradical power of the tested antioxidant.

The DPPH assay was first described by Marsden Blois in 1958;[6] however, the current form of the assay is most like that described in 1995 by Brand-Williams et al.[5–8] The assay is used universally to measure the efficacy of antioxidants used in the food industry to prevent food spoilage. In addition, it has found great utility in the cosmetic industry as noted by many examples in the literature.[9–12]

It is noteworthy, however, that the DPPH assay is not useful in experiments with blood plasma, since proteins present in the plasma tend to participate as a result of the alcohol used as the solvent medium in the DPPH assay.[13,14]

2,2′-AZINO-*BIS*(3-ETHYLBENZOTHIAZOLINE-6-SULFONIC ACID) ASSAY

Like the DPPH assay, the 2,2′-azino-*bis*(3-ethylbenzothiazoline-6-sulfonic acid) (ABTS) assay, also known as the Trolox equivalent antioxidant assay (TEAC), finds widespread use

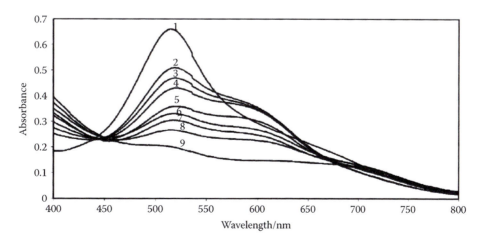

Figure 6.3 UV/vis spectra of DPPH· in methanol treated with various concentrations of aniline. Spectra 1-9 correspond to increasing quantities of aniline added to the medium (0, 0.051, 0.254, 0.505, 0.754, 1.00, 1.962, 2.429, and 2.886 mg). (Reprinted from *Curr. Appl. Phys.*, 4, Gizdavic-Nikolaidis, M. et al., Evaluation of antioxidant activity of aniline and polyaniline, 343–346, Copyright 2004, with permission from Elsevier.)

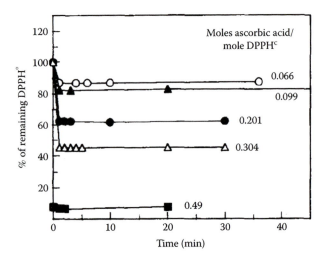

Figure 6.4 Amount of DPPH remaining when reacted with ascorbic acid, based on absorption maxima readings at 520 nm as a function of reaction time. (Reprinted from *Lebensm-Wiss u-Technol.*, 28, Brand-Williams, W. et al., Use of a free radical method to evaluate antioxidant activity, 25–30, Copyright 1995, with permission from Elsevier.)

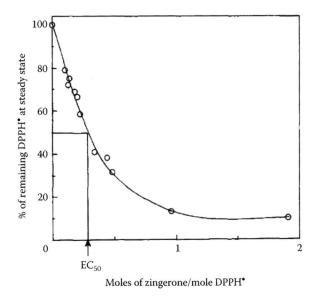

Figure 6.5 Amount of DPPH remaining when reacted with zingerone, based on steady-state readings of plots such as those shown in Figure 6.4. (Reprinted from *Lebensm-Wiss u-Technol.*, 28, Brand-Williams, W. et al., Use of a free radical method to evaluate antioxidant activity, 25–30, Copyright 1995, with permission from Elsevier.)

in testing in vitro antioxidant efficacy for biological systems as well as many finished formulations used in the food and cosmetic industries.[15–18] The assay is actually based on changes in the absorbance spectrum of the radical form of ABTS, which we will refer to as ABTS$^{•+}$ (Figure 6.6). As discussed in the following, ABTS$^{•+}$ absorbs in the visible region

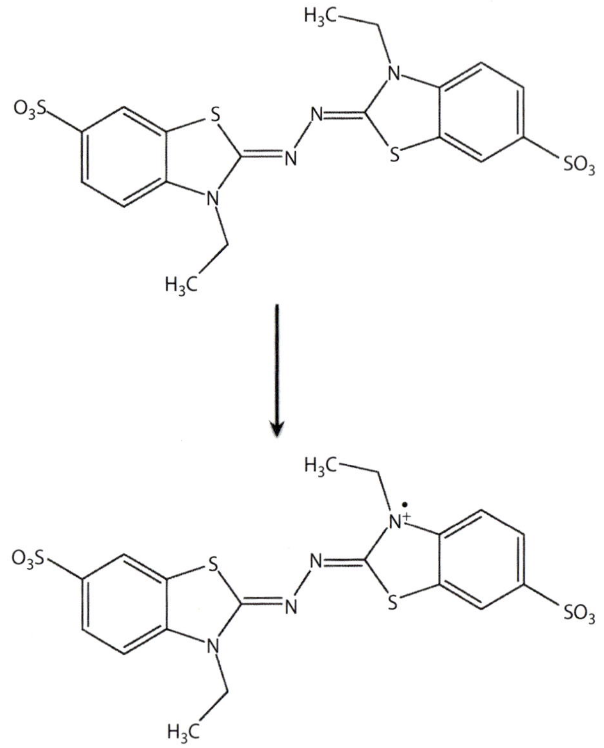

Figure 6.6 Conversion of ABTS to its radical cationic form, ABTS$^{•+}$.

of the electromagnetic spectrum, whereas ABTS does not. In this assay, the radical, ABTS$^{•+}$, reacts with the antioxidant of interest and produces ABTS. The experiment begins with ABTS, which one may purchase from a specialty chemical supplier. The radical, ABTS$^{•+}$, is then generated by utilizing one of the systems shown in Table 6.1, which are allowed to react with ABTS.

Throughout the years, the ABTS assay has undergone various revisions.[19–23] However, the form of the assay that has prevailed is often referred to as a decolorization assay.[24] this is because the radical, ABTS$^{•+}$, absorbs visible light (Figure 6.7); however, as ABTS$^{•+}$ reacts with the antioxidant of interest the reduced form (ABTS), which has negligible absorbance in the visible region, is produced. Often, this method is referred to as the aforementioned TEAC because the results obtained for the antioxidant of interest are compared to results obtained when the water-soluble vitamin E derivative, Trolox, is utilized in this assay.

When conducting the ABTS assay there are several different experimental approaches one may take. These were

Table 6.1 Systems for generating ABTS$^{•+}$ from ABTS.

Metmyoglobin/H_2O_2
Horseradish peroxidase/H_2O_2
MnO_2
Potassium persulfate ($K_2O_8S_2$)
2,2′-azo-*bis*(2-aminopropane) (ABAP)

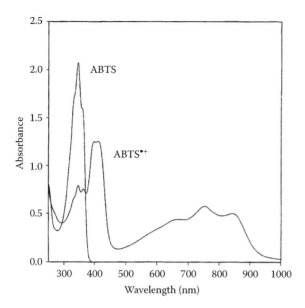

Figure 6.7 Absorbance spectra of ABTS$^{•+}$ and its reduced form (ABTS). (From Arnao, M.B. et al.: Estimation of free radical-quenching activity of leaf pigment extracts. *Phytochemical Analysis*. 2001. 12. 138–143. Copyright Wiley-VCH Verlag GmbH & Co. KGaA. Reproduced with permission.)

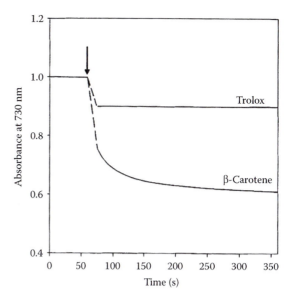

Figure 6.8 Absorbance of ABTS$^{•+}$ at 730 nm for two antioxidants, trolox and beta-carotene. The radical generating system was horseradish peroxidase-H$_2$O$_2$. The arrow represents the time at which the antioxidants were added to the reaction medium. (From Arnao, M.B. et al.: Estimation of free radical-quenching activity of leaf pigment extracts. *Phytochemical Analysis*. 2001. 12. 138–143. Copyright Wiley-VCH Verlag GmbH & Co. KGaA. Reproduced with permission.)

outlined originally by Miller and Rice-Evans, who were pioneers of the ABTS assay:[20]

1. *Decolorization assay*: The radical, ABTS$^{•+}$, is formed by one of the selected methods and it is allowed to reach a steady-state concentration. Once the radical is formed, the antioxidant to be tested may be added to the reaction assembly. As a result, ABTS$^{•+}$ is converted to ABTS resulting in a change in the absorption spectrum—a color loss. Normally, the loss in absorbance at a particular wavelength is followed and this is used as a measure of the total antioxidant activity.

2. *Inhibition assay*: In order to generate the radical, ABTS$^{•+}$, the metmyoglobin–H$_2$O$_2$ system is used. First, ABTS and H$_2$O$_2$ are added to the reaction vessel. Metmyoglobin is later added, triggering the conversion of ABTS to ABTS$^{•+}$. At a fixed point in time, key properties are measured.

3. *Inhibition assay*: All compounds are added to the reaction vessel simultaneously, resulting in the onset of the conversion of ABTS to ABTS$^{•+}$. Again, the metmyoglobin–H$_2$O$_2$ system is used to generate the radical. Various antioxidants can be compared on the basis of reaction rates.

4. *Lag time measurement assay*: As earlier, all compounds are added to the vessel simultaneously resulting in the initiation of ABTS to ABTS$^{•+}$ conversion. In this experiment, one measures the time required to reach a steady-state concentration of ABTS$^{•+}$.

Of the four different types of assay guidelines, the decolorization assay has come to be considered the most reliable. This is because the radical is formed first, until a steady-state concentration is reached. Then, the antioxidant to be tested is added. Problems incur when all compounds are added simultaneously at the start of the reaction since the antioxidant can react with the species (or intermediates) whose job is to generate ABTS$^{•+}$.

An example of data collected utilizing the decolorization assay is provided in Figure 6.8. Reported in the figure is the absorbance of ABTS$^{•+}$ at 730 nm as a function of time after a selected antioxidant, either Trolox or beta-carotene, is added to the reaction vessel. From this plot, one can determine the absorbance before the antioxidant is added and after a steady-state concentration is reached. Thus, if several experiments are conducted at various antioxidant concentrations, a dose-dependence plot for the antioxidant of interest may be obtained (Figure 6.9).

RADICAL TRAPPING PARAMETER ASSAY

In its original form, the total (peroxyl) radical trapping parameter (TRAP) assay was designed, and used almost universally, to measure the antioxidant capacity of blood plasma and other biological fluids. The concept behind this assay is that it measures the total antioxidant capacity offered by all of the protective antioxidants present in the biological fluid, as they act independently and synergistically. These include small-molecule antioxidants, such as ascorbic acid and vitamin E, as well as enzymatic antioxidants. Overall, the TRAP assay has been one of the most used assays to examine the effects of disease or dietary antioxidants on the total antioxidant capacity of plasma. Thus, current scientific

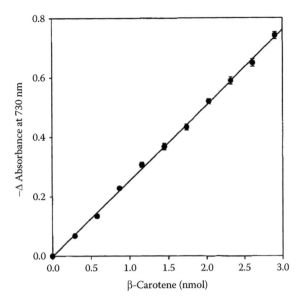

Figure 6.9 Change in absorbance of ABTS·+ at 730 nm when beta-carotene is used as the antioxidant in the assay. The radical generating system was horseradish peroxidase–H_2O_2. (From Arnao, M.B. et al.: Estimation of free radical-quenching activity of leaf pigment extracts. *Phytochemical Analysis*. 2001. 12. 138–143. Copyright Wiley-VCH Verlag GmbH & Co. KGaA. Reproduced with permission.)

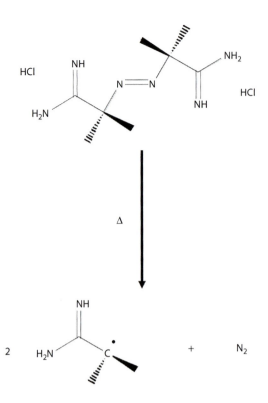

Figure 6.10 Structure of AAPH and its thermal decomposition to a free radical species. It is also known under the synonyms: 2,2′-azo*bis*(2-methylpropionamidine) dihydrochloride and 2,2′-azo*bis*(isobutyramidine) dihydrochloride.

evidence indicates that knowledge of the total antioxidant capacity of plasma could serve as a predictable indicator of the state of health and well-being of an individual.

The TRAP assay measures the antioxidant status of plasma by reporting the concentration (µmol) of peroxyl radicals that are trapped by one liter of plasma.[25] The design of the assay relies on the generation of peroxyl radicals by thermal decomposition of the water-soluble azo initiator 2,2′-azo-*bis*(2-amidinopropane) dihydrochloride (Figure 6.10). Once the initiator has been added to plasma, the oxygen consumed is measured using an oxygen electrode. The oxygen consumption is directly related to the oxidation of susceptible substrates in the plasma. Initially, oxygen consumption is hindered by antioxidants present in the biological fluid that is being tested. However, this initial lag phase (induction period) is followed by an increase in oxygen consumption, which is believed to indicate that all of the antioxidants have been depleted and oxidation is occurring to lipids, resulting in the formation of lipid peroxyl radicals. Figure 6.11 contains a plot obtained from a typical experiment in which the concentration of O_2 is monitored.

As stated earlier, during the initial induction period for the plasma (τ_{plasma}), the rate of oxygen consumption is slow due to antioxidant protection. After the antioxidants in plasma have been depleted, there is a drastic change in the slope of the curve as a result of lipid peroxidation. Further along in the

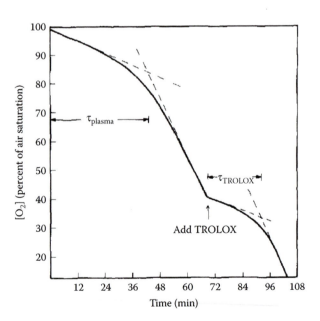

Figure 6.11 Plot of O_2 concentration as a function of time for a TRAP experiment. (Reprinted from *Biochim. Biophys. Acta*, 924, Wayner, D.D.M. et al., The relative contributions of vitamin E, urate, ascorbate and proteins to the total peroxyl radical-trapping antioxidant activity of human blood plasma, 408–419, Copyright 1987, with permission from Elsevier.)

plot, we see that Trolox is added as a standard, permitting the determination of an induction period for Trolox (τ_{Trolox}).

The TRAP value is calculated using the following equation, originally derived from Wayner et al.:[26]

$$\mathrm{TRAP} = \frac{2 \cdot [\mathrm{Trolox}] \cdot \tau_{plasma}}{\tau_{Trolox} \cdot f} \quad (6.4)$$

The stoichiometric factor of 2 in Equation 6.4 represents the number of peroxyl radicals trapped per added molecule of antioxidant. The induction period for plasma and Trolox is given by τ_{plasma} and τ_{Trolox}, respectively. Finally, the concentration of Trolox must be factored into the calculation of TRAP as well as dilution factor, f, in the event that the sample is prepared in a buffer solution.

The original TRAP assay has undergone many revisions since it was originally reported by the Ingold group in 1985.[27] For example, it was found that using an oxygen electrode in the original assay was disadvantageous, because the electrode was not stable over the course of the entire experiment.[28] As a result, this led to the introduction of the fluorescent protein, beta-phycoerythrin (ex. 495 nm; em. 575 nm).[29] Thus, as before, the initiator initially reacts with residence antioxidants, and once these have been depleted continues by damaging the fluorescent probe. The decrease in fluorescence of the probe is analogous to original experiments in which the oxygen concentration was monitored. Another frequently used modification to the TRAP assay is to use luminol-enhanced chemiluminescence.[30] Luminol, a molecule frequently used in crime scene investigations to detect blood, exhibits chemiluminescence when it undergoes oxidation. It is believed that peroxyl radicals react with luminol and its chemiluminescence may be monitored using a luminometer. The experimental design is slightly different from the original TRAP assay; however, one may still calculate a TRAP value.

The TRAP assay is not only limited to measuring the antioxidant capacity of biological fluids, such as blood plasma.[31,32] It has also been applied to the study of olive oil, wine, solid food extracts, and plant extracts.[33–35] To the best of this author's knowledge, there have been no reports in the literature where the TRAP assay has been used to study the effects of antioxidants in skin. However, one possible application of this assay might be to investigate the effect of topical antioxidant treatment in skin on the antioxidant status of blood plasma.

FERRIC REDUCING ABILITY OF PLASMA ASSAY

Similar to the TRAP assay, the original FRAP assay was designed to measure the ferric reducing ability of plasma (FRAP).[36] However, the assay has undergone revisions and is now commonly employed to measure the antioxidant capacity of substances other than plasma, especially extracts that can easily be dissolved in a suitable solvent.[37–43] The assay is carried out using a complex of 2,4,6-tripyridyl-s-triazine (TPTZ) and the ferric (Fe^{3+}) form of iron. Figure 6.12 contains the structure of the organic ligand, TPTZ, in which case two moles of TPTZ complex with one Fe^{3+} atom. At low pH, the ferric iron present in this complex may be reduced to ferrous iron (Fe^{2+}) in the presence of antioxidants, as shown in Equation 6.5:

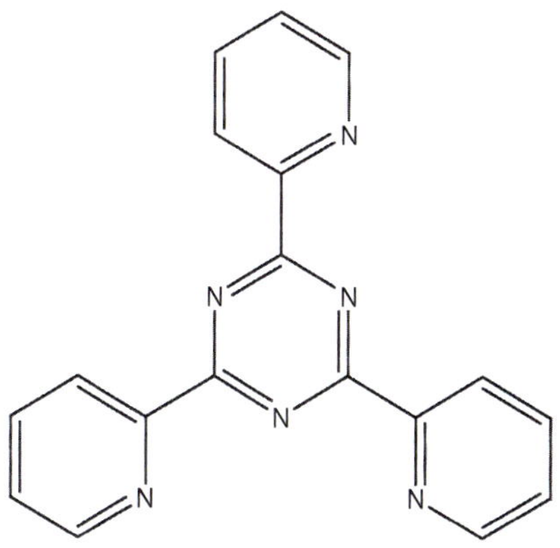

$$Fe^{3+}(TPTZ)_2 + AOH \rightarrow Fe^{2+}(TPTZ)_2 + AOH^{+\bullet} \quad (6.5)$$

As a result of the conversion of Fe^{3+} to Fe^{2+}, the complex develops an intense blue color with an accompanying absorption at 593 nm. Thus, by monitoring the change in absorption as a function of reaction time, a steady state value may be obtained. Figure 6.13 includes the

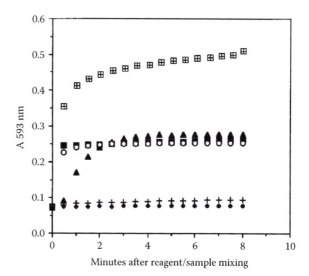

Figure 6.12 The structure of the organic ligand, TPTZ.

Figure 6.13 Reaction kinetics for FRAP experiments with various antioxidants: bilirubin (crossed squares), ascorbic acid (filled squares), uric acid (triangles), alpha-tocopherol (open circles), albumin (plus sign), and reagent alone (diamonds). (Reprinted from *Anal. Biochem.*, 239, Benzie, I.F.F. and Strain, J.J., The ferric reducing ability of plasma [FRAP] as a measure of *antioxidant power*: The FRAP assay, 70–76, Copyright 1996, with permission from Elsevier.)

reaction kinetics for various antioxidants tested by Benzie and Strain.[36] From the plot, the change in absorbance ($\Delta A_{593\,nm}$) can be determined for each tested antioxidant by taking the difference between the last absorbance reading and the initial reading obtained for an Fe^{2+} standard solution. Further, by using Equation 6.6 the FRAP value (µmol/L) for each antioxidant can be calculated:

$$\text{FRAP} = \frac{\Delta A_{\text{sample}}}{\Delta A_{\text{standard}}} \times \text{FRAP}_{\text{standard}} \quad (6.6)$$

OXYGEN RADICAL ABSORBANCE CAPACITY ASSAY

The oxygen radical absorbance capacity (ORAC) assay is another in vitro assay, which uses a fluorescent probe that is susceptible to damage by free radical species. Historically, beta-phycoerythrin, which is a light-harvesting protein from the red algae *Porphyridium cruentum*, was used as the fluorescent probe in this assay. It is known to undergo damage by peroxyl radicals, resulting in a decrease in its intrinsic fluorescence. An initiator is utilized to generate a radical species that eventually leads to the evolution of peroxy radicals. In a typical experiment, one may monitor the fluorescence as a function of time (fluorescence decay curve) for a control system (initiator + fluorescent probe) and a corresponding system that contains an antioxidant (initiator + fluorescent probe + antioxidant). Ideally, the system containing the antioxidant should inhibit the fluorescence decay induced by the peroxy radicals.

As shown in Figure 6.14, two plots are obtained for each system, allowing the calculation of the area under the curve for the fluorescence decay curve.[44] By comparing the area under the curve values of the test system with the standard, antioxidant efficacy can be determined. Typically, results are reported as ORAC units, which are given in Trolox equivalents, and correspond to the concentration of Trolox that has the same antioxidant activity as one liter of test solution. The ORAC value can be calculated as shown by Equation 6.7:

$$\text{Relative ORAC value} = \frac{S_{\text{sample}} - S_{\text{blank}}}{S_{\text{Trolox}} - S_{\text{blank}}} \times \frac{[\text{Trolox}]}{[\text{Sample}]} \quad (6.7)$$

where S is the area under the fluorescence curve for the samples and Trolox.[45] The concentrations of Trolox and the sample also need to be factored into the equation for calculating the ORAC value.

Similar to the TRAP assay, the peroxyl radical is generated using the heat-labile, water-soluble initiator, AAPH (Figure 6.10), in which slightly elevated temperatures result in the scission of the nitrogen double bond and, further, formation of the carbon-centered radical. By reacting with O_2, the carbon-centered radical can form a peroxy radical. As stated earlier, the formation of the AAPH radical allows the protein—traditionally beta-phycoerythrin or R-phycoerythrin are used—to undergo oxidation resulting in a loss of its fluorescence emission. Thus, when an antioxidant is introduced into the system, we are in fact measuring its ability to scavenge the AAPH radical.

The ORAC assay is based on initial work completed by Glazer's group; however, in later years considerable contributions were made by Cao et al.[29,46–48] Throughout time the ORAC assay has undergone several modifications, the most notable was the substitution of fluorescein for the fluorescent protein, phycoerythrin.[45] This was in part due to lot-to-lot variability and interactions that occur between phycoerythrin and polyphenols, which quench the protein's fluorescence.[44] Further, phycoerythrin is susceptible to photobleaching when used with microplate readers (plate readers)—devices used to analyze an aliquot located in a microtiter plate well.[44] Thus, shown in Figure 6.15 is the contemporary employed fluorescent probe, fluorescein, which undergoes oxidation by reaction with the AAPH-induced peroxyl radicals, resulting in the formation of a nonfluorescent, leuco-form of the probe.

As with many of the antioxidant capacity assays, the ORAC assay was initially designed to measure the antioxidant capacity of plasma. It has, of course, been extended to study other systems, which have complex antioxidant compositions.[49–51] For example, it is often utilized for analyzing various types of food groups including fruits, vegetables, chocolate, and tea.[1,52–55] It has also been employed to examine antioxidant status of tissues as well as bioavailability studies of various antioxidants.[1] This assay may very easily be adapted to applications related to cosmetics. It is extremely useful for determining the antioxidant efficacy of extracts or complex formulations containing various antioxidants, which may act synergistically.

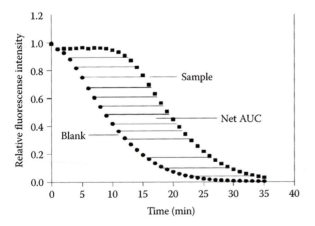

Figure 6.14 Determination of the ORAC value. See text for explanation. (Reprinted with permission from Huang, D. et al., *J. Agric. Food Chem.*, 50, 4437–4444, 2002. American Chemical Society.)

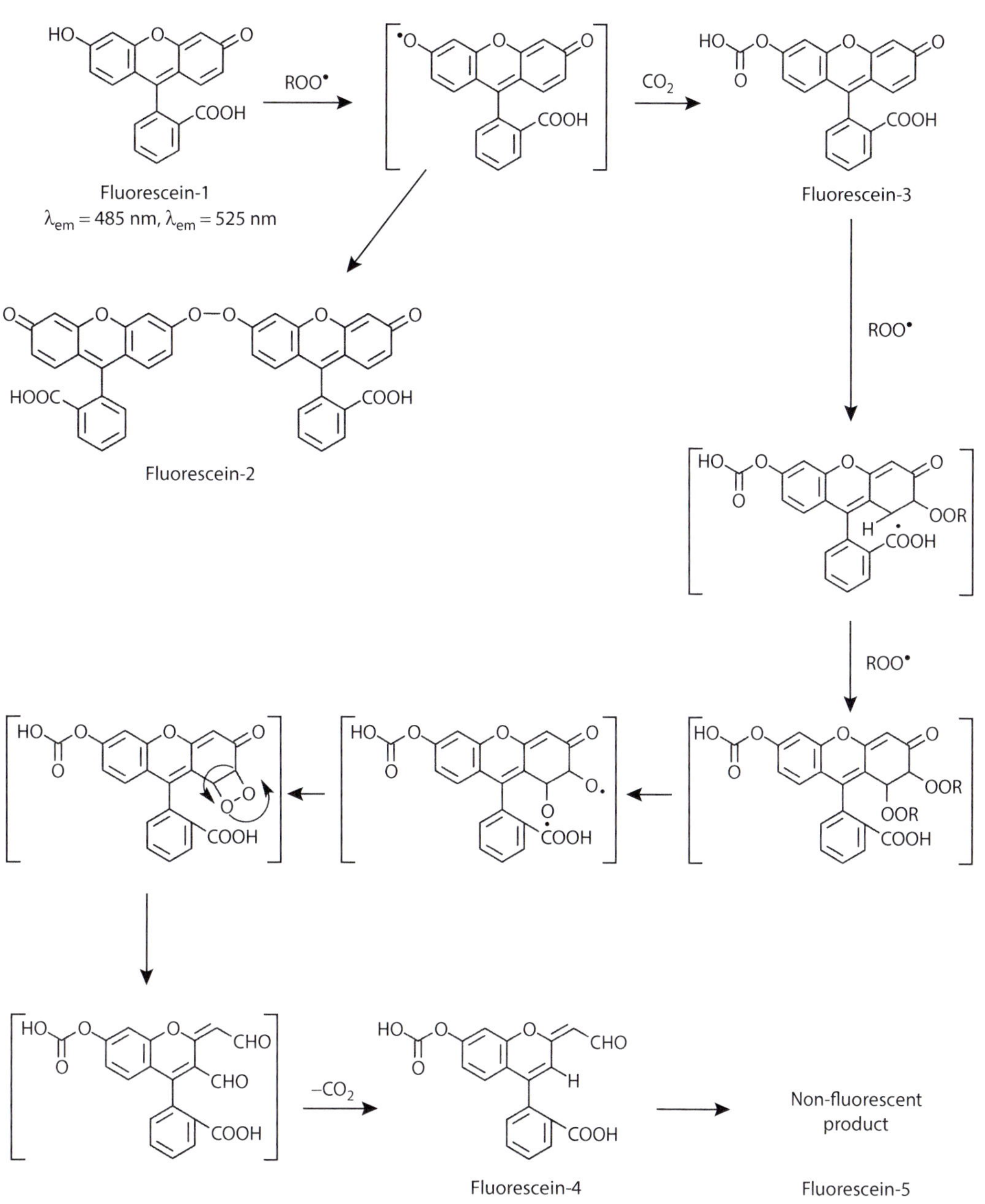

Figure 6.15 Reaction of fluorescein (utilized in the modern-day ORAC assay) with a peroxy radical, forming the non-fluorescent (leuco-form) of the probe. (Adapted from Ou, B. et al., *J. Agric. Food Chem.*, 49, 4619–4626, 2001.)

DEOXYRIBOSE ASSAY

This assay is the one of the most applied tests to measure the HO• scavenging potential of various antioxidants. It is considered an inexpensive alternative to performing pulse radiolysis experiments. After generation of HO•, the radical is allowed to react with 2-deoxyribose (DR), which results in the formation of various molecular fragments of DR (Figure 6.16).[1] The DR degradation products may then be heated at low pH to produce malondialdehyde (MDA), which when allowed to react with thiobarbituric acid produces a pink chromophore [(TBA)$_2$-MDA chromogen] with λ_{max} = 532 nm (see the thiobarbituric acid assay section in Chapter 5.). Therefore, one may determine the efficacy of a radical scavenger antioxidant by measuring the rate of (TBA)$_2$-MDA chromogen production in the presence of added antioxidant. Thus, added antioxidant will compete with DR to scavenge HO• resulting in less (TBA)$_2$-MDA chromogen formation and, hence, less damage to DR.[56]

In the deoxyribose assay, radical generation is accomplished by utilizing Fenton chemistry to produce the HO•. Ferric chloride (FeCl$_3$) and ethylenediamine tetra-acetic

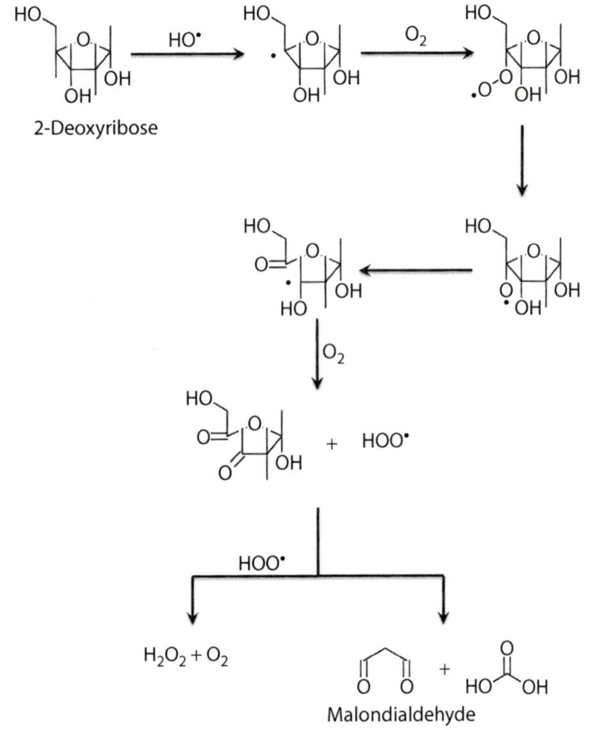

Figure 6.16 Reaction of 2-deoxyribose with HO· ultimately resulting in the formation of MDA. (Adapted from Cheeseman, K.H. et al., *Biochem. J.*, 252, 649–653, 1988.)

acid (EDTA) generate the Fe(II)-EDTA complex in the presence of ascorbic acid. The Fe(II)-EDTA complex can then undergo the Fenton reaction in the presence of H_2O_2 to produce Fe(III)-EDTA and HO·.

$$Fe^{2+}\text{-EDTA} + O_2 \rightarrow Fe^{3+}\text{-EDTA} + O_2^{\bullet-} \quad (6.8)$$

$$2O_2^{\bullet-} + 2H^+ \rightarrow H_2O_2 + O_2 \quad (6.9)$$

$$Fe^{2+}\text{-EDTA} + H_2O_2 \rightarrow HO^- + HO^\bullet + Fe^{3+}\text{-EDTA} \quad (6.10)$$

Once the hydroxyl radical has been generated, it then reacts with DR resulting in the production of deoxyribose fragments, which further undergo decomposition to MDA, and upon heating, reacts with TBA to produce a pink chromophore.

$$HO^\bullet + \text{Deoxyribose} \rightarrow \text{Fragments} \rightarrow \text{MDA} \quad (6.11)$$

$$2\text{TBA} + \text{MDA} \rightarrow \text{Chromogen} \quad (6.12)$$

Typically, these experiments are carried out by measuring the reaction kinetics associated with the process described previously. The absorbance at 532 nm is measured at the end of the experiment (after 1 hour) and corresponds to the rate of the reaction between HO· and DR, which also happens to be the rate-limiting step. The final absorbance reading (*A*) is read for various concentrations of free radical scavenger (*S*) to obtain a plot of $1/\text{Abs}_{532}$ versus [*S*]. Using Equation 6.13, the rate of the reaction between S and HO· may be determined (see Halliwell et al. for derivation):[57]

$$\frac{1}{A} = \frac{1}{A^O}\left(1 + \frac{k_s[S]}{k_{DR}[DR]}\right) \quad (6.13)$$

A and A^O are the absorbance readings in the presence and absence, respectively, of a free radical scavenger. The concentration of DR is constant in this experiment and the reaction rate between HO· and DR is obtained from pulse radiolysis experiments (3.1×10^9 M^{-1} s^{-1}). Thus, by calculating the slope ($k_s/k_{DR}[DR]A^O$) of the $1/\text{Abs}_{532}$ versus [*S*] plot, the rate constant (k_s) for the reaction of HO· and the scavenger may be determined.

The deoxyribose assay has been used extensively to test the ability of various types of antioxidants to scavenge HO·. In particular, it has been extensively used to measure the hydroxyl radical scavenging ability of biologically important antioxidants as well as numerous antioxidants found in foods.[1,58]

The author would like to acknowledge that much of the information provided in this section was garnered from the original work reported by Halliwell et al.[57] The reader is also referred to a report by Aruoma in the *Methods in Enzymology* series.[59]

EVALUATION OF POTENTIAL SKIN CARE ANTIOXIDANTS

Numerous studies, with the intention of determining antioxidant efficacy for skin care applications, use antioxidant assays, especially as a first step to gain a better understanding of antioxidant behavior. Typically, it is recommended to use several different assays and to investigate a range of antioxidants.[60] In the respective sections for each assay outlined in this chapter, selected references are noted for assays employed to specifically probe the behavior of antioxidants intended for skin care use. Nevertheless, all of the assays may be used to determine the efficacy of prospective skin care antioxidants.

CONCLUDING REMARKS

The literature abounds with studies regarding the various antioxidant assays discussed in this chapter. In this text, we make an attempt to cover the most widely used assays and to provide a fundamental and practical explanation of their use. To provide the reader with an appreciation of the number of studies concerning or using the assays, Table 6.2 includes key review articles and benchmarking studies related to the present discussion. The studies cited in the table are mostly aimed at those working in the food industry or in some aspect of biological oxidation. Their use, however, in some cases has been, and in all cases could be, extended to skin care.

Table 6.2 Review and benchmarking studies of antioxidant assays. Please note that some of the studies also discuss lipid peroxidation assays, which are not included in the table.

Study	Assays reviews
Antolovich et al.[13]	ABTS; FRAP; TRAP; and phycoerythrin
Buenger et al.[2]	DPPH; ABTS; dichlorofluoroscein-diacetate; and luminol photoluminescence
Cao and Prior[61]	ORAC; ABTS; and FRAP
Collins[62]	ABTS and FRAP
Hoelzl et al.[63]	FRAP; ABTS; and total free radicals in plasma
Huang et al.[64]	TRAP; ORAC; TEAC; DPPH; N, N-dimethyl-p-phenylenediamine; total phenols assay by Folin-Ciocalteu reagent; Cu(II) reduction capacity; H_2O_2 scavenging capacity, HO$\cdot$ scavenging; peroxynitrite (ONOO$^-$) scavenging; and singlet oxygen scavenging
Prior and Cao[65]	FRAP; TEAC; ORAC; luminol-based assays; dichlorofluoroscein-diacetate; total oxyradical scavenging capacity; crocin based assays; and phycoerythrin based assays
Sánchez-Moreno[1]	TRAP; ORAC; TEAC; DPPH; scavenging of radical cation from N, N-dimethyl-p-phenylenediamine; and scavenging assays for HO$\cdot$; H_2O_2, HOCl; and peroxyl radical
Schlesier et al.[14]	TRAP; FRAP; TEAC; DPPH; 2,2-diphenyl-l-picrylhydrazyl assay; N, N-dimethyl-p-phenylendiamine assay; and photochemiluminescence assay
Thaipong et al.[66]	ABTS; DPPH; FRAP; and ORAC

REFERENCES

1. Sánchez-Moreno C. *Food Sci Tech Int.* 2002;8:121–137.
2. Buenger J et al. *Int J Cosmet Sci.* 2006;28:135–146.
3. Kušar A et al. *Hum Exper Toxic.* 2006;25:599–604.
4. Gizdavic-Nikolaidis M et al. *Curr Appl Phys.* 2004;4:343–346.
5. Brand-Williams W et al. *Lebensm-Wiss u-Technol.* 1995;28:25–30.
6. Blois MS. *Nature.* 1958;181:1199–1200.
7. Bondet V et al. *Lebensm -Wiss u-Technol.* 1997;30:609–615.
8. Molyneux P. *Songklanakarin J Sci Technol.* 2004;26:211–219.
9. Bonina F et al. *Int J Cosmet Sci.* 1998;20:331–342.
10. Bonina F et al. *J Cosmet Sci.* 2002;53:321–335.
11. Ley JP. Phenolic acid amides of phenolic benzylamines against UVA-induced oxidative stress in skin. *Int J Cosmet Sci.* 2001;23:35–48.
12. Rudolph T et al. *IFSCC Mag.* 2006;9:211–216.
13. Antolovich M et al. *Analyst.* 2002;127:183–198.
14. Schlesier K et al. *Free Rad Res.* 2002;36:177–187.
15. Arnao MB et al. *Phytochem Anal.* 2001;12:138–143.
16. Cano A et al. *Phytochem Anal.* 1998;9:196–202.
17. van der Berg R et al. *Food Chem.* 1999;66:511–517.
18. Villaño D et al. *Talanta.* 2004;64:501–509.
19. Arnao MB et al. *Anal Biochem.* 1996;236:255–261.
20. Miller NJ, Rice-Evans CA. *Free Radical Res.* 1997;26:195–199.
21. Miller NJ et al. *Clin Sci.* 1993;84:407–412.
22. Rice-Evans CA, Miller NJ. *Meth Enzymol.* 1994;234:279–293.
23. Erel O. *Clin Biochem.* 2004;37:277–285.
24. Re R et al. *Free Radic Biol Med.* 1999;26:1231–1237.
25. Ghiselli A et al. *Free Rad Biol Med.* 1995;18:29–36.
26. Wayner DDM et al. *Biochim Biophys Acta.* 1987;924:408–419.
27. Wayner DDM et al. *FEBS Lett.* 1985;187:33–37.
28. Alho H, Leinonen J. *Meth Enzymol.* 1999;299:3–15.
29. DeLange RJ, Glazer AN. *Anal Biochem.* 1989;177:300–306.
30. Lissi E et al. *Free Rad Biol Med.* 1995;18:153–158.
31. Aejmelaeus R et al. *FEBS Lett.* 1996;384:128–130.
32. Aejmelaeus RT et al. *Free Rad Biol Med.* 1997;23:69–75.
33. Gorinstein S et al. *J Nutr Biochem.* 2003;14:154–159.
34. Pellegrini N et al. *J Nutr.* 2003;133:2812–2819.
35. Polydoro M et al. *Life Sci.* 2004;74:2815–2826.
36. Benzie IFF, Strain JJ. *Anal Biochem.* 1996;239:70–76.
37. Benzie IFF, Strain JJ. *Meth Enzymol.* 1999;299:15–27.
38. Gardner PT et al. *Food Chem.* 2000;68:471–474.
39. Maksimović Z et al. *Bioresour Technol.* 2005;96:873–877.
40. Niemeyer HB, Metzler M. *J Food Eng.* 2003;56:255–256.
41. Szöllősi R, Szöllősi-Varga I. *Acta Biol Szeged.* 2002;46:125–127.
42. Then M et al. *Acta Biol Szeged.* 2003;47:115–117.
43. Tsai P et al. *Food Res Int.* 2002;35:351–356.
44. Huang D et al. *J Agric Food Chem.* 2002;50:4437–4444.
45. Ou B et al. *J Agric Food Chem.* 2001;49:4619–4626.
46. Glazer AN. *Meth Enzymol.* 1990;186:161–168.
47. Cao G, Prior RL. *Meth Enzymol.* 1999;299:50–62.
48. Cao G et al. *J Agric Food Chem.* 1996;44:3426–3431.
49. Prior RL et al. *J Agric Food Chem.* 2003;51:3273–3279.
50. Wang H et al. *J Agric Food Chem.* 1997;45:304–309.
51. Wu X et al. *J Agric Food Chem.* 2004;52:4026–4037.
52. Guo C et al. *J Agric Food Chem.* 1997;45:1787–1796.
53. Kalt W et al. *J Agric Food Chem.* 1999;47:4638–4644.
54. Wang H et al. *J Agric Food Chem.* 1996;44:701–705.

55. Wang SY, Lin H-S. *J Agric Food Chem.* 2000;48:140–146.
56. Cheeseman KH et al. *Biochem J.* 1988;252:649–653.
57. Halliwell B et al. *Anal Biochem.* 1987;165:215–219.
58. Halliwell B, Gutteridge JMC. *Free Radicals in Biology and Medicine*, 5th ed. Oxford, UK: University Press; 2015.
59. Aruoma OI. *Meth Enzymol.* 1994;233:57–66.
60. Chen L, Wang S. *Photodermatol Photoimmunol Photomed.* 2012;28:228–234.
61. Cao G, Prior RL. *Clin Chem.* 1998;44:1309–1315.
62. Collins AR. *Am J Clin Nutr.* 2005;81 Supp:261S–271S.
63. Hoelzl C et al. *J Physiol Pharmacol.* 2005;56(Supp 2):49–64.
64. Huang D et al. *J Agric Food Chem.* 2005;53:1841–1856.
65. Prior RL, Cao G. *Free Rad Biol Med.* 1999;27:1173–1181.
66. Thaipong K et al. *J Food Compos Anal.* 2006;19:669–675.

Electron spin resonance of skin

Life in electron paramagnetic resonance (EPR) could be tedious and frustrating, but it was exciting and it was fun and I reckon it still is.

—Neil Atherton
Electron Paramagnetic Resonance: A Practitioner's Toolkit

Electron spin resonance (ESR), also known as electron paramagnetic resonance (EPR), is a unique research tool that can directly identify free radicals and measure their concentration. It is a technique based on fundamental quantum physics that has found widespread application in the analysis of skin. In most studies, skin biopsies or homogenates are used for analysis. However, in vivo data may be collected by making special adjustments during the operation of the ESR instrument. Regardless, far less work has been completed in vivo—probably due to limited sensitivity. ESR can directly detect endogenous long-lived (persistent) free radicals in skin, such as the ascorbate and melanin radicals. By monitoring their concentration, we can subject the sample, directly in the instrument, to treatments or stresses such as UV irradiation and monitor the formation or reduction of radical species. Moreover, ESR can provide information about the overall redox state of skin—for example, how many radicals are present. ESR can also furnish data regarding the degree of oxygenation of tissues (oximetry) and the biophysical properties of lipid membrane structures.[1] In most cases, this type of data is generated using nitroxide probes (nitroxyl spin labels)—stable radicals that are not easily metabolized. Thus, they react with and incorporate themselves into the structure of radical biological species and serve as an indicator of the redox state of the tissue.

This chapter discusses the fundamental theory behind the operation of an ESR, as well as providing a better understanding of ESR spectra. In addition, the concept of spin traps is introduced—persistent radicals that are used to trap (react with) extremely short-lived radical species (e.g., superoxide anion [$O_2^{-\cdot}$] or hydroxyl radical [$HO\cdot$]). Detection of these radicals would otherwise be impossible without the use of a spin trap. A review of some ESR applications in skin is provided along with a discussion of ESR imaging.

ELECTRON SPIN RESONANCE THEORY

The identity and quantity of a free radical present in a sample may be determined by ESR. It is the only technique that directly measures the concentration of free radicals present in a sample—it is unlike other methods and assays, which rely on indirect approaches to quantify radical concentrations. As a resonance technique, ESR is based on principles similar to those of the more familiar and more common nuclear magnetic resonance (NMR). However, with ESR the interactions of an unpaired electron—which has a magnetic moment—are monitored with other particles in a molecule that also has a magnetic moment, most often protons.

Molecules are often described as either diamagnetic or paramagnetic. In the first case, all electrons in the sample are arranged in pairs, while in the latter one or more unpaired electrons are present. An electron can adopt one of two spin orientations and resides in one of the spin orbitals associated with an electronic energy level ($m_s = +\frac{1}{2}$ or $m_s = -\frac{1}{2}$). Typically, an electron has no preference for one state or the other since both spin states are degenerate (equal in energy). However, in the presence of a magnetic field, an energy gap between the two states emerges in which $m_s = -\frac{1}{2}$ becomes the lower energy state. This phenomenon is illustrated in Figure 7.1, where the electron spin state energy is plotted as a function of applied magnetic field strength.

The Lorentzian curve at the bottom of Figure 7.1 indicates absorption as a result of electron promotion from a lower to higher energy state. In most ESR experiments, an external magnetic field is applied to the sample and swept over a suitable field range. When electrons are subjected to a magnetic field they tend to align their magnetic moments with the applied magnetic field vector. The electrons that align their magnetic moment with the magnetic field will actually precess about the magnetic field analogous

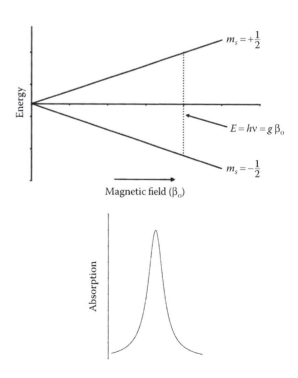

Figure 7.1 Effect of an applied magnetic field on the spin states of a free electron.

to the motion of a spinning top. Depending on an electron's neighboring environment—for example, protons on adjacent carbons (alpha- or beta-carbon)—that electron will have a characteristic precessional frequency, which is proportional to the energy difference between the two spin states. While the magnetic field is swept in an ESR experiment, the sample is exposed to microwave radiation. At a particular magnetic field strength, the difference in energy between the electron spin states is equivalent to the photon energy of the incoming microwaves, which induces a transition from the $m_s = -\frac{1}{2}$ state to the $m_s = +\frac{1}{2}$ state. The frequency and applied magnetic field strength at which this transition takes place is where resonance occurs between the sample and the microwave radiation. As a result, energy is absorbed by the sample, resulting in a signal in the ESR spectrum. Further, the transition energy from one spin state to the other is proportional to the precessional frequency, magnetic field, and local environment of the radical species.

$$\Delta E = g\beta H = h\nu \quad (7.1)$$

The energy absorbed by the sample when going from the $m_s = -\frac{1}{2}$ to $m_s = +\frac{1}{2}$ electron spin state is given by ΔE. The value, g, represents the Landé factor, which is analogous to the magnetogyric ratio (γ) used to describe a proton in NMR. The value of g is dependent on the radical's environment and causes an electron to precess at slightly different frequencies. For a free electron, g has a value of 2.0023, while in most organic samples g values of 1.9–2.1 are usually observed.[2] Planck's constant is denoted by h and the electron precessional frequency by ν. The applied magnetic field is given by H and β is the Bohr magneton, which is the magnetic moment of a free electron and given by:

$$\beta = eh/2m_e \quad (7.2)$$

where m_e and e are the mass and charge of an electron, respectively, and $\hbar$ is equal to $h/2\pi$.

Similar to the phenomenon experienced in NMR, the unpaired electron in a radical sample can undergo coupling in which the electron is split by neighboring magnetic nuclei. This occurs because the electron magnetic field can interact with or is disrupted by other magnetic nuclei, such as protons. When this occurs, the two energy levels that were originally split by the applied magnetic field are each further split ($n + 1$ times) for each interaction between the unpaired electron and another magnetic nuclei in the sample. This means if two protons interact with one electron, the original two spin energy levels will be split, resulting in three energy levels for $m_s = +\frac{1}{2}$ and three energy levels for $m_s = -\frac{1}{2}$. Figure 7.2 contains an energy level diagram to explain this phenomenon. The arrows to the right of the electron spin states in the figure indicate the possible electron spin orientations. Energy transitions can occur between like states, resulting in three possible transitions with an absorption

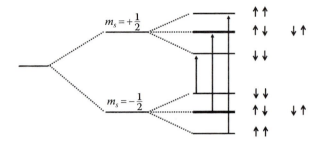

Magnetic field

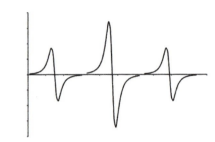

Figure 7.2 Interaction of an unpaired electron with two equivalent protons.

peak occurring on the ESR spectrum for each transition. It is noteworthy that the absorption peaks—represented in the spectrum in Figure 7.2—resulting from lower energy transitions are at lower magnetic field strengths (down field) than higher energy transitions, which is in accordance with Equation 7.1. Before moving on, it is also worth mentioning that ESR spectra are typically displayed as first- or second-derivative absorption curves. This is done for practical purposes—reasons beyond the scope of this review—and will not be expounded upon herein. Figure 7.3 provides a typical Lorentzian-shaped absorption curve with the corresponding first- and second-derivative representations.

As fundamental examples, the spectra for the methyl radical ($CH_3^\bullet$) and the ethyl radical ($CH_3CH_2^\bullet$) are included in Figures 7.4 and 7.5.[3,4] In the case of $CH_3^\bullet$, three equivalent protons interact with the unpaired electron, resulting in ($n + 1$), a quartet of energy transitions, represented as a first-derivative spectrum in the figure. It is worth mentioning, similar to multiplets in an NMR spectrum, the peak intensities in an ESR spectrum follow the rules of Pascal's triangle. Also included in Figures 7.4 and 7.5 is the hyperfine splitting constant, usually denoted by the symbol, a. The hyperfine splitting constant, analogous to the coupling constant in NMR, provides the magnetic field spacing between absorption peaks for energy transitions occurring between equivalent nuclei and the electron. The value of the hyperfine coupling constant depends on the location within the molecule of the radical and the interacting nuclei. In the case of $CH_3^\bullet$, all three protons are considered equivalent. A slightly more complex spectrum is observed for

Electron spin resonance theory 105

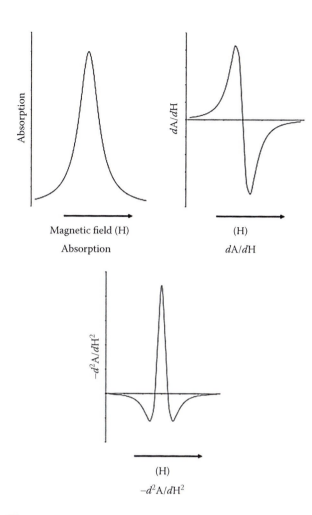

Figure 7.3 Signal representation in ESR.

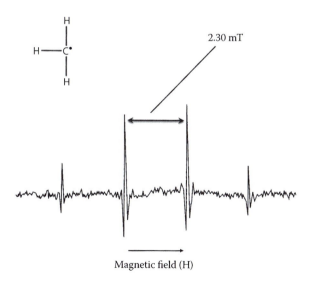

Figure 7.4 ESR spectrum of the methyl radical. (Reprinted with permission from Fessenden, R.W. and Schuler, R.H., *J. Chem. Phys.*, 39, 2147–2195. Copyright 1963 by the American Institute of Physics.)

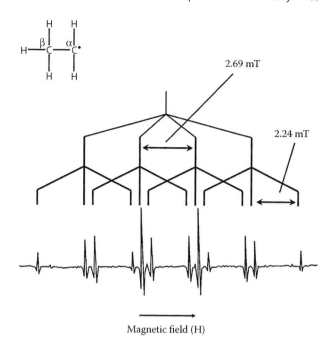

Figure 7.5 ESR spectrum of the ethyl radical. (Reprinted with permission from Fessenden, R.W. and Schuler, R.H., *J. Chem. Phys.*, 39, 2147–2195. Copyright 1963 by the American Institute of Physics; Stick diagram redrawn from Lowry, T.H. and Richardson, K.S., *Mechanism and Theory in Organic Chemistry*, Harper & Row, New York, 1987.)

$CH_3CH_2\cdot$ (Figure 7.5), which illustrates the splitting effect in which the interaction of the three protons on the β carbon results in a quartet, and the two protons on the α carbon a triplet. As a result, the overall spectrum contains a quartet of triplets. A stick diagram is also included in the figure in order to resolve the peaks (lines) occurring from each type of electron-nuclear interaction. This type of diagram is commonly employed to aid in the characterization of a spectrum. One point that these model examples do not address is the difficulty that is often encountered when attempting to identify free radical species in an ESR spectrum. For example, overlap of two or more signals is just one case in which peak assignments can be a rather arduous task.

In a thorough treatise on the applications of ESR in biology, Borg outlines five key points in regard to the characteristics of an ESR spectrum.[5]

1. The position (magnetic field strength) where resonance occurs on the spectrum is primarily determined by the spectroscopic splitting factor (*g*). This is given by the relationship shown in Equation 7.1.
2. As stated earlier, the number of spectral lines (peaks) is directly proportional to the number of interactions between the unpaired electron and local magnetic fields.
3. The spacing between peaks (the hyperfine splitting constant, *a*) is indicative of the nuclear hyperfine interaction strength.

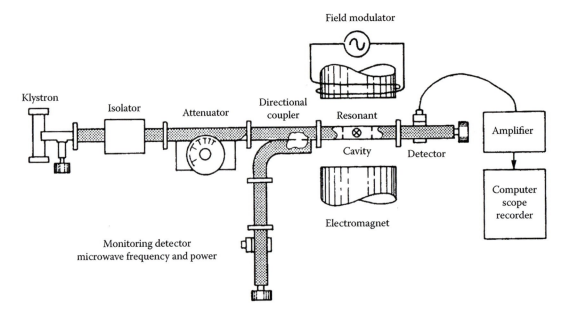

Figure 7.6 Schematic of an ESR spectrometer. (From Weil, J.A. and Bolton, J.R., *Electron Paramagnetic Resonance*, 2nd ed. 2007. Copyright Wiley-VCH Verlag GmbH & Co. KGaA. Reproduced with permission.)

4. The width and shape of the spectral peaks, if due to experimental, as opposed to instrumental, factors, contains information about the relaxation and lifetime of a transition.
5. Peak intensity or, more importantly, peak area is directly proportional to the free radical concentration in a given sample.

As already stated, during most ESR experiments the microwave frequency is kept constant while the magnetic field is swept over a particular range. This is normally done using microwave energy with wavelengths ranging from a few millimeters to a few centimeters.[3] Klystron tubes are universally employed as a source of microwave radiation; however, they have a very narrow frequency range, which is why the radiation is usually kept constant while the magnetic field is varied. Most modern spectrometers are able to detect radicals with a concentration as low as 10^{-8} M, although 10^{-6} M is probably a more correct estimation of detection limit.[6] For illustration, a schematic of a typical X-band ESR instrument is provided in Figure 7.6. Aside from the Klystron source and the field modulator, other key components of the instrument include those elements that amplify the signal and enhance sensitivity. A more thorough discussion of the instrumental components found in an ESR instrument is provided in Weil and Bolton.[7]

SPIN TRAPPING

The direct detection of endogenous persistent radicals in skin, specifically the ascorbyl and melanin radicals, has been accomplished at room temperature.[8-10] However, more reactive radical species, such as $O_2^{-\bullet}$, $HO^\bullet$, alkoxyl radicals ($RO^\bullet$), and sulfhydryl radicals ($S^\bullet$), have extremely short spin relaxation times, resulting in broad signals (line width), not allowing for proper characterization. Therefore, in order to detect the more reactive radicals in skin, it is necessary to employ a suitable spin trapping agent.[11]

A spin trapping agent reacts with a radical, by way of an addition reaction, to form a spin adduct, which is a much more stable (persistent) radical. In regard to the formed spin adduct, the spin trapping agent is referred to as the spin trap and the radical portion of the newly formed compound as the radical addend. The resulting spin adduct is a much more long-lived radical than the highly reactive species we wish to detect, thereby allowing detection of this radical (spin adduct) using conventional ESR techniques. Generally, nitrones and nitroso compounds are used as spin traps, which become nitroxides upon electron donation (oxidation) to the radical species.[1] Figure 7.7 provides several examples for the addition of a radical to a nitrone spin trap. Nitroxides are fairly stable, because the unpaired electron is resonance stabilized. N-*tert*-butyl alpha-nitrone (PBN) was one of the original spin traps that were used to detect carbon- and oxygen-centered radicals. Later, alpha-(4-pyridyl-1-oxide)-N-*tert*-butyl-nitrone (POBN) was developed as an analog to PBN, which had better trapping capabilities. The spin trap, 5,5-dimethyl-1-pyrroline-N-oxide (DMPO), which is the most universally used for biological samples, can trap carbon-, oxygen-, and sulfur-centered free radicals.[1] An example spectrum, demonstrating the use of the DMPO spin trap in skin is provided later in Figure 7.12.

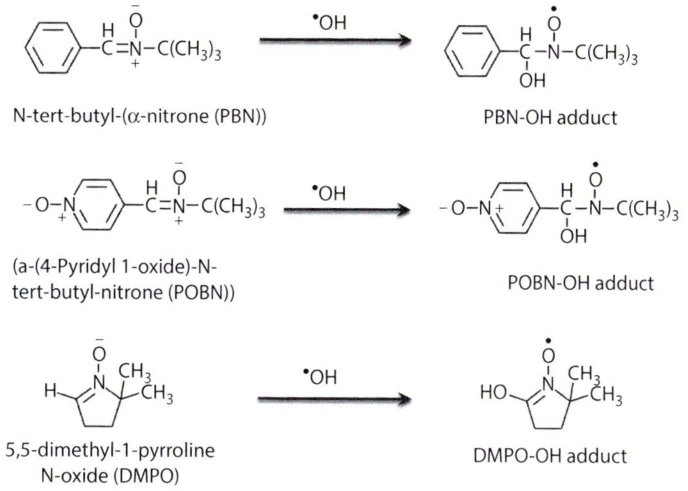

Figure 7.7 Spin trapping of radical species.

DETECTION OF FREE RADICALS IN SKIN BY ELECTRON SPIN RESONANCE

Many of the studies conducted on skin with ESR focus on gaining a better understanding of the mechanism of radical formation in skin, as well as other phenomena related to antioxidant mechanisms of defense.[9,12–14] Due to skin's inherent vulnerability to oxidative damage, the majority of studies deal with UV-induced production of radicals in skin.[15–23] Some analyses demonstrate the protective role (against UV damage) of treatment with antioxidants.[24–26] The concentration of endogenous ascorbate or a trapped free radical can be used as a probe of oxidative damage. Thus, lower concentrations of the monitored radical species will correspond to antioxidant protection. One may also follow free radical production in the presence of sunscreens and self-tanning agents.[27] This is of particular concern since some cosmetic products are believed to generate free radicals when subjected to UV exposure.[28,29] Further, certain cosmetics, such as essential oils, may have free radical scavenging activity, which may also be monitored by ESR.[30] In addition, many phenomena with melanin may be monitored by ESR, including elucidation of melanin's mechanistic role as a free radical scavenger and the formation of free radicals as a result of melanin synthesis.[31,32] From a slightly alternative perspective, Plonka et al. investigated hair growth with ESR.[33]

In addition, ESR studies can be used to divulge conformational information about lipid bilayers—that is, the order/disorder of the alkyl chains—by using special ESR probes. Several studies were conducted on stratum corneum membranes and isolated stratum corneum sheets/biopsies to discern stratum corneum lipid dynamics in skin.[34–36] Stratum corneum lipid conformation can also be monitored from tape-stripping experiments in conjunction with ESR after treatment with surfactants, such as sodium dodecyl sulfate (SDS).[37] In addition, considerable efforts have been expended to understand how/where antioxidants incorporate themselves into skin cell membranes[38] as well as to determine UV-induced damage to important biological molecules in skin.[39–42]

Due to ESR's potential for in vivo measurements, great efforts have been made to research the irritation potential of spin traps.[43–47] The use of anthralin for the treatment of psoriasis is also of great concern from a free radical perspective due to its activation by UV. Therefore, ESR is particularly suited to study the formation and activity of anthralin free radicals.[48,49]

Almost all ESR studies are carried out on a selection of substrates consisting of skin homogenates, biopsies, isolated stratum corneum, and stratum corneum membranes. While often the source of skin is typically of murine origin (normally the dorsal region), punch biopsies and glue-extracted stratum corneum may be obtained from live human volunteers. Further, in vivo testing is now also employed in ESR investigations, especially ESR imaging, which is discussed in the section *ESR Imaging of Skin* of this chapter.

THE USE OF ELECTRON SPIN RESONANCE TO MEASURE EXOGENOUS ANTIOXIDANT EFFICACY IN SKIN

One approach to monitoring the oxidative stress in skin with ESR is to measure the level of ascorbate free radical (Asc$^{\bullet-}$) present, which serves as an internal non-invasive probe. Ascorbic acid serves as terminal reductant in skin leaving its radical form behind, which implies that higher concentrations of Asc$^{\bullet-}$ will be found in samples that have undergone oxidative stress. Several studies have been published on this topic.[8,20,50] According to the findings from these studies, Asc$^{\bullet-}$ is detectable at room temperature and is found at low levels, which have been shown to increase upon UV-irradiation within the ESR chamber. A representative example of the Asc$^{\bullet-}$ spectrum is shown

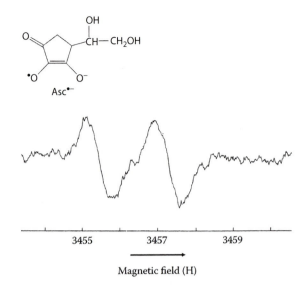

Figure 7.8 ESR spectrum of the ascorbate radical in skin. (Reprinted from *J. Invest. Dermatol.*, 104, Jurkiewicz, B.A. et al., Effect of topically applied tocopherol on ultraviolet radiation-mediated free radical damage in skin, 484–488, Copyright 1995, with permission from Elsevier.)

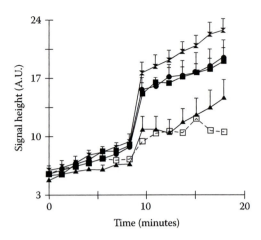

Figure 7.9 Asc$^{\cdot-}$ ESR signal height as a function of irradiation time for various samples. □, IPA vehicle treated-skin exposed to room light only; ■, IPA vehicle-treated skin; ●, tocopherol acetate-treated skin; ✶, alpha-tocopherol-treated skin, and ▲, tocopherol sorbate-treated skin. (Reprinted from *J. Invest. Dermatol.*, 104, Jurkiewicz, B.A. et al., Effect of topically applied tocopherol on ultraviolet radiation-mediated free radical damage in skin, 484–488, Copyright 1995, with permission from Elsevier.)

in Figure 7.8, in which case two relatively broad spectral lines are observed corresponding to the resonance-stabilized radical where a hyperfine splitting constant (a^{H4}) of 1.8 G was found. Also included in the figure is the structure of Asc$^{\cdot-}$ as proposed by Bors and Buettner.[51] To demonstrate the utility of the Asc$^{\cdot-}$ technique in measuring the efficacy of antioxidant treatments in skin, Jurkiewicz et al. monitored the Asc$^{\cdot-}$ level in untreated skin with skin that had been treated with various tocopherol derivatives following UV irradiation.[25] Their findings, shown in Figure 7.9, demonstrate that treatment with the tocopherols, especially tocopherol sorbate, decreased the amount of Asc$^{\cdot-}$ detected by ESR.

Other work, also completed by Jurkiewicz and Buettner, demonstrated the use of the POBN spin trap to detect a carbon-centered radical in skin upon exposure to UV irradiation.[20] The POBN-radical adduct ESR spectrum is provided in Figure 7.10, where the asterisks (*) identify the spectral components associated with spin trap adduct and the carats (^) denote the signal attributed to Asc$^{\cdot-}$. Such methodology may be used to demonstrate the deleterious effects of UV radiation as well as the free radical scavenging activity of an antioxidant. Figure 7.11 provides a plot of POBN signal intensity as a function of UV irradiation time. As expected, there is no increase for the non-irradiated sample during the course of the experiment. In contrast, subjecting the sample to UV irradiation results in a monotonic increase in the POBN-radical adduct signal as a function of time. Treatment with Desferal—an iron chelator, which prevents the formation of free radicals—reduces the intensity of the POBN-radical adduct signal, indicating that less radical is present in the antioxidant treated sample.

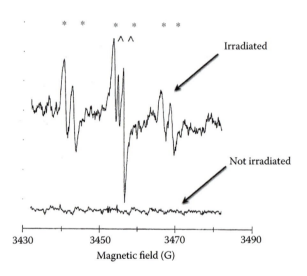

Figure 7.10 ESR spectrum of UV radiation-induced POBN radical adducts in skin. The asterisk (*) is used to designate the location of the POBN-radical adduct signal and the carat (^) the ascorbate radical signal. (From Jurkiewicz, B.A. and Buettner, G.R.: EPR detection of free radicals in UV-irradiated skin: Mouse versus human. *Photochemistry and Photobiology*. 1996. 64. 918–922. Copyright Wiley-VCH Verlag GmbH & Co. KGaA. Reproduced with permission.)

Another example is shown in Figure 7.12, which provides spectra of skin biopsies treated with the DMPO spin trap, resulting in the formation of DMPO-radical adducts. The biopsies in both spectra were exposed to UV radiation. In the lower spectrum, the signal intensity of the DMPO-radical adduct is greater than the upper spectrum. Such a

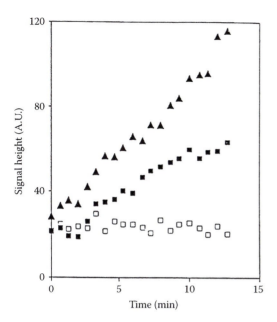

Figure 7.11 POBN-radical adduct signal in skin as a function of irradiation time. □, control-not irradiated; ■, irradiated and treated with Desferal; ▲, irradiated. (From Jurkiewicz, B.A. and Buettner, G.R.: Ultraviolet light-induced free radical formation in skin: an electron paramagnetic resonance study. *Photochemistry and Photobiology.* 1994. 59. 1–4. Copyright Wiley-VCH Verlag GmbH & Co. KGaA. Reproduced with permission.)

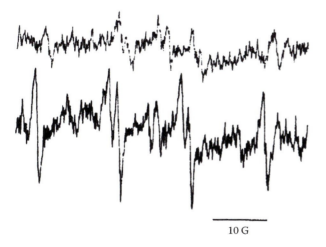

Figure 7.12 ESR spectra of human skin biopsies exposed to UV irradiation in situ utilizing the DMPO spin trap. Untreated skin (lower spectrum) reveals a more intense DMPO-radical adduct signal. The upper spectrum is of skin treated with Desferal, in which case the DMPO-radical adduct signal is less intense, indicating the presence of less free radicals. (From Jurkiewicz, B.A. and Buettner, G.R.: EPR detection of free radicals in UV-irradiated skin: Mouse versus human. *Photochemistry and Photobiology.* 1996. 64. 918–922. Copyright Wiley-VCH Verlag GmbH & Co. KGaA. Reproduced with permission.)

result is expected, since the lower spectrum is for the untreated skin sample (containing more radicals, hence greater spin trap-radical adduct signal) and the upper spectrum is for skin treated with Desferal, thus, resulting in fewer radicals and a lower intensity signal emitted from the sample.

In recent years, researchers have continued to carry out studies in which ESR was used to measure the efficacy of antioxidant treatments.[52–54] Typically, such studies are accomplished with ex vivo skin samples or in vitro cell culture systems. In addition to testing pure antioxidants, one may also measure the protective properties of sunscreen formulations.[55] One group of researchers even proposed the calculation of a radical skin protection factor and antioxidant power based on ex vivo ESR studies of skin treated with sunscreens containing antioxidants.[56]

ELECTRON SPIN RESONANCE IMAGING OF SKIN

ESR imaging (also referred to as EPR imaging) allows for measurement of the spatial distribution of radicals in skin samples. In the early 1990s, there was a lot of interest in this topic among dermatological researchers working with ESR technology. Early studies by Kristel et al. demonstrated the utility of ESR imaging to monitor the distribution of exogenous nitroxides and nitroxide-labeled drugs in skin biopsies.[57] Soon afterwards, a significant amount of work was completed by J. Fuchs et al. throughout the 1990s and into the twenty-first century, which brought ESR imaging of skin to its current state of development.[1,6,23,58–63]

Normal ESR measurements are usually conducted at X-band (9.5 GHz) frequency. To conduct ESR imaging experiments, one must carefully manipulate the frequency (for example, from X-band to S band [3.0 GHz]), magnetic field strength, and the field gradient.[64] X-band spectroscopy can be employed for ESR imaging of skin biopsies; however, low frequencies (S band or L band) are required for in vivo measurements. Data, in the form of images, can be collected as the spatial distribution of the radical (1D, 2D, or 3D images) or spectral-spatial images also as 1D, 2D, or 3D images.[64]

In skin, ESR imaging has primarily been used to monitor the redox state. For example, treatment with nitroxides allows us to monitor their depth of penetration and concentration. If the nitroxide concentration decreases, this indicates that more free radicals are present in this tissue. Figure 7.13 provides an example of a skin biopsy treated with the nitroxide, 3-carboxy-2,2,5,5-tetramethylpyrrolidine-1-oxyl (PCA). PCA is a persistent radical, detectable by ESR imaging, which will react with resident radicals. Therefore, its concentration will decrease in the presence of free radicals. In Figure 7.13a, the ESR image was collected after PCA was allowed to penetrate to the deep layers (>1.5 mm) of skin. There are three major bands corresponding to PCA and its distribution is equal throughout the depth (various layers) of skin. When the skin is exposed to UV light, the amount of PCA in the upper layers of skin is depleted (Figure 7.13b) due to the increased quantity of free radicals in this region. Thus, UV penetration is confined

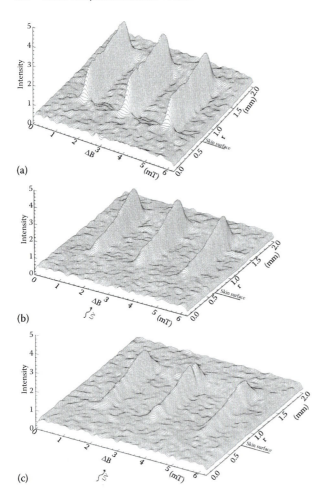

Figure 7.13 ESR spectral-spatial image utilizing PCA as a probe. In (a) PCA was allowed to penetrate for 5 minutes allowing for equal distribution throughout the skin. After UV irradiation for 5 minutes (b) PCA is depleted in the upper layers of skin. Further consumption in the uppermost portion of skin is observed after (c) 20 minutes of UV exposure. (Reprinted from *Free Rad. Biol. Med.*, 35, Herrling, T.E. et al., UV-induced free radicals in the skin detected by ESR spectroscopy and imaging using nitroxides, 59–67, Copyright 2003, with permission from Elsevier.)

to the epidermis. After further UV exposure (20 minutes), the amount of PCA in the epidermis decreases even more (Figure 7.13c).

Another notable application of ESR imaging to skin is the penetration of nitroxide-labeled drugs, such as retinoic acid or dihydrolipoate.[59,65] From these studies, it can be clearly distinguished which molecules are able to mitigate barrier function of skin. ESR imaging is also used frequently in drug delivery research.[66,67] It has even been reported as a metric device for characterizing the various stages of melanoma.[68]

CONCLUDING REMARKS

Over the last three decades, a great deal of research has been conducted that used ESR to investigate phenomena in skin. Such circumstances owe to the importance of free radicals in skin—especially UV-induced radicals—and their management by endogenous antioxidants or exogenous treatments such as sunscreens or antioxidants. Unlike any other technique, ESR offers us many possibilities to understand free radical mechanisms and behavior in skin. For further reading on the topic of ESR and skin, the reader is referred to an excellent book chapter written by Fuchs et al.[1] and several reviews that have appeared in the literature.[69,70] For general reading, the classics can still be found in used book stores[71–73] as well as some of the more easily available, up-to-date treatises on the subject.[7,74,75]

REFERENCES

1. Fuchs J et al. Detection of free radicals in skin: A review of the literature and new developments. In: Thiele J, Elsner P (Eds.). *Oxidants and Antioxidants in Cutaneous Biology, 29*. Basel, Switzerland: Karger; 2001, pp. 1–17.
2. Barrow GM. *Physical Chemistry*, 6th ed. New York: McGraw-Hill College; 1996.
3. Fessenden RW, Schuler RH. *J Chem Phys*. 1963;39:2147–2195.
4. Lowry TH, Richardson KS. *Mechanism and Theory in Organic Chemistry*. New York: Harper & Row; 1987.
5. Borg DC. Applications of electron spin resonance in biology. In: Pryor WA (Ed.). *Free Radicals in Biology, 1*. New York: Academic Press; 1976.
6. Fuchs J et al. *J Invest Dermatol*. 1992;98:713–719.
7. Weil JA, Bolton JR. *Electron Paramagnetic Resonance*, 2nd ed. Hoboken, NJ: John Wiley & Sons; 2007.
8. Buettner GR, Jurkiewicz BA. *Free Rad Biol Med*. 1993;14:49–55.
9. Herrling T et al. *Spectrochim Acta Part A*. 2008;69:1429–1435.
10. Herrling T et al. *SÖFW*. 2007;133(9):26–32.
11. Buettner GR. *Free Rad Biol Med*. 1987;3:259–303.
12. Guo Q, Packer L. *Red Rep*. 1999;4:105–111.
13. Fuchs J et al. *Meth Enzymol*. 1990;186:670–674.
14. Fuchs J et al. *J Invest Dermatol*. 1989;93:633–640.
15. Kagan V et al. *Free Rad Res Commun*. 1992;16:51–64.
16. Nishi J et al. *J Invest Dermatol*. 1991;97:115–119.
17. Herrling T et al. *Spectrochim Acta Part A*. 2006;63:840–845.
18. Takeshita K et al. *Free Rad Biol Med*. 2006;40:876–885.
19. Takeshita K et al. *J Invest Dermatol*. 2004;122:1463–1470.
20. Jurkiewicz BA, Buettner GR. *Photochem Photobiol*. 1996;64:918–922.
21. Ogura R et al. *J Invest Dermatol*. 1991;97:1044–1047.
22. Moll K-P et al. *Chem Med Chem*. 2008;3:653–659.
23. Herrling TE et al. *Free Rad Biol Med*. 2003;35:59–67.
24. Kobayashi S et al. *Photochem Photobiol*. 1998;67:669–675.
25. Jurkiewicz BA et al. *J Invest Dermatol*. 1995;104:484–488.
26. Kitazawa M et al. *Photochem Photobiol*. 1997;65:355–365.

27. Jung K et al. *Spectrochim Acta Part A.* 2008;69: 1423–1428.
28. Xia Q et al. *Toxicol Lett.* 2007;168:165–175.
29. Murrary AR et al. *Chem Res Toxic.* 2007;20:1769–1777.
30. Ao Y et al. *J Clin Biochem Nutr.* 2008;43:6–12.
31. Tada M et al. *J Clin Biochem Nutr.* 2010;46:224–228.
32. Tada M et al. *J Clin Biochem Nutr.* 2010;47:162–166.
33. Plonka PM et al. *J Dermatol Sci.* 2008;49:227–240.
34. Nakagawa K et al. *Spectrochim Acta Part A.* 2006;63:816–820.
35. Alonso A et al. *Chem Phys Lipids.* 2000;104:101–111.
36. Nakagawa K. *Lipids.* 2010;45:91–96.
37. Yagi E et al. *J Cosmet Sci.* 2010;61:39–48.
38. Pawlikowska-Pawlęga B et al. *Biochim Biophys Acta.* 2012;1818:1785–1793.
39. Metreveli N et al. *J Photochem Photobiol B Biol.* 2008;93:61–65.
40. Jiang S et al. *Free Rad Biol Med.* 2010;48:1144–1151.
41. Haywood R et al. *Free Rad Biol Med.* 2008;44: 990–1000.
42. Haywood R et al. *Photochem Photobiol.* 2011;87: 117–130.
43. Fuchs J et al. *Toxicology.* 2000;151:55–63.
44. Kitagawa S, Ikarashi A. *Chem Pharm Bull.* 2001;49: 165–168.
45. Fuchs J et al. *Free Rad Biol Med.* 1997;22:967–976.
46. Fuchs J et al. *Toxicology.* 1998;126:33–40.
47. Fuchs J et al. *Free Rad Biol Med.* 1998;24:643–648.
48. Fuchs J, Packer L. *J Invest Dermatol.* 1989;92:677–682.
49. Mäder K et al. *J Invest Dermatol.* 1995;104:514–517.
50. Jurkiewicz BA, Buettner GR. *Photochem Photobiol.* 1994;59:1–4.
51. Bors W, Buettner GR. The vitamin C radical and its reactions. In: Packer L, Fuchs J (Eds.). *Vitamin C in Health and Disease.* New York: Marcel Dekker; 1997.
52. Kawai S et al. *Free Rad Res.* 2010;44:267–274.
53. Meinke M et al. *Eur J Pharm Biopharm.* 2012;81: 346–350.
54. Piao M et al. *Int J Mol Sci.* 2011;12:8146–8160.
55. Haywood R et al. *Free Rad Res.* 2012;46:265–275.
56. Wang S et al. *J Am Acad Dermatol.* 2011;65:525–530.
57. Kristel J et al. *Drug Dev Ind Pharm.* 1989;15:1423–1440.
58. Fuchs J et al. *Free Rad Res Commun.* 1991;15:245–253.
59. Freisleben H-J et al. *Arzneim-Forsch/Drug Res.* 1994;44: 1047–1050.
60. Herrling TE et al. *Appl Magn Reson.* 1996;11: 471–486.
61. He G et al. *J Magn Reson.* 2001;148:155–164.
62. Herrling T et al. *J Magn Reson.* 2002;154:6–14.
63. He G et al. *Free Rad Biol Med.* 2004;36:665–672.
64. Fuchs J et al. *Meth Enzymol.* 1994;233:140–149.
65. Michel C et al. *Int J Pharm.* 1993;98:131–139.
66. Kempe S et al. *Eur J Pharm Biopharm.* 2010;74:55–66.
67. Gabrijelčič V et al. *Int J Pharm.* 1990;62:75–79.
68. Godechal Q et al. *Exp Dermatol.* 2012;21:341–346.
69. Plonka PM. *Exp Dermatol.* 2009;18:472–484.
70. Hochkirch U et al. *Spectroscopy.* 2006;20:1–17.
71. Ingram DJE. *Free Radicals as Studied by Electron Spin Resonance.* London, UK: Butterworths Scientific; 1958.
72. Alger RS. *Electron Paramagnetic Resonance.* New York: Wiley Interscience; 1968.
73. Atherton NM. *Principles of Electron Spin Resonance.* New York: Ellis Horwood; 1993.
74. Rieger P. *Electron Spin Resonance: Analysis and Interpretation.* Cambridge, UK: Royal Society of Chemistry; 2007.
75. Lund A et al. *Principles and Applications of Electron Spin Resonance.* Dordrecht, Netherlands: Springer; 2008.

Treatment of skin with antioxidants

> By controlling free radicals, antioxidants can make the difference between life and death, as well as influence how fast and how well we age.
>
> —Lester Packer and Carol Coleman
> *The Antioxidant Miracle*

Awareness of the beneficial effects of antioxidants has evolved from a growing body of research, which has demonstrated that many diseases are, in part, a result of free radical damage. For example, cardiovascular disease and cancer have definitively been linked with the deleterious actions of free radicals. In fact, one of the theories of aging purports that free radicals are primarily responsible for the degenerative processes that our body suffers over a lifetime.[1] Free radicals are, in effect, a normal part of the body's metabolic processes and pose significant danger when our own antioxidant defense system becomes overwhelmed by an abundance of these radicals. Through their harmful action, free radicals damage lipids, proteins, and DNA. Free radicals have both internal and external origins, the latter constituting UV light, ozone, and air pollution, among others, all of which can potentially cause damage to the skin. In addition to photoaging, UV irradiation is also responsible for squamous and basal cell carcinomas and immune suppression.

The use of antioxidants in various skin treatments is a concrete approach to improve the overall health state of skin. This statement is supported by a wealth of research conducted over the last several decades toward better understanding how antioxidants mitigate the effects of solar radiation. Topical application of antioxidant-containing products reduces the deleterious effects of UV radiation, which lead to photoaging, photoimmunosuppression, and photocarcinogenesis. While some antioxidants may offer some photoprotection as a solar filter, the majority of their mechanisms are through their antioxidant capacity or immunomodulating effects. This chapter will review some of the most common antioxidants used in skin care formulations, starting with the most fundamental species: vitamin E, vitamin C, and coenzyme Q. Historically, these were probably the most studied antioxidants due to their importance in the endogenous antioxidant system (Chapter 3). Equally important are a vast majority of botanical extracts, which contain many phytoantioxidants. In recent years, research has focused on understanding the antioxidant behavior of polyphenols in an attempt to harness their protective properties for skin. In some cases, specific polyphenols are used in formulation, while in others the extract is directly added. With further regard to the utilization of antioxidants to treat skin, other important factors to consider are differences between oral supplementation and topical treatment and delivery of antioxidants to targeted tissue.

Recent advances in carrier technologies, such as emulsions, lipid vesicles, and solid lipid particles, now allow for the efficient delivery of antioxidants, oftentimes increasing permeation efficacy and decreasing irritation. Finally, it should be noted that antioxidants represent an important component of most commercial sunscreen formulations, offering protection against the formation of free radicals that cannot be achieved with UV filters alone.

VITAMIN E

Vitamin E, commonly obtained through diet, is an essential ingredient, and also an important lipid-soluble antioxidant that protects against lipid peroxidation in plasma and tissues, notably skin. There are eight isomeric forms of vitamin E (Chapter 9) that are classified into two groups, tocopherols and tocotrienols, which differ in their hydrophobic moieties. The most prevalent forms in skin are alpha-tocopherol (RRR-alpha-tocopherol) (~90%) and gamma-tocopherol (~10%).[2] The long phytyl chain of vitamin E allows this antioxidant to embed itself in membranes, leaving the chromanol ring, which contains the free radical neutralizing hydroxyl group, at the lipid-aqueous interface. In nature, vitamin E is found in many foods and plant oils where it confers protection against oxidative damage (Figure 8.1). Endogenous alpha-tocopherol

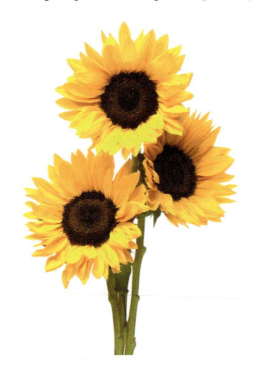

Figure 8.1 Sunflower seeds are one of the best whole food sources of vitamin E. It is also found in many other food sources including almonds, peanuts, green vegetables, pine nuts, and olives.

is found in the various skin layers, and notably, a role for it has been elucidated from studies that proved sebum escorts alpha-tocopherol to the skin's surface to provide protection at the interface of the body and the environment (for further discussion, Chapter 1).

Due to its important role in skin health and well-being, there is a great deal of interest in the personal care industry to fortify skin with alpha-tocopherol. Unfortunately, there are formulating/stability issues that sometimes hamper the successful delivery of biologically active alpha-tocopherol to skin. For this reason, various esterified forms of the antioxidant have become available in the specialty chemicals market, which provide formulators with a longer shelf life of their finished product. Esterification is normally carried out at the hydroxyl group position on the chromanol ring (see, e.g., tocopheryl acetate and tocopheryl phosphate in Figure 8.2). This has the unfortunate disadvantage of rendering the antioxidant inactive, since it is unable to donate a proton from the hydroxyl group. However, studies have shown that once the synthetic form of the antioxidant is delivered to skin during penetration, particularly in the case of tocopheryl acetate, hydrolysis of the acetate group returns the antioxidant to its bioactive form, able to exert its antioxidant action.[3-10] However, bear in mind that the conversion of vitamin E acetate to vitamin E in skin is still a very controversial subject.[11] Table 8.1 contains a list of other tocopherol derivatives that are utilized in cosmetic preparations; by no means exhaustive, this list provides a general scope of the modified forms of tocopherol available. The Personal Care Products Council website (www.personalcarecouncil.org) provides a more thorough listing.

A considerable amount of evidence suggests an integral role for topically applied vitamin E in the protection of skin from lipid peroxidation, photoaging, and UV-induced immunosuppression (Table 8.2 bears a list of example studies).[12-16] While protection against lipid peroxidation seems fairly obvious—by impeding free radical propagation—the mechanism by which photoimmunosuppression and photoaging are prevented is less clear.[17]

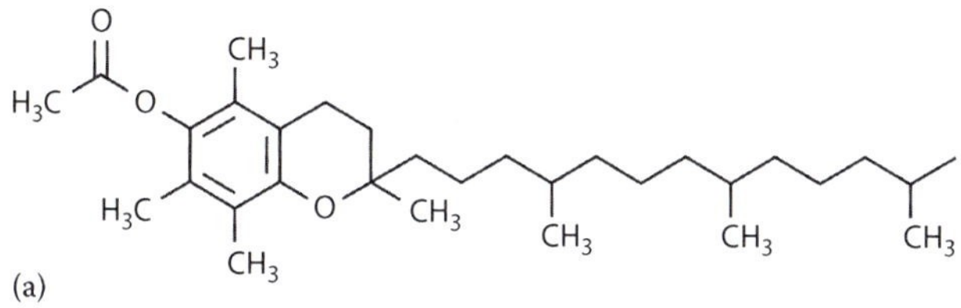

Table 8.1 Commercially available tocopherol derivatives.

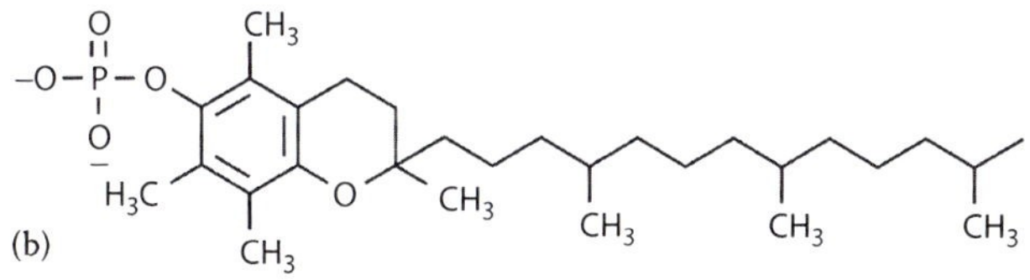

Tocopheryl acetate
Tocopheryl dimethylglycinate
Tocopheryl ethyl succinate ethyldimonium ethosulfate
Tocopheryl ferulate
Tocopheryl glucoside
Tocopheryl linoleate/oleate
Tocopheryl nicotinate
Tocopheryloxypropyl trisiloxane
Tocopheryl phosphate
Tocopheryl phosphocholine
Tocopheryl retinoate
Tocopheryl succinate
Tocopheryl succinate methylglucamide
Tocopheryl tranexamate HCl

The protective effect of vitamin E against photoaging could, in part, be due to its inhibition of matrixmetalloproteinase (MMP) expression—an enzyme responsible for the breakdown of collagen.[18] Studies have even demonstrated a protective role of vitamin E in photocarcinogenesis.[19-22] Mechanistically, vitamin E protects DNA against UV-induced cyclobutane pyrimidine dimers.[23,24] Further, numerous studies have demonstrated its potential to reduce UV-induced erythema and edema.[25-29] It is important to note that the isomeric form of vitamin E chosen for an application plays an important role in its efficacy against UV-induced damage.[30,31]

As already noted, there has been considerable interest in understanding possible conversions of vitamin E when it is administered in vivo. In mammalian tissues, vitamin E is known to lose its potency as an antioxidant in vivo as compared to its properties in cell culture. One reasonable explanation for such a phenomenon could stem from the conversion of alpha-tocopherol to alpha-tocopheryl phosphate, which occurs due to the activity of a tocopherol kinase and, possibly, other enzymes. While losing antioxidant potency, one has to recognize the positive attributes of alpha-tocopheryl phosphate, which is believed to play an important role in cell signaling. While alpha-tocopherol has some activity related to the modulation of cell proliferation, alpha-tocopheryl phosphate was shown to inhibit cell growth of THP-1 monocytes—a cell culture line derived from cells of leukemia patients. In terms of gene expression, alpha-tocopheryl phosphate was shown to be much more potent than alpha-tocopherol.[32]

For all its benefits, vitamin E has some inherent problems with topical treatment, resulting in contact dermatitis in some individuals.[33,34] In some cases, such findings may have originated from the overuse of vitamin E to prevent scar formation as a result of injury. Perhaps the diminishment of scars by vitamin E is an urban legend or merely anecdotal evidence. Regardless, it is still an active area of debate in the literature.[35-37] It is also suggested that vitamin E by itself can

Figure 8.2 Molecular structure of (a) tocopheryl acetate and (b) tocopheryl phosphate. For comparison to the structure of alpha-tocopherol and other vitamin E isomers, see Chapters 3 and 9.

Table 8.2 Summary of studies demonstrating in vivo photoprotection due to topical treatment with vitamin E and its derivatives.

Compound(s)	Species	Endpoint(s)	Efficacy	Year	Reference
Vitamin E and derivatives	Rabbit	Erythema (MED)	Vitamin E protective; Vitamin E acetate not protective	1979	324
Vitamin E and derivatives	Human, rabbit	PUVA-induced erythema and changes in mechanoelectrical properties of skin	Vitamin E and derivatives with short chain protective; vitamin E acetate not protective	1984	26
Vitamin E	Mouse	Lipid peroxidation	Protective	1988	325
Vitamin E acetate	Mouse	Lipid peroxidation and DNA synthesis	Protective	1991	28
Vitamin E acetate	Mouse	Erythema, edema, and skin sensitivity	Protective	1992	29
Vitamin E and derivatives	Human	Erythema (skin color)	Moderate protection of vitamin E and vitamin E acetate when applied occlusively after UVR exposure	1995	326
Vitamin E acetate	Mouse	Skin tumor incidence and immunosuppression	No protection	1996	31
Vitamin E	Mouse	Lipid peroxidation	Protective	1998	13
Vitamin E	Mouse	Erythema, pigmentation, skin tumor incidence	Protection after prolonged application	2000	25

Source: Thiele, J. and Dreher, F., Antioxidant defense systems in skin, In: Elsner, P. and Maibach, H., (Eds.), *Cosmeceuticals and Active Cosmetics: Drugs Versus Cosmetics*, Taylor & Francis Group, Boca Raton, FL, pp. 37–87, 2005.

act as a pro-oxidant.[2] In any event, formulation parameters ultimately govern the efficacy and delivery of the antioxidant.[38] Oftentimes, several different antioxidants are formulated together. To this end, much effort has been put forth to understand the behavior of combinations of various antioxidants and any possible synergies that may exist, especially with respect to vitamins E and C.

VITAMIN C

Ascorbic acid, or vitamin C, is the major water-soluble antioxidant in skin and most other body tissues. It is likewise found in a variety of fruits and vegetables (Figure 8.3) and is often obtained via diet or through vitamin supplements. Vitamin C is integral in managing the free radical levels in the aqueous and interfacial zones of skin. It is also key to vitamin E activity, as it recycles the oxidized form of alpha-tocopherol back to its active form (Chapter 3). In addition, vitamin C is a cofactor important for the synthesis of collagen and maintenance of sustainable MMP levels.[12,39,40] It specifically acts as a cofactor for prolyl hydroxylase and lysyl hydroxylase in the synthesis of collagen (Chapter 3). A lack of dietary vitamin C results in the degenerative disease scurvy, which was especially prevalent among European sailors between the sixteenth and nineteenth centuries.[41] In recent years, ascorbic acid derivatives have been used as skin whitening agents, whereby they act as inhibitors of tyrosinase activity, thereby impeding melanin synthesis.[42]

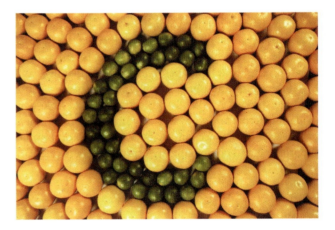

Figure 8.3 Citrus fruits, such as oranges, tangerines, grapefruits, and limes, are most commonly associated as a good vitamin C source. It is also found in other fruits and vegetables, such as strawberries, broccoli, potatoes, cantaloupe, and tomatoes.

Unlike vitamin E, which has an absorption profile in the UVB range, vitamin C does not act as a solar filter. Its mechanism of protective action against photo-induced processes is primarily antioxidative in nature.[11] Topical application of vitamin C prevents UV-induced photoimmunosuppression, photoaging, and

Table 8.3 Summary of studies demonstrating in vivo photoprotection due to topical treatment with vitamin C and its derivatives.

Compound(s)	Species	Endpoint(s)	Efficacy	Year	Reference
Vitamin C	Mouse	Skin wrinkling, skin tumor incidence, and histology	Protective	1992	327
Vitamin C palmitate	Human	Erythema (skin color)	Poor protection when applied occlusively after UVR protection	1995	326
Vitamin C	Yorkshire pig	Sunburn cell formation	No protection against UVR-induced damage; protective against PUVA-induced damage	1996	328
Vitamin C	Human	Erythema (skin color and blood flow)	Poor protection	1998	329

Source: Thiele, J. and Dreher, F., Antioxidant defense systems in skin, In: Elsner, P. and Maibach, H., (Eds.), *Cosmeceuticals and Active Cosmetics: Drugs Versus Cosmetics*, Taylor & Francis Group, Boca Raton, FL, pp. 37–87, 2005.

erythema.[43–46] It also acts as an anti-inflammatory agent, evidenced by its mitigating action resulting in a decrease in erythema, even when it is applied after sunburn.[11] In terms of photoaging, the tyrosinase inhibitory activity of vitamin C prevents the formation of solar lentigines, while its stimulation of collagen synthesis and inhibition of elastin synthesis prevents solar elastosis.[11,47] Table 8.3 summarizes several studies seeking to determine the efficacy of topically applied vitamin C. In comparison to vitamin E, far fewer studies of vitamin C have been conducted on skin or shown such promising results.

Despite all of its positive benefits, ascorbic acid tends to burden formulators with inherent problems due notably to its instability. The stability of ascorbic acid is pH and temperature dependent, with more acidic, lower temperature mediums providing greater stability.[48] Ascorbic acid stability is also affected by the type of vehicle employed. For example, ascorbic acid is more stable in emulsified systems than aqueous solutions, and this stability increases with the complexity of the emulsion (e.g., water-in-oil versus water-in-oil-in-water).[49] In light of its formulation issues, many ascorbic acid derivatives are available for use in skin care preparations, which increase long-term stability. The most popular of these are magnesium ascorbyl phosphate and ascorbyl-6-palmitate; however, a host of others are available. Figure 8.4 contains structures for several commercial examples of ascorbic acid derivatives. Unlike the case of the vitamin E analogues, most derivatives of ascorbic acid are not metabolized in the skin and thus should be expected to have less or no antioxidant activity if substituent groups are placed where the antioxidant active hydroxyl groups were present in the original ascorbic acid molecule (Figure 3.12 in Chapter 3).[11,46]

Overall, ascorbic acid can mitigate via delivery a variety of skin health issues resulting from exposure to UV light. In most efficacy studies, the effective concentration levels

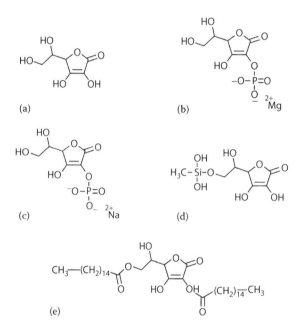

Figure 8.4 Molecular structure of (a) ascorbic acid and several commercially available derivatives including (b) magnesium ascorbyl phosphate, (c) sodium ascorbyl phosphate, (d) methylsilanol ascorbate, and (e) ascorbyl dipalmitate.

of ascorbic acid typically range from 5%–15%.[11] Lower pH levels (~3.5) eliminate the ionic charge of ascorbic acid and allow it to be optimally delivered to the skin.[46] At any rate, numerous studies have demonstrated the efficacy of topically applied ascorbic acid in protecting skin against UV radiation and its resulting implications, including photo-immunosuppression, erythema, pigment darkening, and photoaging. Further, it has proven clinical efficacy in the prevention and reversal of photoaging.[11]

VITAMIN A

Vitamin A is a group of lipid-soluble compounds that includes retinol, retinal, retinoic acid, and retinyl esters, known collectively as retinoids (Figure 8.5). This group affects a number of physiological functions including vision, immune function, and reproduction.[50] Retinoids are obtained via diet and usually from dairy products, liver, and some fish oils. In addition to the retinoids, several carotenoids are also commonly categorized within the vitamin A group, most notably beta-carotene and beta-cryptoxanthin. These carotenoids are obtained by consuming fresh fruits and vegetables; beta-carotene is notably sourced from sweet potatoes and carrots, as well as green leafy vegetables. Carotenoids within the vitamin A group are metabolized in the body to form retinoids. Curiously, not all carotenes (e.g., lycopene and lutein) fall within the vitamin A class, since they do not undergo the same conversion reactions to retinoids and, therefore, do not participate in retinoid physiological functions such as sight.

Retinoids are commonly used to treat acne vulgaris or photodamaged skin. Topical treatment is normally achieved with retinol, retinal, or retinyl esters (e.g., retinyl palmitate).[51] By enzymatic activity, these molecules are converted in skin to the active form, *trans*-retinoic acid. Most of present knowledge of the mechanism and function of *trans*-retinoic acid in skin deals with the epidermis.[52] It binds to retinoic acid and retinoid X receptors, triggering a series of biochemical events and ultimately stimulating keratinocyte proliferation and increasing the thickness of the epidermal layer. In addition, retinoids affect the dermis by such action on fibroblasts as the down regulation of collagenase, an enzyme that breaks down peptide bonds in collagen, which would ultimately lead to damaged structural collagen fibrils in the dermis and alteration of skin mechanical properties and visual aesthetics.[53]

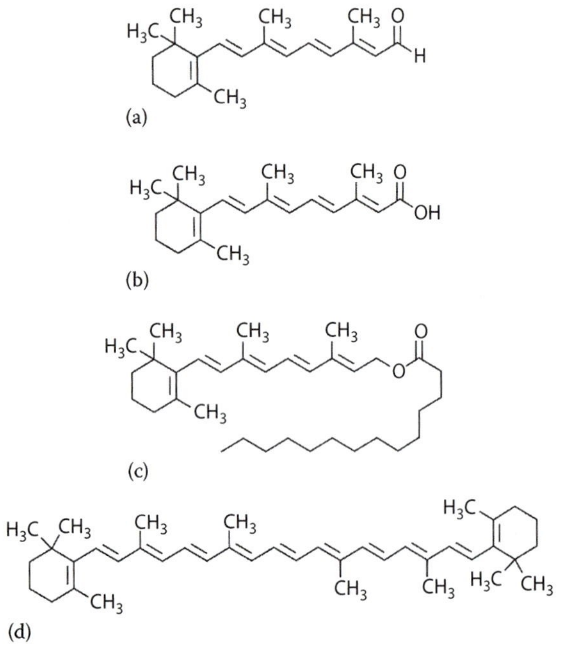

Retinyl derivatives do not act as antioxidants in skin; however, carotenoids that fall into the retinoid class are antioxidants inasmuch as they act as quenchers of singlet oxygen ($^1O_2$). Appreciable levels of beta-carotene and lycopene are found in skin, although, as already stated, lycopene is not a retinoid. Carotenoids in skin are depleted by solar radiation; therefore, it would seem reasonable that topical treatment with beta-carotene should supplement the antioxidant network. Studies have shown, however, that topical treatment with beta-carotene is less effective than dietary supplements in fortifying skin.[54] Topical treatments are probably not as robust in this case, since they can be easily shed with desquamating skin or physically removed by interaction of skin with fabric (from clothing) or other objects. Interestingly, it was shown that topically applied beta-carotene does protect skin from infrared-induced free radicals. Again, it should be emphasized that topically applied beta-carotene in skin is less stable than that obtained from the diet or applied creams containing a complex mixture of antioxidants.[55] In fact, most studies investigating the protective effects of beta-carotene against UV radiation administer dietary supplementation as a means of antioxidant delivery to the skin. Indeed, dietary beta-carotene does incorporate itself in skin. At high enough doses, skin develops a yellow coloration (known as hypercarotenodermia), which is particularly noticeable in the palms of the hands and soles of the feet. Over the last several decades, a significant amount of research was completed to investigate the possible role of beta-carotene in protection of skin against UV-induced ailments.[56-62] Regarding UV-induced erythema, there are conflicting results in the literature; in some cases, beta-carotene was found to reduce erythema,[56,61] while in others it was found to have minimal impact.[57,58] Similar conflicting evidence exists for investigations of a possible role of beta-carotene in reducing UV-induced immunosuppression,[59,60] although differences may be attributed to the use of humans in some studies versus animals in others. Early studies of animal models indicate a protective effect of beta-carotene in the prevention of UV-induced and carcinogen-induced skin tumors.[63] Unfortunately, ensuing studies on humans failed to show any beneficial effects of beta-carotene supplementation on nonmelanoma skin cancer prevention.[64,65] In part, conflicting findings between humans and animal models might be explained by anatomical differences, especially those that exist in fatty tissue where beta-carotene is stored.

Beta-carotene is often used to treat a number of dermatological disorders. It is frequently prescribed as a prescription drug for erythropoetic protoporphyria—a photosensitivity disease of the skin. Moreover, it is utilized for many diseases either caused by UV light or where heightened sensitivity to UV light is developed, such as solar urticaria, polymorphic light eruptions, hydroa vacciniforme, lupus erythematosus, and photoallergic drug reactions.[66] In one study, topically applied beta-carotene was effective in treating patients with

Figure 8.5 Molecular structure of (a) retinal, (b) retinoic acid, (c) retinyl palmitate, and (d) beta-carotene.

melasma—a pigmentary disorder resulting in patches of brown discoloration in skin.[67] In addition to its medical uses, beta-carotene has also found its way into many sunscreen formulations as a secondary sun protectant—often leaving skin with a desirable golden brown tone. By itself, however, beta-carotene does not provide sufficient SPF to protect skin from solar radiation.[66] It should also be pointed out that beta-carotene increases cancer incidence in individuals who are susceptible to lung cancer.[68-71] The mechanism of this phenomenon is not yet known; evidently, however, beta-carotene might act as a pro-oxidant. While the carotenoids that fall under the retinoid class of molecules offer hope of antioxidant intervention of free radical processes in skin, retinyl derivatives do not act as de facto antioxidants in skin. They may provide other benefits in the treatment of skin damaged by free radical activity.

SELENIUM

Selenium is a trace element that plays a pivotal role in several metabolic pathways, antioxidation, and immune system function. It is found in soil and is commonly introduced to the human body via plant stuffs in the diet. Most of the selenium in our diet comes from bread, cereal, meat, and poultry.[72] In proteins, selenium exists in the selenocysteine form that serves as the active site for many biochemical reactions (Figure 8.6). The most important selenoproteins, in terms of antioxidants, are glutathione peroxidase and thioredoxin reductase (both discussed in Chapter 3). As an enzyme cofactor in the antioxidant glutathione peroxidase, selenocysteine is instrumental in the breakdown of H_2O_2 and fatty acid hydroperoxides. Similarly, thioredoxin reductase (another antioxidant enzyme) decomposes lipid hydroperoxides with the help of a selenocysteine active site, in addition to the regeneration of several important antioxidants, such as ascorbic acid and lipoic acid.

Selenium generated considerable interest in the medical community when it was discovered that patients with higher serum levels of selenium demonstrated a reduced risk for developing certain types of cancer.[73] As early as the 1980s, epidemiological studies found a similar correlation between blood plasma levels of selenium and skin cancer incidence.[74] Moreover, subjects living in selenium-rich areas were found to be less likely to develop many other types of cancer.[75] Unfortunately, a large-scale, long-term study failed to show the same trend with regard to nonmelanoma skin cancers, although overall lower cancer rates in the group of patients who orally administered selenium were observed.[11,76,77] However, it is important to note that these patients had a history of squamous or basal cell carcinoma, which is certainly a much different situation than patients with no previous history of skin carcinomas. Despite the implications of this study, there is still much interest in utilizing selenium for topical treatment of skin.

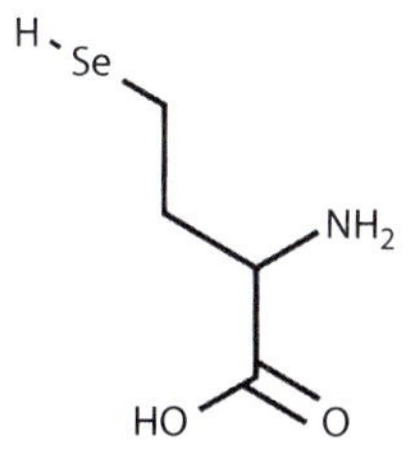

Topical L-selenomethionine was shown to increase minimal erythemal dose, thereby conferring greater UV-resistance to skin.[78] In a study of UV-induced pigmentation in a mouse model, L-selenomethionine, administered orally and topically, reduced pigmentary effects.[79] Initially, topical treatment was less efficacious than oral supplementation; however, after an extended period of treatment (16 weeks) both oral administration and topical treatment resulted in equal inhibition of UV-induced pigmentation. In the same study, investigators also monitored the development of UV-induced skin cancer in the mice over a 50-week period.

After 16 weeks, topical treatment and oral administration of L-selenomethionine led to the development of fewer tumors than the placebo. This trend continued; however, after 36 weeks and until the end of the study (week 50), topical treatment with L-selenomethionine was more efficacious than oral supplementation.

Typically, selenium is available for topical delivery in the form of selenium sulfide (SeS_2 or Se_2S_6) and L-selenomethionine.[12] In personal care products, selenium sulfide is mostly used in shampoos to treat seborrheic dermatitis or dandruff.[80,81] While selenium sulfide does not penetrate skin, topical administration of L-selenomethionine leads to effective incorporation into the skin's structure.[82]

UBIQUINONE DERIVATIVES

As discussed in Chapter 3, coenzyme Q (coQ), or ubiquinone-10, is a lipid-soluble antioxidant that protects membrane lipids from lipid peroxidation and is usually located in the mitochondrion where it plays a major role in aerobic cellular respiration (bioenergetics of oxidative phosphorylation), resulting in the generation of adenosine triphosphate, a key energy source. From a redox standpoint, coQ is a special case as it has three oxidation-reduction states: fully reduced, radical semiquinone, and fully oxidized (refer back to Figure 3.18 in Chapter 3). Such redox properties allow coQ to carry out its dual role as an electron transfer agent in the inner mitochondrial membrane and as an antioxidant. It is instrumental in recycling oxidized alpha-tocopherol back to its reduced, active antioxidant form; however, it can also behave as a pro-oxidant inasmuch that the radical semiquinone forms hydrogen peroxide and superoxide anion ($O_2^{\bullet-}$).[83]

In skin, mitochondrial function is directly linked to the aging process of the cell. As part of the mitochondrial electron transport chain, the proper functioning of coQ

Figure 8.6 Molecular structure of L-selenocysteine.

is imperative for healthy skin cells. As part of the aging process, skin cells undergo a decline in mitochondrial function, as was clearly shown in a study of skin biopsies indicating there are age-dependent differences in the mitochondrial function of keratinocytes.[84]

Coenzyme Q is increasingly found in personal care products where it is typically used as an antiaging or anti-wrinkling active ingredient.[83] Molecular biology studies on fibroblast cell culture systems demonstrated that coQ inhibits the UV-induced upregulation of MMPs, melanin synthesis, and production of inflammatory cytokines.[85–88] In addition to its influence on key transcription factors and the upregulation of matrix proteins, coQ is believed to influence skin aging by antioxidant mechanisms, which have yet to be elucidated.[89] Indeed, the penetration of coQ into the viable layers of the epidermis of porcine skin was shown by a technique known as weak photon emission.[90] Moreover, there are even clinical in vivo results available that purport to reduce wrinkles upon coQ treatment (after about 5 months), although these were evaluations by a dermatologist and not objective data.[88] Fortunately, other researchers investigated the clinical implications of topical coQ treatment on skin and also found a reduction in wrinkle depth.[90]

In addition to the use of coQ in cosmetic formulations, a number of quinone analogues are available to skin care formulators. Figure 8.7 contains some representative structures of molecules offered by specialty chemical manufacturers. One should bear in mind, however, that not all coQ derivatives will behave similarly in cell culture or in vivo. Despite the successes of coQ, some of its analogue forms, especially molecules with a shorter hydrophobic tail (fewer isoprene units), were found not to be efficacious in terms of supplementing lost coQ in the mitochondrial electron transport chain and preventing cellular oxidation.[91] With some structural similarities, hydroquinone,

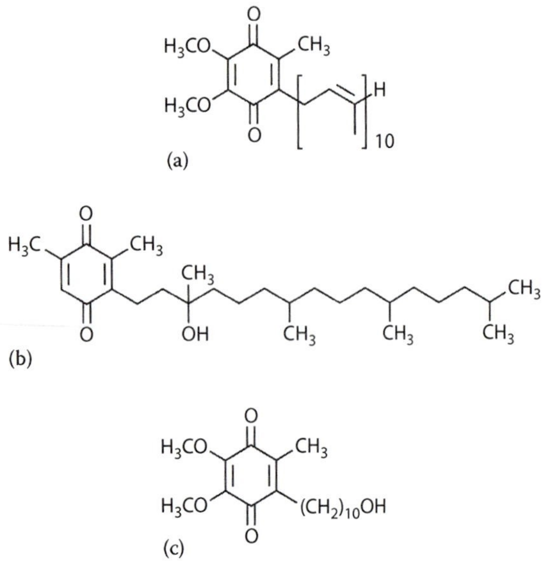

a skin lightening agent that was used for many years in industry, was banned in 2001 due to toxicological issues.[92] Nevertheless, coQ treatment of skin remains a viable approach to prevent oxidative processes, proven by both in vitro biochemical techniques and in vivo studies.

THIOL-BASED ANTIOXIDANTS

Chapter 3 devotes considerable detail to the antioxidant properties of glutathione, a thiol-containing compound. Glutathione works in conjunction with glutathione peroxidase to break down lipid hydroperoxides to their corresponding alcohols, and to rid the cell of H_2O_2, converting it to H_2O. At the cellular level, many thiol-containing compounds play an integral role in maintaining cell homeostasis. They function by a variety of mechanisms, including: (1) quenchers of free radicals, (2) redox reaction substrates, (3) chelating agents, (4) buffer systems, and (5) reductants of disulfide bonds in proteins.[93] Given the protective role played by thiol-containing molecules, there is much interest in skin supplementation with similar exogenous species. Some of the best-known examples include derivatives of glutathione, cysteine, N-acetyl cysteine, and lipoic acid. Note, however, that care must be taken to avoid toxic thiols, of which there are many. Often, they become involved in a redox cycling mechanism between the thiol and disulfide, resulting in the formation of thiyl radicals and active oxygen species, which can damage tissue.[94]

Alpha-lipoic acid is an endogenous antioxidant that exists as a protein-bound cofactor for several important mitochondrial enzymes. Its free form is used as an exogenous dietary supplement for general health and well-being, as well as a topical agent for skin. It is known as a *universal antioxidant*, because it functions in lipophilic regions such as lipid membranes, and aqueous environments such as the cytosol. As shown in Figure 8.8, alpha-lipoic acid exists as a redox couple, either in the lipoic acid (disulfide) or the dihydrolipoic acid form. The redox potential for this couple is −0.32 V, as compared to endogenous glutathione/glutathione disulfide at −0.24 V. Much interest in alpha-lipoic acid stems from its unusually high redox potential, which could allow it to participate as a key component of the endogenous antioxidant system.[95] Due to its redox potential, alpha-lipoic acid can, in fact, reduce glutathione disulfide to glutathione—a recycling mechanism that allows oxidized glutathione (glutathione disulfide) to return to its antioxidant active state (glutathione). As discussed in Chapter 3, glutathione participates in the recycling of vitamin C, which then recycles vitamin E, or glutathione can directly recycle vitamin E. Such events would provide alpha-lipoic acid with a direct link to the endogenous antioxidant system.

Various in vitro and in vivo tests have been carried out to fully understand the potential of alpha-lipoic acid in skin care applications. Podda et al. carried out several studies in culture on normal human keratinocytes and in vivo on murine skin,[95] and were able to establish that alpha-lipoic acid converts to its more active form, dihydrolipoic acid, upon introduction to keratinocyte cultures

Figure 8.7 Molecular structure of (a) coQ, (b) tocoquinone, and (c) hydroxydecyl ubiquinone.

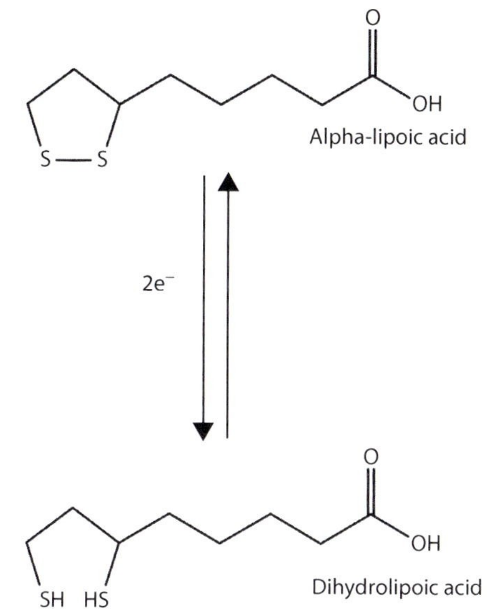

Figure 8.8 Molecular structure of alpha-lipoic acid and dihydrolipoic acid, a redox couple.

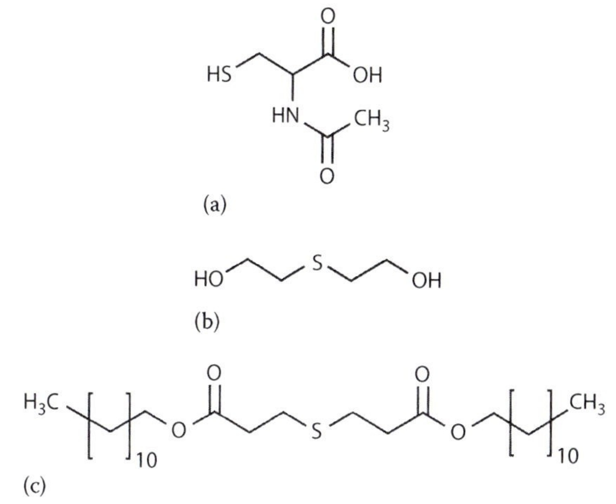

Figure 8.9 Molecular structure of (a) N-acetyl cysteine, (b) thiodiglycol, and (c) dilaurylthiodipropionate.

and after topical treatment in mice—5% alpha-lipoic acid in propylene glycol was applied to skin and converted within 2 hours.[96] Further, introduction of alpha-lipoic acid to keratinocyte cell cultures prevents the loss of lipid-soluble antioxidants and inhibits the activation of the redox-sensitive transcription factor, nuclear factor-kappa B.[95] In fibroblasts, alpha-lipoic acid increases the biosynthesis of collagen.[97] Furthermore, alpha-lipoic acid (5% use level in a cream) also prevents photoaging in skin, based on clinical studies of human volunteers.[98]

Although there is little guidance in the literature in the formulation of alpha-lipoic acid, a report of its stability in emulsions appeared a number of years ago.[99] It was reported to be unstable in the studied formulation and was unable to be stabilized by vitamin E; however, vitamin A did provide stability. As already mentioned, alpha-lipoic acid has the advantage of being active in both lipid and aqueous environments. In formulation this may present some challenges, especially if alpha-lipoic acid migrates to the aqueous-lipid interface where oxidation is most likely to occur.

In addition to lipoic acid, there are a number of thiol-containing compounds available in the personal care specialty chemicals market (Figure 8.9). Unfortunately, there is very little information available in the literature as to the mechanism and efficacy of these antioxidants, or even their suggested applications. Most work focuses on the utility of N-acetyl cysteine as a topical treatment. In a pair of studies, its function in UV-exposed fibroblasts was examined by looking at its influence on the level of endogenous glutathione and its protective properties of DNA.[100,101]

Despite their potential benefits, there is often a reluctance to use thiol-containing molecules in skin care preparations due to their overwhelming odor. It should also be noted, however, that glutathione and other thiol-containing molecules have proven efficacy as depigmentation agents.[102]

SACCHARIDE-CONTAINING ANTIOXIDANTS

Studies have shown that polysaccharides can have anti-hyperglycemic, immunomodulating, anti-inflammatory, and antioxidant activities.[103] Normally, the antioxidant activity does not come from the saccharide portion of the molecule, but rather a pendant phenolic/polyphenolic moiety. In fact, many polyphenols exist in plants and fruits with a saccharide component, probably providing a more harmonious structure within the botanical's morphology. While there are a handful of saccharide-based antioxidants available in the Personal Care Products Council's *Ingredient Dictionary*, there is limited information in the literature as to their efficacy for the treatment of skin. This is unfortunate since saccharides are very compatible with skin. One of the most utilized saccharide antioxidants in personal care products is arbutin, which in most cases is employed as a skin whitening agent. Table 8.4 contains a list of some common saccharide-based antioxidants.

For illustration, the structure of hesperidin, a flavanone glycoside that is found in citrus fruits, is provided in Figure 8.10. Bear in mind that some saccharidic antioxidants would actually be better categorized as polyphenols, especially in the case of hesperin. Most phytoantioxidants exist in nature as the saccharide form. Regardless of the categorization, understanding the mechanism of action and most functional form is of utmost importance.

Table 8.4 Common saccharide-containing antioxidants used in personal care products.

Arbutin
Chlorogenic acid
Hesperidin methyl chalcone
Isoquercitin
Sorbityl furfural

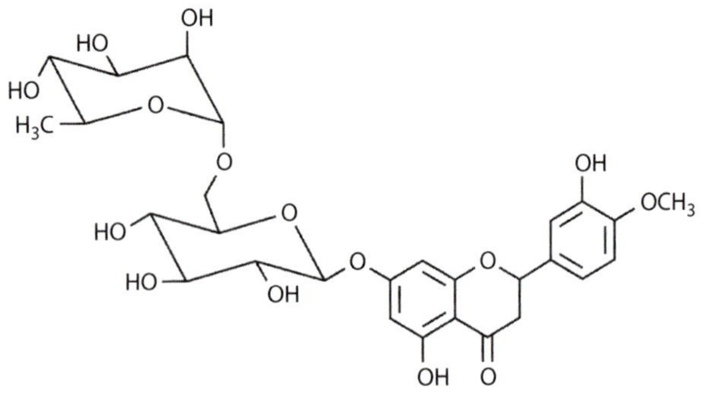

Figure 8.10 Molecular structure of hesperidin, a flavanone glycoside found in citrus fruits.

Interestingly, some compounds derived from carbohydrates also have free radical scavenging activity. For example, mannitol—a sugar alcohol and medication normally used to decrease intracranial and eye pressure—has reported antioxidant benefits and is often used in combination with hyaluronic acid fillers, commonly employed for aesthetic surgery to increase volume of the skin as well as ameliorate lines and wrinkles. The use of mannitol in the fillers is two-fold as it helps to reduce inflammation during the filling procedure as well as to provide long-term protection to the injected hyaluronic acid filler from free radical decomposition.[104]

POLYPHENOLS

The next time you are at a dinner party, listen carefully to the echoes in the room and you might hear discussions divulging the health benefits offered by a glass of 1996 Bordeaux wine or a fine piece of Belgian chocolate. Wine and chocolate, as well as many plants, fruits, vegetables, and nuts contain polyphenols, a group of molecules that plants have evolved to create in order to protect themselves from the harsh elements of the environment. Polyphenols are antioxidants that have become increasingly recognized as possible combatants of the dangerous free radicals that threaten the well-being of the human organism. In studies of skin, many of them have been found to also exhibit anti-inflammatory, immunomodulatory, and chemopreventive properties.[105–110]

Description of polyphenols

Many plant-derived molecules that have biological activity belong to the large family of compounds known as phytochemicals. Polyphenols represent an expansive group therein, and, according to current estimates, their number of known members exceeds several thousand. The polyphenol category of molecules is typically further divided into four primary classes: phenolic acids, flavonoids, lignans, and stilbenes. Of these groups, phenolic acids and flavonoids are the most prevalent groups in nature and, accordingly, the most studied. The table in Figure 8.11 contains a selected list of many of the compounds that belong to the flavonoid class. In general, all of the molecules structurally share the same common feature of multiple aromatic rings as well as attached hydroxyl groups. Figure 8.12 gives an example specific to the flavonoids. The hydroxylation and saturation of the central ring varies between each of the flavonoid groups in the figure. Rings A and C can contain one or more hydroxyl groups, giving rise to various molecules within each group. The antioxidant action

Flavonoids

Flavones	Flavanols	Isoflavonoids	Anthocyanidins
	Flavan-4-ol	Isoflavanes	Cyanidin
Flavones Apigenin Luteolin Tangeritin	Flavan-3-ol Catechin Catechin-3-gallate Epicatechins Epigallocatechin Epicatechin-3-gallate Epigallocatechin-3-gallate Gallocatechin Gallocatechin-3-gallate	**Isoflavones** Daidzein Genistein Glycitein	Delphinidin Malvidin
Flavonols Diosmin Kaempferol Myricetin Quercetin Quercitrin Rutin			
Flavanones Butin Hesperetin Hesperidin Naringin Sakuranin	Flavan-3,4-diol Proanthocyanidins	Phytoestrogens	Peonidin Petunidin

Figure 8.11 Selected members of the flavonoid class of molecules. The most common groups and subgroups are shown. Neoflavonoids are not shown.

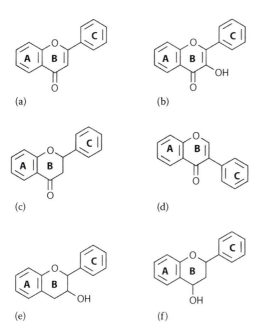

Figure 8.12 General skeletal structural features of groups of molecules in the flavonoid class: (a) flavone, (b) flavonol, (c) flavanone, (d) isoflavone, (e) flavan-3-ol, and (f) flavan-4-ol. Rings A and C can contain one or more hydroxyl group (-OH) substitutions.

of polyphenols is exerted by the proton donating ability of the hydroxyl group, which is able to neutralize a free radical and form a much more stable polyphenolic radical. Normally, the reaction proceeds by the general pathway shown in Equation 8.1, in which case the antioxidant donates a proton to the free radical species.

$$A\text{-}OH + R^{\bullet} \rightarrow A\text{-}O^{\bullet} + RH \qquad (8.1)$$

In this equation, A-OH represents a polyphenol, $R^{\bullet}$ a free radical, $A\text{-}O^{\bullet}$ a stable polyphenolic radical, and RH an inactivated radical. The chemical nature of the polyphenols, with their highly conjugated electronic structure, renders a stable, persistent radical that is not very reactive.

Aside from antioxidant activity, polyphenols also carry out other biological functions. It has been known for some time that this diverse group of molecules interacts with proteins. In fact, some of the original interest in polyphenols stems from their *anti-nutritional* capabilities, in which they bind with food proteins, resulting in decreased absorption in the gastrointestinal tract.[111] Equally interesting, the astringency associated with eating and drinking various fruits and beverages can be attributed to insoluble precipitate formed by the complexation of saliva proteins with the ingested polyphenols.[111] Further, many polyphenols act as anti-inflammatory agents. Current research suggests that the anti-inflammatory property of polyphenols arises from their ability to inhibit various cytokines and other proteins that are involved in cellular signaling.[11,112–118] In the paragraphs that follow, several types of polyphenols—recipients of a considerable amount of interest in skin research, evidenced by a plethora of academic literature—are outlined. In general, there are countless studies on the biological activity of polyphenols, most of which are interested in the anti-carcinogenic properties of polyphenols with special reference to various organs such as skin, lungs, stomach, esophagus, liver, pancreas, colon, and prostate.[111] In the sections below, we investigate the protection of skin by various polyphenols.

Phenolic acids

Caffeic and ferulic acids are frequently used in skin care preparations. They are hydroxycinnamates, or phenolic acids, found in grains, fruits, vegetables, and beverages where they are associated with saccharidic components.[117,119] As shown in Figure 8.13, each compound is structurally characterized by a phenolic and acrylic functional group. There has been considerable interest in the personal care industry to exploit the health benefits of these compounds in skin. Studies of ex vivo pig skin (with a Franz diffusion cell) and in vivo mouse tissue provide a strong case that ferulic and caffeic acid cross the stratum corneum barrier when topically applied.[120,121] In in vivo studies of humans, both phenolic compounds were found to reduce UV-induced erythema.[122] Caffeic acid has even found promise as an active ingredient for wound treatment in in vitro cell culture studies and in vivo in mice,[123] where it was found to downregulate important markers of inflammation and reduce free radical activity. In terms of formulation stability, ferulic acid has temperature- and pH-dependent instabilities that interfere with its incorporation into formulation.[124] Its stability, however, can be improved by including dypropylene glycol in the final formulation.

Gallic acid is another important phenolic acid that is found in gallnuts, green tea, red wine, and certain types of bark. It is a biologically active molecule that has antioxidant, antimicrobial, anti-inflammatory, and anticarcinogenic properties. Its anticarcinogenic and antimutagenic properties were demonstrated in mouse models, where

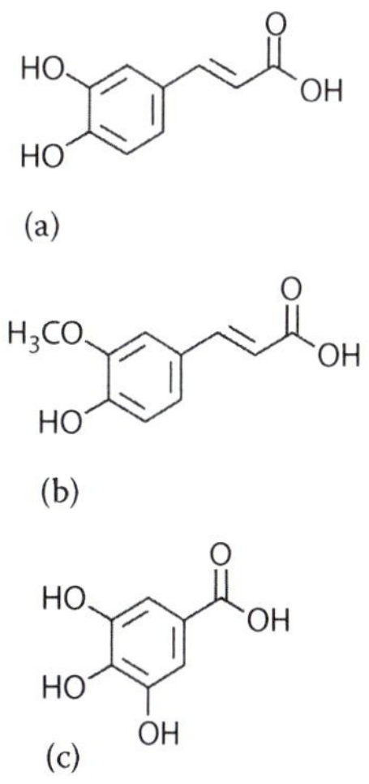

Figure 8.13 Molecular structure of (a) caffeic acid, (b) ferulic acid, and (c) gallic acid.

the detrimental biological effects of the tumor promoting chemical, 12-O-tetradecanoyl-phorbol-13-acetate (TPA), on in vivo mouse skin were inhibited.[125] It was also found to inhibit three biochemical markers of skin tumor promotion: ornithine decarboxylase activity, hydroperoxide production, and DNA synthesis. Recent work has shed light on the possible utility of gallic acid as an agent against the migration and invasion of melanoma cells.[126] In other work, gallic acid-loaded niosomes formulated into a gel enhanced penetration/absorption of gallic acid.[127] In a follow-up study, the same system was shown to reduce skin aging as indicated by a reduction in elastic recovery, extension, and roughness of skin.[128] Gallic acid and its derivatives have even been shown to have antimelanogenic (skin whitening) properties that function by a mechanism that inhibits tyrosinase activity.[129]

Tea polyphenols

Who hasn't heard someone say, "I prefer tea—no coffee for me please." Whether that person knows it or not, he or she is making a judicious decision to drink the more antioxidant rich beverage. Black, green, and oolong teas come from the same plant, *Camellia sinensis*, and are rich with various types of polyphenols. The difference between the three teas results from their manufacturing processes and, consequently, their antioxidant compositions are different. For example, green tea undergoes a milder preparation process and is chock-full of catechins, which belong to a class of polyphenols known as the flavanols (Figure 8.14). The four principle catechins in green tea consist of epicatechin, epigallocatechin, epicatechin-3-gallate, and epigallocatechin-3-gallate. Epigallocatechin-3-gallate is the most abundant of the catechins in green tea and, accordingly, the most studied.[130] Black tea, like oolong tea, is subjected to an enduring fermentation process that converts the epicatechins to condensed forms of polyphenols, which predominantly contains the theaflavin and thearubigin (Figure 8.15).

Over the years, a significant amount of research has been conducted in which the effect of tea on skin has been investigated, most notably green tea.[113,118,130] These studies

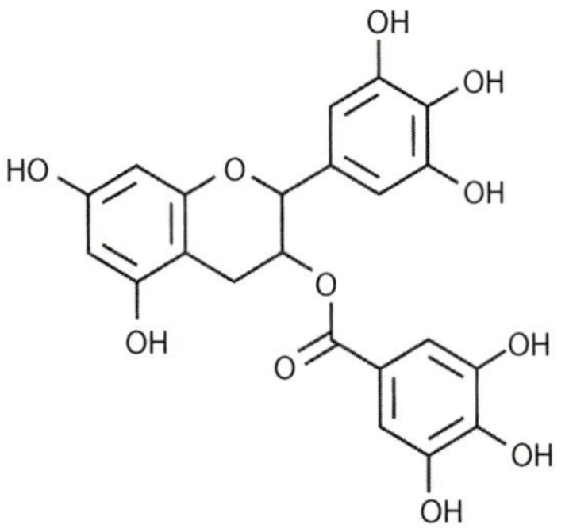

Figure 8.14 Molecular structure of epigallocatechin-3-gallate, one of the most abundant and biologically active green tea polyphenols. See Chapter 9 for the structures of the other catechins.

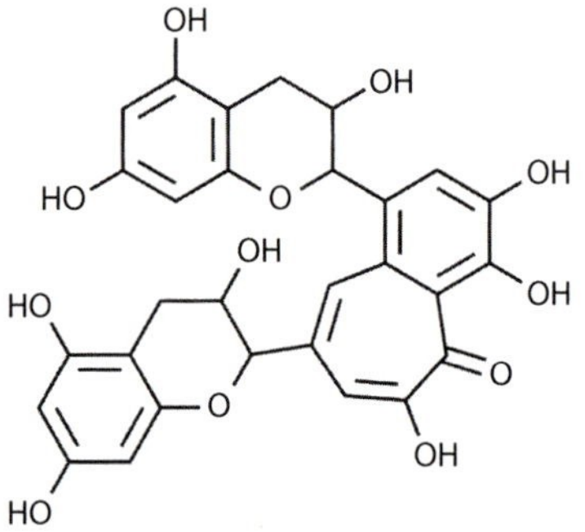

Figure 8.15 Molecular structure of the black tea polyphenol, theaflavin. See Chapter 9 for the structure of thearubin.

not only included oral administration of the extracts, but also topical application in skin care formulations. Overall, the tea polyphenols serve several different functions in protecting the skin. Due to their aromaticity, they absorb harmful UV rays, thus, preventing tumorigenesis. As antioxidants, they scavenge free radicals, preventing damage to cellular proteins, lipids, and DNA. Further, UV light also initiates numerous signal transduction pathways in skin cells (keratinocytes and fibroblasts) that lead to inflammation. Green tea polyphenols are known regulators of these signal transduction pathways, thereby acting as anti-inflammatory agents. Moreover, green tea polyphenols aid in wound healing by promoting keratinocyte differentiation. In brief, an extensive amount of research has demonstrated the numerous protective effects of green tea when topically applied to the skin. Table 8.5 includes a summary of studies aimed at elucidating the mechanisms behind the protective effects of green tea. Much effort has gone into understanding how tea polyphenols prevent photocarcinogenesis. Current evidence indicates possible modulation of DNA repair systems.[131] Of course, we would be remiss not to mention the inhibition of UV-induced immunosuppression by green tea polyphenols, which we know to be intimately linked with the development of carcinomas.[132] In terms of treatment, topical application of green tea polyphenols is more efficacious than oral administration as far as its protection of skin from UV radiation.[133] Aside from one report of minor irritation, topical treatment with green tea polyphenols has no known side effects.[134] Green tea and other tea polyphenols have also been reported to reduce sebum production and as treatment-modality for acne vulgaris.[135]

Soy isoflavones

The soybean plant is native to Eastern Asia and has been an integral part of the diet in these countries for many years. Due to its extraordinary nutritional benefits, soy is the recipient of much interest by both Eastern and Western cultures. Dietary intake of soy has been thought, in part, to be responsible for the low incidence of cardiovascular disease and certain types of cancers in many Asian countries. In addition to being a good source of omega-3 fatty acids, soy contains the polyphenolic compounds known as

Table 8.5 Selected studies investigating the protective effects of green tea polyphenols on skin.

Species	Endpoint(s)	Efficacy	Year	References
Mouse	Skin tumorigenecity – topical treatment	Protective	1988	330
Mouse	Photocarcinogenesis (number of tumors) – topical treatment and oral administration	Protective	1989 1991	331,332
Human	Erythema; histological examination – topical treatment	Protective	2001	333
Mouse	UVB-induced oxidation of lipids and proteins, depletion of endogenous antioxidants, and inhibition of MAPK proteins – topical treatment	Protective	2003	133
Mouse	UV-induced immunosuppression – topical treatment	Protective	2006	131
Mouse	UV-induced immunosuppression – oral administration	Protective	2010	132

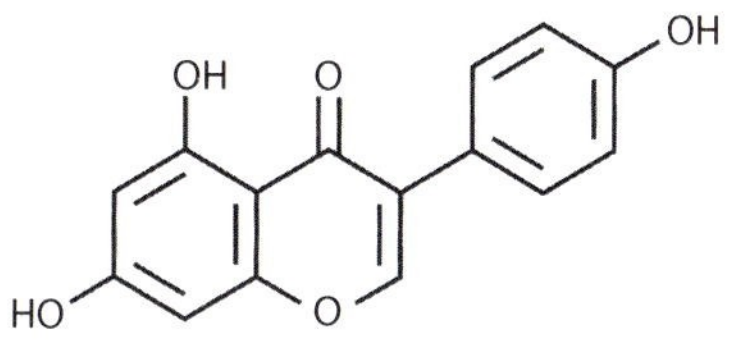

Figure 8.16 Molecular structure of genistein.

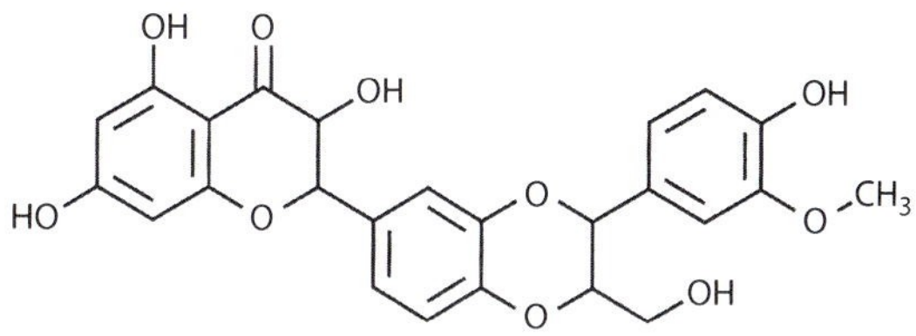

Figure 8.17 Molecular structure of silibinin.

isoflavones. The most abundant isoflavone in soy is genistein (Figure 8.16), which has been the subject of many research accounts investigating the positive health benefits of soy.[11,112,115,117] The protective action of genistein in skin, and in other tissues, has primarily been elucidated through studies that have demonstrated its anti-carcinogenic properties, which are believed to involve cellular signaling pathways.[136] Most of these studies have been carried out using the hairless mouse as a model.

Silymarin

The milk thistle plant (*Silybum marianum*), originally native to the Mediterranean region and parts of the Middle East and Asia, is a potent herbal remedy for diseases of the liver such as cirrhosis, jaundice, and hepatitis.[137] The extract of the milk thistle plant, known as silymarin, contains three notable flavonolignans: silibinin, silydianin, and silychristine. Of the three flavonoids, silibinin is considered the most biologically active and most abundant antioxidant in silymarin (Figure 8.17 for the structure of silibinin). A significant amount of research has been conducted as to the effects of topical treatment of silymarin on UV-induced damage in skin.[114] It has demonstrated effectiveness in preventing tumorigenesis in mouse models and as an anti-inflammatory agent and modulator of cellular signaling proteins. Further, silymarin has proven effective in preventing lipid peroxidation. In the prevention of photocarcinogenesis, a great deal of effort has gone into understanding the mechanisms by which silymarin functions as an antioxidant, anti-inflammatory, and immunomodulatory agent.[138] Figure 8.18 provides a summary of the molecular mechanisms that are modulated by silymarin during UV exposure based on in vivo and in vitro studies.

Treatment with silymarin inhibits the depletion of key endogenous antioxidants, such as glutathione, glutathione peroxidase, and catalase. Further, it results in decreased levels of H_2O_2, mitogen-activated protein kinases (MAPKs), nuclear factor-kappa B, and other reactive oxygen species (ROS)—all factors associated with oxidative stress in the skin. MAPKs and nuclear factor-kappa B are molecular signaling pathways that have been implicated in the development of skin tumors.[138] In terms of inflammation, silymarin decreases edema, hyperplasia (cell proliferation), and migration of leukocytes (a source of oxidative stress) to the skin. It reduces cyclooxgenase-2 and prostaglandin activity (biochemical markers of inflammation), and myeloperoxidase expression (an indicator of infiltrating leukocytes). Finally, silymarin modulates the immune system,

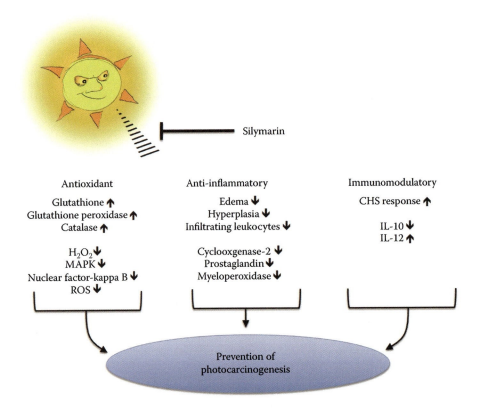

Figure 8.18 Protective effects of silymarin against photocarcinogenesis. Treatment with silymarin of UV irradiated in vivo skin and in vitro skin cells results in the upregulation (↑) and downregulation (↓) of various important biochemical markers.

resulting in downregulation of interleukin-10 (IL-10), an immunosuppressive cytokine, and upregulation of interleukin-12 (IL-12), an immunostimulant. During UV exposure the contact hypersensitivity response (CHS) is greater when silymarin is used as a therapeutic agent as opposed to no treatment. The greater the CHS, the healthier functioning is the immune system. Overall, there are many prospectives for silymarin in the treatment of skin. In the last two decades, numerous studies have been conducted to better understand the photoprotective effects of silymarin on skin. For a comprehensive treatise of this subject, the recent review by Vaid and Katiyar is most helpful.[138]

Curcumin

The Indian spice turmeric has a number of therapeutic uses and has been used since antiquity in the practice of traditional Hindu medicine (Ayurveda). Curcumoids are key components of turmeric, providing its characteristic yellowish color. Curcumin is one of the most important curcumoids in turmeric and is responsible for many of turmeric's medicinal uses.[139] Curcumin is found in the rhizomes (roots) of the turmeric plant, *Curcuma longa* (Figure 8.19). It has been studied extensively over the last fifty years as a potential therapeutic agent in wound healing, diabetes, Alzheimer's disease, Parkinson's disease, cardiovascular and pulmonary diseases, and arthritis.[140] Turmeric

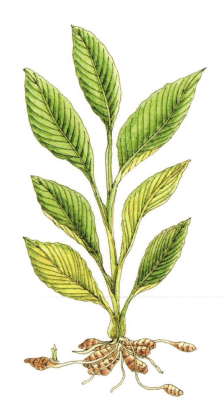

Figure 8.19 Illustration of the turmeric plant (*Curcuma longa*) showing its rhizomes where the curcuminoids are found.

is also an integral component of traditional medicine for its anti-rheumatic properties and to treat insect bites and wounds.[141]

A great deal of research has been conducted in recent years to elucidate the possible benefits of curcumin as a topical skin treatment, especially for psoriasis, scleroderma, and cancer,[142] most of which focused on the inhibition of chemically induced carcinogenesis in mouse models. Its behavior is thought to be anti-inflammatory and antioxidant in nature. In a series of studies, the effect of curcumin on mouse skin containing tumors was studied utilizing the tumor-promoting agent TPA.[143–145] Findings showed that curcumin inhibits tumor promotion in mice subjected to TPA.

In studies of mice (in vivo) and skin culture systems (keratinocytes), curcumin inhibits important cellular processes of inflammation such as nuclear factor-kappa B, cyclooxygenase-2, and lipoxygenase.[144,146] Such findings help explain why curcumin inhibits skin inflammation. Curcumin also decreases TPA-induced ornithine decarboxylase activity (it is usually upregulated in a variety of tumors), epidermal DNA synthesis (prologue to tumor development), hyperplasia (proliferation of cells), formation of c-Fos and c-Jun (these can become oncogenes), H_2O_2, and oxidized DNA (5-hydroxymethyl-2′-deoxyuridine).[145] In addition to its anticarcinogenic properties, curcumin is also a useful wound-healing agent.[142,147,148]

There are a number of considerations for curcumin with regard to stability and formulation. First, curcumin absorbs light in the visible region of the electromagnetic spectrum (408–430 nm) and is also unstable under the influence of UV light. Both factors are important for final packaging of curcumin as a raw ingredient or in a finished formulation. Second, depending on pH curcumin exists in the keto and enol forms (Figure 8.20). The keto form (pH 1–7) is yellow in color, while the enol form (>pH 7.5) presents as orange/red coloration. Third, curcumin is unstable at pH > 7, which may not be as much of an issue in the finished formulation but should be considered in regard to processing. Fourth, curcumin is a photosensitizer, leading to the generation of $^1O_2$, which could lead to its own self-degradation.[141]

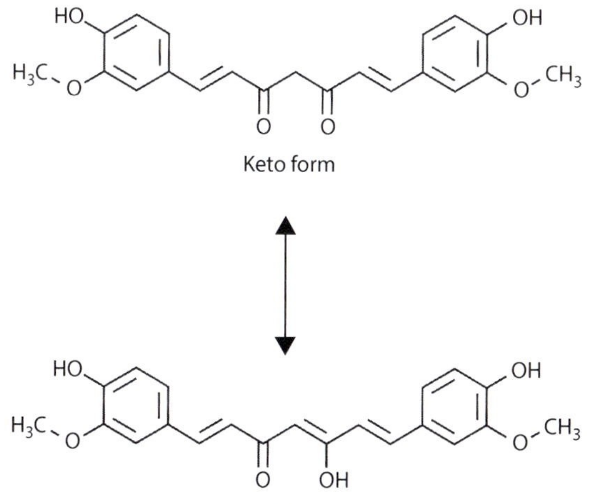

Due to its limited bioavailability by nutritional supplementation, many studies have aimed at delivery modalities for curcumin. By these means, formulators may find a suitable approach for cutaneous delivery by topical application. Such studies focus on encapsulation with biodegradable microspheres (bovine serum albumin and chitosan), polymeric micelles, polymeric nanoparticle encapsulates (allowing curcumin to be soluble in aqueous modalities), cellulosic systems with hydrophobic/hydrophilic components, and gels (carbomer and hydroxypropylcellulose).[149–153]

Curcumin offers much promise and many prospects for future use in skin care. A number of studies have outlined its potential use as an anticarcinogenic agent. While its antioxidant mechanisms are not as well elucidated in skin as some of the more common antioxidants (e.g., vitamin E, vitamin C), further studies in this area should be forthcoming. For recent reviews about curcumin in skin health and personal care applications, the reader is referred to References 141, 154, and 155.

Quercetin

Quercetin is a flavonoid that occurs naturally in fruits, vegetables, seeds, tea, and coffee, though its highest concentrations are found in green and black tea, onions, broccoli, apples, and red wine.[156] Structurally, like other flavones, quercetin contains a heterocyclic pyrone ring, which is connected on both sides to phenolic moieties. Normally, in nature, quercetin most commonly exists in the form of rutin (quercetin-3-rutosinide)—a glycoside containing a disaccharide covalently attached to the quercetin unit (Figure 8.21). Interest in quercetin as a therapeutic agent stems from its pharmacological activity as an antiallergic, anti-inflammatory, and anticarcinogenic agent,[141,157] while its use as an antioxidant stems from studies demonstrating its utility as a free radical scavenging agent ($O_2^{\cdot-}$ and lipid peroxyl species) as well as possible chelating mechanisms with ferrous ions.[158–160]

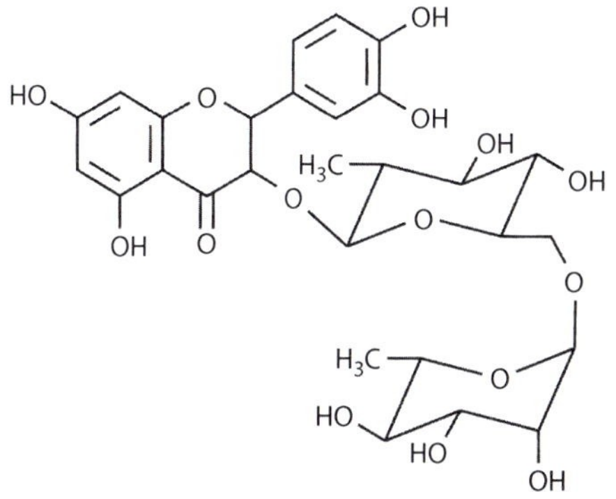

Figure 8.20 Tautomeric structures of curcumin corresponding to its (a) keto and (b) enol forms. The keto form is the stable form of curcumin and persists at low and neutral pH.

Figure 8.21 Molecular structure of rutin, also known as quercetin-3-rutosinide.

In vivo studies administering topical treatment of quercetin to the dorsal skin of mice demonstrated a decrease in UV-induced myeloperoxidase activity (an indicator of peroxidation), inhibition of UV depletion of reduced glutathione (an endogenous antioxidant), and a decrease in total proteinases (enzymes that damage connective tissue) caused by UV exposure.[161] In another in vivo study of rats, quercetin was found to decrease the amount of UV-induced malondialdehyde (a marker of lipid peroxidation) and prevent damage to endogenous antioxidants in skin.[162,163] In addition to quercetin's in vivo activity, in vitro tests of fibroblast cell culture systems shed light on the possibility of a protective mechanism against collagen destruction by impeding the activity of MMPs.[164]

Due to solubility issues in both aqueous and organic systems, much effort has been put forth to increase quercetin's efficiency of delivery.[165] Cutaneous absorption of quercetin occurs when topically applied to skin, although the mode of delivery will greatly influence the amount reaching the interior layers of the epidermis.[166,167] A detailed study of the effects of a transdermal delivery system highlighted propylene glycol monocaprylate and propylene glycol monolaurate as the most efficient vehicles of those tested.[168] The more common dimethylformamide and L-menthol were also evaluated as enhancers in combination with carbomer gel.[169] The combination of L-methanol and carbomer was the most effective system. Delivery by microemulsion was also explored and found to enhance delivery and permit quercetin to prevent lipid peroxidation in the skin.[170] Likewise, a water-in-oil emulsion effectively penetrated and provided protection of the skin against solar radiation.[171] Quercetin was also incorporated in lipid microparticles as yet another alternative for its efficient delivery.[172]

Quercetin has proven stability in formulations designed for topical application.[173] However, the molecule's photostability is an issue for packaging and application concerns since it will often be applied during or prior to exposure to sun.[174] Moreover, quercetin was even proposed as a possible sunscreen agent, by incorporating it into an oil-in-water emulsion at a concentration of 10% (w/w).[175] It provides some absorbance in the UVA range and reaches sufficient SPF values when used in conjunction with other solar protective agents.

Tannins

Tannins are a group of polyphenols found in the leaves, bark, seeds, roots, and rhizomes of several plant species (Table 8.6). Upon consumption, they have a characteristic astringent, bitter taste. Modern medicine had until recently deemed foods rich in tannins to have low nutritional value; nowadays, it is known that consuming high levels of tannins leads to reduced levels of digested nutrients, while lower levels can actually increase bioavailability of nutrients.[176] Their use in traditional medical practices, such as Ayurveda, is common for a variety of therapies. It is now recognized that tannins have antioxidant, anticarcinogenic, and antimicrobial properties.[177]

Table 8.6 Sources of tannins.

Bark	Cinnamon, wild cherry, cinchona, willow, *Acacia mimosa*, oak, and *Hamamelis*
Seed	Cocoa, guarana, kola, and areca
Leaf	*Hamamelis* and green tea
Roots and rhizomes	*Krameria* (*Rhatany*) and fern
Fruits	Berries (cranberries, blueberries, and strawberries), pomegranate, and persimmons
Nuts	Walnuts, hazelnuts, and pecans
Beverages	Beer (from malt and hops) and fruit juices (e.g., apple juice)

Source: Bele, A. et al., *Asian J Plant Sci.*, 9, 209–214, 2010.

Classification of tannins is not based on chemistry, but usually refers to a complex class of polyphenols of high molecular weight that form reversible and irreversible complexes with proteins.[176] They are normally classified into two groups: hydrolyzable and condensed tannins. Hydrolyzable tannins usually contain a carbohydrate backbone with pendant hydroxyl groups that are esterified with phenolic acids such as gallic acid. On the other hand, condensed tannins (also known as proanthocyanidins) are usually higher in molecular weight than the hydrolyzable tannins and are biopolymers composed of flavonoid moieties.

The use of tannins in skin care applications is limited, according to peer-reviewed literature. There is, however, a series of studies by Gali-Muhtasib et al. where the protective effects of tannic acid against photocarcinogenesis in hairless mice are investigated.[178–180] Indeed, their studies found that tannic acid (Figure 8.22) from tara pods (*Caesalpinia spinosa*) provided significant protection to skin against UVB irradiation. Its use resulted in lower levels of UVB

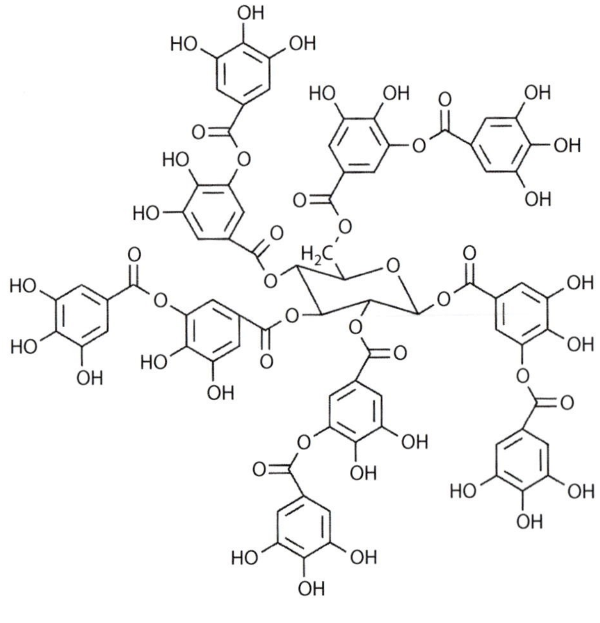

Figure 8.22 Molecular structure of tannic acid.

induced hydrogen peroxide formation (ROS formation), ornithine decarboxylase activity, and DNA synthesis (the latter two being biochemical indicators of tumor formation).[178,179] These researchers continued their studies by comparing the delivery method of tannic acid and found that topical treatment and intraperitoneal injection were successful modalities to deliver the antioxidant and suppress photocarcinogenesis. In contrast, dietary supplementation by force feeding was not effective.[180]

One notable tannin prevalent in the personal care products industry is the emblica antioxidant, derived from the extract of *Phyllanthus emblica*. The extract contains several low molecular weight (<1000) hydrolyzable tannins: emblicanin A, emblicanin B, pedunculagin, and punigluconin.[181] It has antioxidant properties and inhibits MMP-1 and MMP-3 activity in fibroblast cultures. In addition, it markedly reduces UV-induced erythema.[182]

Unfortunately, there is limited information in the literature as to the formulability of tannins. However, it should be noted that they form colloidal structures in water and their solubility ultimately depends on molecular weight. In addition, they are soluble in alcohol and acetone.[177] More than likely, the lower molecular weight hydrolyzable tannins should be easier to incorporate into a final formulation.

Resveratrol

In the last two decades, there has been an explosion of research into the potential health benefits of the polyphenol resveratrol (3,5,4′-trihydroxystilbene) (Figure 8.23). It naturally occurs in the skin of grapes (*Vitis vinifera*), certain berries, peanuts, and medicinal plants, such as Japanese knotweed (*Polygonum cuspidatum*).[183] Resveratrol exists as two isomeric forms (Figure 8.24). Upon exposure to UV light the trans-form is converted to the cis-form. It also exists in nature as a derivative stilbenoid glucoside form known as resveratrol-3-O-beta-D-glucoside (piceid). Resveratrol notoriety is possibly due to its proposed relationship with the *French Paradox*.[184] In a study of men living in Southwestern France with relatively high dietary fat intake, researchers found that these same subjects had much lower incidence of cardiovascular disease than other populations with similar fat intake levels. Higher levels of consumption of red wine was believed to be a key factor in the *French Paradox*. Ever-increasing numbers of discoveries associated with the benefits of resveratrol led the scientific community and general public to associate it with indispensable health benefits.[185] As early as 1997, reports appeared about resveratrol's ability to prevent carcinogenesis in laboratory mice.[186] It has antioxidant, anti-inflammatory, and anti-tumorigenic properties.[183] For these reasons, there is great interest in the dermatological research community to exploit resveratrol as a protective agent for skin, especially in the prevention of UV-induced damage (Table 8.7).[187]

In photocarcinogenesis studies of SKH-1 mice, results indicate that topical treatment with resveratrol inhibits the UVB-induced incidence of tumors and delays the onset of tumor development.[188] In this study, mice were either pretreated 30 minutes prior to each UVB exposure, or 5 minutes afterwards. Interestingly, the post-treatment was equally effective as the pre-treatment, indicating that resveratrol presumably works by mechanisms other than

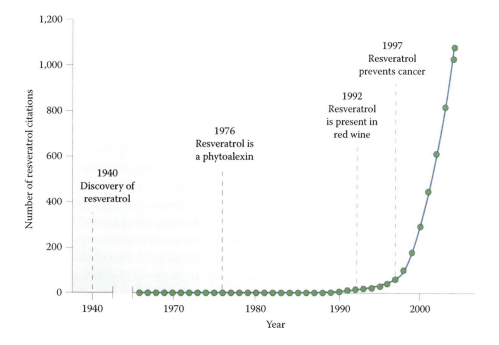

Figure 8.23 Resveratrol citations appearing in PubMed as a function of year. (Reprinted by permission from Nature, *Nat Rev Drug Discov*. Originally published in J. Baur and D. Sinclair, Therapeutic potential of resveratrol: the in vivo evidence, vol. 5.324 Copyright [2006]).

those of a sunscreen. Further studies by the same group demonstrated that resveratrol prevents the development of photocarcinogenesis by inhibiting the action of survivin—a molecule that prevents normal apoptosis from occurring.[189] Resveratrol was also found to prevent UVB-induced expression of cyclooxygenase and ornithine decarboxylase enzyme activities, which are known indicators of tumor promotion in skin.[190,191] There is also significant evidence that resveratrol mitigates cellular signaling mechanisms associated with photoaging, including MAPKs, nuclear factor-kappa B, and MMPs.[191–193] In addition, resveratrol was shown to increase the activity of superoxide dismutase and glutathione peroxidase when HaCaT keratinocytes were irradiated with UVA light.[194] Even in the most recent studies, there are still attempts to elucidate the protective mechanisms of resveratrol in skin.[195–198]

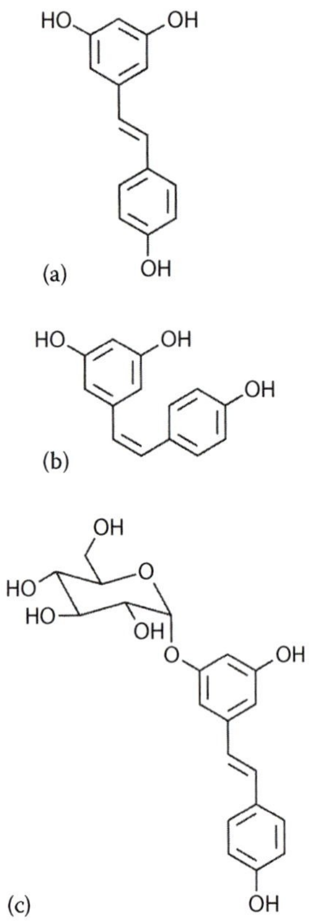

The bioavailability of orally administered resveratrol is too low for it to provide systemic protection. Therefore, alternative approaches such as topical or transdermal delivery offer much greater probability for therapeutic intervention. In a study that examined a variety of delivery vehicles for resveratrol, it was found that aqueous buffer systems at lower pH levels resulted in the greatest permeation.[199] Hydrogel delivery systems were also very efficient; however, the amount of permeation into the viable epidermis depended on the viscosity of the hydrogel. Overall, it was found that the stratum corneum did not impede delivery of resveratrol to the viable epidermis and dermis.

To close polyphenols...

The vast number of polyphenolic compounds found in nature have great potential influence on human health and well-being. Within the scientific community, much of this interest has focused on systemic supplementation with polyphenols and the biological effects on various bodily tissues, organs, and cell types. Promise has been shown in the area of topical skin treatment, especially for the polyphenols reviewed in this chapter; however, many polyphenols still require further elucidation, in terms of their in vivo antioxidant activity, cutaneous delivery, and mechanism of biochemical action.

Figure 8.24 Molecular structures of isomeric and glucoside forms of resveratrol: (a) *trans*-resveratrol, (b) *cis*-resveratrol, and (c) resveratrol-3-*O*-beta-D-glucoside (piceid).

Table 8.7 In vivo studies of resveratrol topically applied to skin.

Species	Brief description	Result	Year	Reference
CD-1 mice	Anti-cancer activity of 4 wine polyphenols	*trans*-Resveratrol reduced the amount of DMBA-induced skin tumors and was absorbed more effectively than the other polyphenols	2002	334
SKH-1 mice	Assess the involvement of survivin in UVB-mediated skin cancer induction	Resveratrol inhibited UVB-mediated skin cancer development by inhibition of survivin and associated apoptotic proteins	2005	189
SKH-1 mice	UVB radiation-mediated skin tumorigenesis	Resveratrol reduced the incidence of tumors and delayed tumorigenesis	2005	188
SirT1-null mice	Chemopreventive effects in SirT1-null mice	Topically applied resveratrol reduced tumorigenesis more effectively in normal Sirt1 genotype mice.	2009	335

Source: Ndiaye, M. et al., *Arch Biochem Biophys.*, 508, 164–170, 2011.

BOTANICAL EXTRACTS

The use of natural materials in personal products has increased significantly in the last decade. Extracts of natural products are often chock-full of polyphenols and other phytonutrients that are used to treat skin. Botanicals evolved to produce these ingredients in order to protect themselves from environmental insults, including harmful UV radiation. Many botanicals have been used for millennia in traditional Chinese medicine and Ayurveda. Nowadays, there is a flurry of activity in the skin care market with similar types of ingredients, due to a growing body of scientific evidence demonstrating their utility as skin therapeutic agents. Among other things, botanical ingredients have shown promise as anti-inflammatories for skin to treat rosacea,[200] preventative agents against melanoma,[201] bioactives for the treatment of skin aging,[202] and protective agents against UV-induced immunosuppression and photocarcinogenesis.[203] This section outlines the properties of several botanical extracts important in skin care. This list is by no means exhaustive but provides significant insight on the use of botanical extracts in skin care. Table 8.8 contains a more extensive list of extracts, which have also been identified as protective agents against UV-induced damage.

Ginkgo biloba extract

Native to China, *Ginkgo biloba* is the oldest living tree species on Earth.[214] Individual trees can age 2,500 years. The extract of its leaves has been used in Chinese medicine since antiquity to treat various ailments. As one of the most commonly used herbal dietary supplements in the United States, it is a very common remedy to improve blood circulation and memory, and to relieve depression. The biological activity of *Ginkgo biloba* consists of free radical scavenging, lowering oxidative stress, reducing neural damage, reducing platelet aggregation, anti-inflammation, anti-tumor activity, and anti-aging.[215] Clinically, it is used to treat central nervous system disorders, such as Alzheimer's disease.[216]

The extract of *Ginkgo biloba* leaves contains flavonoids and terpene tri-lactones. The flavonoids consist of flavone and flavonol glycosides, acylated flavonol glycosides, biflavonoids, flavane-3-ols, and proanthocyanidins. Of the flavonoids, the flavonol glycosides are the most abundant group in the *Ginkgo biloba* extract and often contain derivatives of quercetin, kaempferol, and isorhamnetin with glucose or rhamnose.[217] The terpene tri-lactones, or ginkgolides, are also an important group of active ingredients that are unique to *Ginkgo biloba* extract (Figure 8.25). They are cage-like structures consisting of six five-membered rings: a spiro[4.4]-nonane carbocyclic ring, three lactones, and a tetrahydrofuran ring.[218]

Table 8.8 Botanical extracts utilized in skin care applications for their antioxidant benefits.

Botanical extract	Biological actives	Efficacy studies
Capparis spinosa flower buds	Quercetin derivatives Kaempferol derivatives Caffeic acid Ferulic acid *p*-Cumaric acid Cinnamic acid	Antioxidant activity and inhibition of UV-B-induced erythema;[204] antihistaminic; and antiallergic[205]
Culcitium reflexum H.B.K. leaf	Cinnamic acid Quercetin derivatives Isorhamnetin derivatives Kaempferol	Antioxidant activity and inhibition of UVB-induced erythema[206]
French maritime pine bark (pycnogenol)	Procyanidins Benzoic acid Cinnamic acid Ferulic acid	Inhibition of UVB-induced erythema and expression of nuclear factor-kappa B[206,207]
Pomegranate fruit	Anthocyanins Hydrolyzable tannins	Modulates molecular signaling pathways in keratinocytes, such as nuclear factor-kappa B and mitogen-activated protein kinases;[208,209] inhibits tumorigenesis[210]
Red orange	Anthocyanins Hydroxycinnamic acids Flavanones Ascorbic acid	Antioxidant activity and inhibition of UVB-induced erythema[211]
Sanguisorba officinalis L. root	Hydrolyzable tannins	Inhibition of photoaging[212]
Sedum telephium L. leaf	Flavonol glycosides Polysaccharides	Antioxidant activity and inhibition of UVB-induced erythema[213]

Source: Svobodová, A. et al., *Biomed Papers.*, 147, 137–145, 2003.

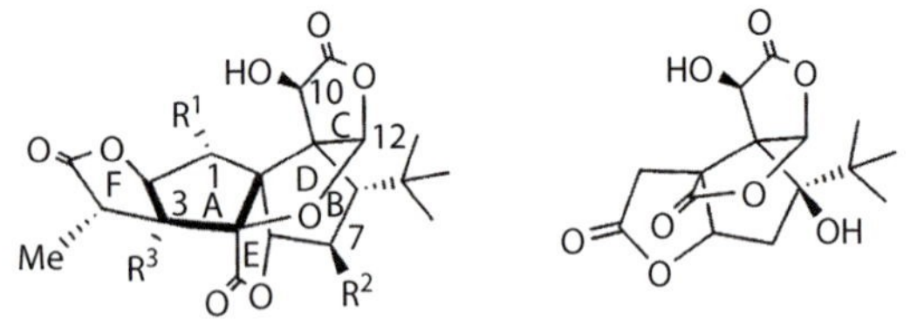

	R¹	R²	R³
Ginkgolide A (GA, 1)	H	H	OH
Ginkgolide B (GB, 2)	OH	H	OH
Ginkgolide C (GC, 3)	OH	OH	OH
Ginkgolide J (GJ, 4)	H	OH	OH
Ginkgolide M (GM, 5)	OH	OH	H

Bilobalide (BB, 6)

Figure 8.25 Structures of terpene tri-lactones (five ginkgolides and bilobalide) found in *Ginkgo biloba* leaf extract. (From Strømgaard, K. and Nakanishi, K.; Chemistry and biology of terpene trilactones from Ginkgo biloba. *Angew Chem Int Ed.* 2004, 43, 1640–1658. Copyright Wiley-VCH Verlag Gmbh & Co. KGaA. Reproduced with permission.)

In vitro studies using Franz diffusion cells demonstrated the permeation efficacy of key components (epigallocatechin-3-gallate and quercetin) of *Ginkgo biloba* extract from cosmetic formulations.[219] It has been used as an antiwrinkle agent and was found to improve skin moisturization.[220] Orally administered, *Ginkgo biloba* extract has even been successfully used in the treatment of vitiligo vulgaris.[221] Surprisingly, there are few studies investigating its photoprotective properties. In one such study, topical treatment with *Ginkgo biloba* extract resulted in a reduction in UV-induced erythema and sunburn cell formation.[222]

Grape seed extract

After preparation of wine or juice, grape seeds (*Vitis vinifera*) are often utilized to prepare grape seed extract. After extraction, the final product is normally dried and purified, yielding an extract of extremely potent antioxidant activity. Grape seed extract mostly contains flavonoids; oligomeric proanthocyanidins represent the largest member of this group. Proanthocyanidins are oligomers of flavan-3-ols such as catechin, epicatechin, and epicatechin-3-*O*-gallate (Figure 8.26). In skin care, topical treatment and dietary intake of grape seed extract inhibits photocarcinogenesis.[223–227] In vitro studies shed light on some of the mechanisms involved, with MAPKs and nuclear factor-kappa B signaling mechanisms playing an integral role—two pathways mitigated by UV-induced oxidative stress.[228,229]

Prunis persica flower extract

This extract comes from the flower buds of the peach tree, which is native to Eastern Asia. The tree bears a fruit with a hairy skin, which we know as a peach. *Prunis persica* flower belongs to the family *Rosaceae*. This extract has been used in Chinese medicine since ancient times to treat various skin conditions. Present day interest in *Prunis persica* flower extract stems from its potential as a skin protectant against UV-induced damage. In vitro studies of *Prunis persica* flower extract demonstrate protection to keratinocytes by

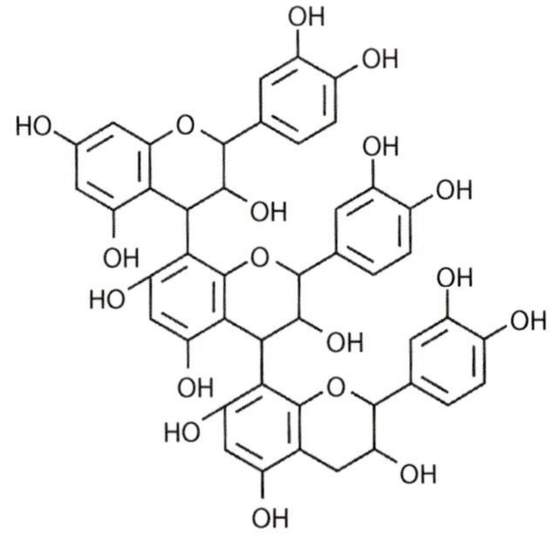

Figure 8.26 Structure of proanthocyanidin C1—an epicatechin trimer—found in grape seed extract.

inhibiting the amount of UV-induced arachidonic acid—a marker of inflammation and oxidative stress.[230] Further, studies of fibroblast cultures revealed protection by the flower of *Prunis persica* against UV-induced DNA damage and lipid peroxidation.[231] In vivo, the extract was not only effective in inhibiting UV-induced erythema (80% inhibition at 0.3 mg/cm²) in guinea pigs and ear edema in mice (49% inhibition at 3.0 mg/ear), but also at preventing skin photocarcinogenesis.[231,232]

FULLERENES AND THEIR USE IN COSMETICS

Fullerenes represent one type of allotrope of carbon. Allotrope refers to possible crystalline forms of a molecule. For example, allotropes of carbon consist of diamond, fullerenes, and graphite. The most common form of fullerene is a C_{60} molecule containing a hollow molecular sphere that is characterized by its highly conjugated structure consisting of 30 carbon double bonds (Figure 8.27). Fullerenes were discovered in 1985 by researchers at Rice University in Houston, TX (United States), who later won the Nobel Prize in Chemistry.[233]

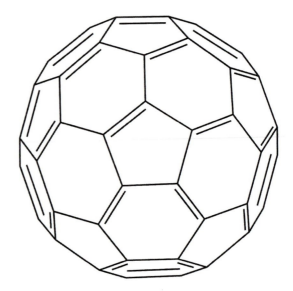

Figure 8.27 Molecular structure of C_{60} fullerene.

The fullerenes became known as Buckminster Fullerenes, or Buckyballs, and received their name due to their structural resemblance to a geodesic sphere, specifically the Montréal Biosphère, which was designed by the American Architect, Buckminster Fuller.

Fullerenes are prepared by vaporizing carbon, which takes place by generating a current between two carbon rods, and then allowing it to condense in an inert gas. They have unique physicochemical properties and offer much promise in biomedical applications. The conjugated nature of the fullerene sphere provides it with free radical scavenging properties allowing it to act like a free radical sponge.[234] Its antioxidant properties have been exploited in several studies focused on understanding how fullerenes can combat free radical damage in keratinocyte cell cultures exposed to UV radiation.[235-237] Interestingly, it has also been shown that during exposure to ultraviolet light, fullerenes undergo photosensitization reactions (transition to a long-lived excited triplet state) and react with molecular oxygen ($^3O_2$), resulting in the formation of $^1O_2$ and $O_2^{\cdot -}$.[234] In turn, these ROS may react with a number of biological targets or even cause a cascade of molecular signaling events that could be harmful to the cell. Nevertheless, more studies are required to determine if the dual nature of fullerenes could hamper their use as free radical scavenging agents in applications involving exposure to solar radiation.

Since C_{60} is very hydrophobic, a focus of contemporary fullerene research is to increase the degree of hydrophilicity of the molecule to make it more biologically available. One approach is to functionalize the outer surface of the fullerene sphere with hydroxyl groups—yielding compounds known as fullerenols (polyhydroxylated fullerenes). Additional chemical modifications that increase the hydrophilicity of fullerenes include the introduction of poly(ethylene glycol) units to the outer surface of the molecule, or the incorporation of the fullerene into a poly(vinylpyrrolidone) or gamma-cyclodextrin shell. Finally, encapsulation of fullerenes into liposomes is yet another approach to increasing the solubility of fullerenes in water. All of these avenues have been successful at increasing the efficacy of fullerene in preventing free radical damage in keratinocyte cell culture systems.[235-237]

Several other studies have actually examined the penetration of C_{60} fullerene derivatives into the skin. For example, utilizing confocal Raman microscopy, researchers from North Carolina State University and Rice University observed the penetration into ex vivo skin of C_{60} fullerene modified with small peptide sequences on its outer shell.[238]

In the early 1990s, toxicological assessment of C_{60} fullerene demonstrated that acute and chronic exposure to the molecule does not result in DNA damage and subsequent development of tumors when topically applied to mouse skin.[239] Additional evidence emerged in the late 1990s that application of fullerenes to skin does not provide an appreciable allergic response in humans.[240] Further studies on functionalized fullerenes also did not reveal any toxicological issues.[241] It should be noted, however, that some controversy exists as to the safe and effective use of fullerenes on skin. In a 2006 article in *Chemical and Engineering News*, Bethany Halford challenged fullerene manufacturers and finished goods companies to provide more data and testing as to the toxicological acceptability of fullerenes in skin care preparations.[242]

More recent research demonstrated the utility of fullerenes in treating acne vulgaris.[243] It has also been shown that fullerenes inhibit the formation of ROS in skin subjected to laser therapy regimens.[244] Not surprisingly, there has been considerable interest in the personal care industry to develop products utilizing fullerene technology to take advantage of its therapeutic properties.[245,246]

EFFECTS OF DIETARY INTAKE OF ANTIOXIDANTS ON SKIN HEALTH

In many industrialized nations, such as the United States, Germany, and the United Kingdom, public health officials recommend daily dietary intake of five servings of fruits and vegetables. This has become known as the *5-a-Day* program. This recommendation is based on the World Health Organization's suggestion that each person consume at least 400 grams of vegetables per day.[247] Furthermore, the U.S. Department of Agriculture (USDA) recommends 2–4 servings of fruit and 3–5 servings of vegetables daily.[248] One strategy for conferring inherent protection to the integument against solar radiation is to supplement diet with antioxidants (Table 8.9). By this approach, antioxidants are metabolized in the gut and distributed to various tissues as needed. This approach has certain advantages over topical application, such as convenience, necessity to maintain a robust protective layer, and time spent applying sunscreen.[249] There are four types of mechanisms by which a supplemental approach could confer protection against the sun: (1) shielding skin from solar radiation (similar to a sunscreen); (2) competition between an antioxidant and another molecular species, which could potentially become damaged, for the damaging species (e.g., a free radical); (3) restoration of damaged targets (e.g., nucleotide excision repair of DNA); and (4) suppression of the inflammatory response.[249] This section assesses the efficacy of selected antioxidants by their potential to prevent non-melanoma skin cancer.

A great deal of work has been carried out on understanding the photoprotective mechanisms of dietary supplementation with butylated hydroxytoluene.[250-254] Overall, these studies demonstrated that dietary intake of the antioxidant by mouse models led to a reduction in photodamage of skin, especially in terms of non-melanoma carcinogenesis. As an example, mice fed a daily diet consisting of 0.5% butylated hydroxytoluene experienced an increase of 65% of the chromophore in the stratum corneum as measured by spectrophotometry. It is difficult to say with certainty whether butylated hydroxytoluene provided protection as a UV absorbing sunscreen or if a free-scavenging mechanism was responsible. Regardless, it is key to note that a large distribution of the antioxidant was found in the stratum corneum.

Table 8.9 Sources of various dietary antioxidants.

Class/component	Source
Carotenoids	
• Beta-carotene	Carrots, various fruits
• Lutein, zeaxanthin	Kale, collards, spinach, corn, eggs, citrus
• Lycopene	Tomatoes and processed tomato products
Flavonoids	
• Anthocyanidins	Berries, cherries, red grapes
• Flavonols—catechins, epicatechins, procyanidins	Tea, cocoa, chocolate, apples, grapes
• Flavanones	Citrus foods
• Flavonols	Onions, apples, tea, broccoli
• Proanthocyanidins	Cranberries, cocoa, apples, strawberries, grapes, wine, peanuts, cinnamon
Isothiocyanates	
• Sulforaphane	Cauliflower, broccoli, Brussel sprouts, cabbage, kale, horseradish
Phenols	
• Caffeic acid, ferulic acid	Apples, pears, citrus fruits, some vegetables
Sulfides/thiols	
• Diallyl sulfide, allyl methyl trisulfide	Garlic, onions, leeks, scallions
• Dithiolthiones	Cruciferous vegetables—broccoli, cabbage, bok choy, collards
Vitamins and minerals	
• Vitamin A	Liver, dairy products, fish
• Vitamin C	Bell peppers, citrus fruits
• Vitamin E	Oils, fortified cereals, sunflower seeds, mixed nuts
• Selenium	Brazil nuts, meats, tuna, plant foods

Source: International Food Information Council Foundation: Media Guide on Food Safety and Nutrition: 2004–2006 and Food and Nutrition Board Institute of Medicine DRI reports.

It should be noted that there was some recent controversy about the use of butylated hydroxytoluene in food products in which consumers questioned the safety and efficacy of synthetic additives, leading a major manufacturer of cereals to remove butylated hydroxytoluene from its products.[255] Regardless of the consumer concerns, butylated hydroxytoluene is considered safe for human consumption at the low concentrations typically employed in food products, which has been substantiated by long-term use studies.[256]

Several decades ago, there was much interest in supplementation with beta-carotene due to promising studies involving mice that demonstrated a protective role against photocarcinogenesis.[257,258,259] It was also shown that high levels of beta-carotene in serum correlated with low incidence of non-melanoma types of skin cancer.[260] More recently, several large clinical studies have brought into question the role of beta-carotene in the prevention of carcinogenesis. With more than 2,000 subjects, both studies found that administration of beta-carotene (30 mg and 50 mg per day, respectively) did not result in decreased incidence of non-melanoma skin cancer.[64,65] Beta-carotene's image is further hampered by a large study published in the *New England Journal of Medicine* that revealed a higher incidence of lung cancer for smokers who administered beta-carotene treatment.[68] Regardless, there is a large body of evidence that correlates high serum levels of beta-carotene with decreased incidence of non-melanoma skin cancer.[249] Unfortunately, the International Agency for Research on Cancer (IARC) issued a statement against recommending beta-carotene for the prevention of cancer:

"Until further insight is gained, beta-carotene should not be recommended for use in cancer prevention in the general population and it should not be assumed that beta-carotene is responsible for the cancer protecting effects of diets rich in carotenoid-containing fruits and vegetables."[261]

Beta-carotene offers promise in the protection of skin against UV-induced damage, although it usually requires long-term supplementation (>10 weeks) to observe inhibition of UV-induced erythema.[262] Nevertheless, the reader is advised to heed the IARC's warning with regard to nutritional supplementation with beta-carotene.

A recent review on the dietary intake of carotenoids in tomatoes was proposed as a possible strategy to combat free radical damage in skin.[262] Four principle carotenoids in tomatoes are beta-carotene (3%), lycopene (100%), phytofluene (10%), and phytoene (10%)—percentages are normalized to lycopene. Various studies have demonstrated the efficacy of tomato-based foods and lycopene as nutritional supplements to protect skin and ward off damage caused by UV-induced processes. In one study, daily administration of tomato paste (10-week study) reduced UV-induced erythema.[263] In another study, synthetic lycopene was compared to tomato extract alone and extract fortified with phytoene and phytofluene.[264] Both extracts were more efficacious, in terms of protection against UV-induced erythema, than synthetic lycopene. It may be that phytoene and phytofluene present in the extracts could act as solar filters incorporated into skin.[262] A mixture of carotenoids and other antioxidants—lycopene (3 mg/day), lutein (3 mg/day), beta-carotene (4.8 mg/day), alpha-tocopherol (10 mg/day), and selenium (75 µg/day)—taken over a period of 12 weeks led to increases in skin thickness and density (as measured by ultrasound), decreases in roughness and scaling, and no change in furrows or wrinkles.[265] In a separate study, lycopene supplementation resulted in an improvement in the wrinkles and furrows in the forehead.[266] Overall, some of the inherent problems of beta-carotene, discussed above, stem from high levels of accumulation in serum. Lycopene, on the hand, is reported not to overaccumulate in serum regardless of nutritional supplement quantity—a strong argument for the use of lycopene over beta-carotene.[262]

The discussion of vitamin A earlier in this chapter outlined the protective properties of retinoids. There have been some positive results demonstrating photoprotection with orally administered retinoids; however, there is conflicting evidence in the literature.

In general, they are not recommended as photoprotective agents for the prevention of squamous and basal cell carcinomas.[249]

Vitamins E and C have warranted a significant amount of attention in studies aimed at preventing UV-induced damage of skin. Oral supplementation with both antioxidants has shown promise in providing photoprotection to the skin.[19,267] However, there have been conflicting results in which vitamin E performed no better than a placebo in terms of clinically assessed sunburn and sunburn cell formation (by examining histological sections).[268] Attempts to fortify the synergistic endogenous antioxidant system can be carried out by administering oral supplementation of both vitamins C and E, thereby permitting a mechanism in which vitamin C replenishes oxidized vitamin E (Chapter 3 has a more thorough discussion of this phenomenon).[269] Indeed, combination therapy of both antioxidants increases the amount of sustainable exposure to solar radiation.[270,271] One should bear in mind that the dosage of antioxidants is not always comparable in studies; in most cases between 20–40 mg per day is administered for human subjects.

As already discussed, topical treatment with the trace element selenium offers promise in photoprotection. Moreover, serum levels in patients with non-melanoma skin cancer were found to contain lower levels of selenium.[74] On the other hand, dietary supplementation with selenium led to no distinguishable differences between the placebo and test group utilizing a dosage of 200 μg.[76] This study was conducted on more than 1,000 subjects from the United States who normally have high plasma levels of selenium. It should be noted, however, that different results in a group of selenium-deficient patients may be observed.[249]

The photoprotective behavior of the nutritional supplementation of epicatechins found in green tea was also the subject of several studies. It is known that intestinal absorption of green tea polyphenols occurs at a fairly rapid pace—normally it takes one to two hours after ingestion before it can be measured in plasma.[272–273] Early studies did not definitively show a correlation between tea intake and inhibition of human cancer development.[274–276] Nevertheless, this does not rule out the possibility of a role for epicatechins in the prevention of other skin-related ailments associated with photodamage, such as photoimmunosuppression and photoaging. In fact, oral administration of epigallocatechin gallate was found to prevent UV-induced erythema.[277] Investigations of similar polyphenols, such as cocoa flavanol supplementation (12-week study), showed reductions in UV-induced erythema.[278] Monitoring photocarcinogenesis, other researchers found that proanthocyanidins from grape seed extract reduced the number and size of carcinomas in hairless mice.[226]

Also of note is the influence of fat intake on non-melanoma skin cancer. In fact, early studies found that high dietary intake of fat reduces the amount of time required for skin tumors to appear in animal models.[279,280] Further, fat intake also influences skin cancer after the initiation phase and during the promotion stage. Indeed, carcinoma can be ameliorated by changing from a high-fat diet to a low-fat diet before the initiation stage. Even more striking, a change in diet prior to the promotion stage can also alleviate tumor promotion. Such findings suggest that even after UV doses capable of inducing a carcinogenic outcome, dietary means may successfully intervene.[249] These studies were conducted using animal models as well as clinical in vivo tests involving more than 100 human patients. In addition to looking at total dietary fat, work was also completed to investigate the nutritional properties of omega fatty acids on mouse skin.[280,281] Diets rich in omega-6 fatty acids correlated with higher incidence of photoimmunosuppression and photocarcinogenesis, while omega-3 fatty acids led to lower rates of carcinogenesis.[282–284] Such results suggest an imperative role for the careful monitoring and scrutinization of diet when conducting nutritional supplementation studies and their effects on skin health.

One would expect that dietary intake would lead to antioxidant distribution deep in tissue and plasma, allowing it to be stored and used for longer periods of time. In remote cases, nutritional supplement provides greater efficacy than topical application. As mentioned, in the case of beta-carotene dietary supplements are more effective at delivery to skin than topical treatment.[54] One reasonable explanation for this phenomenon may be that beta-carotene reaches the skin by sebaceous secretions, which might be a more continuous and robust vehicular delivery route than topical treatment with a formulation. On the other hand, some data in the literature suggest no protection from dietary antioxidant supplementation against UV radiation-induced oxidative stress in skin.[285] Nevertheless, topical treatment with antioxidants remains a quick, effective way to deliver active ingredients to the skin.

Figure 8.28 provides an illustration of the antioxidant capacity of different fruits, vegetables, spices, and nuts. ORAC values, expressed in micromoles of Trolox Equivalents per 100 grams of sample, are plotted for each food type. Interestingly, spices tend to yield the highest ORAC values, probably due to their concentrated nature. ORAC values for berries and nuts are also very high, followed by cruciferous vegetables and other fruits and vegetables. Fruits from the melon family tend

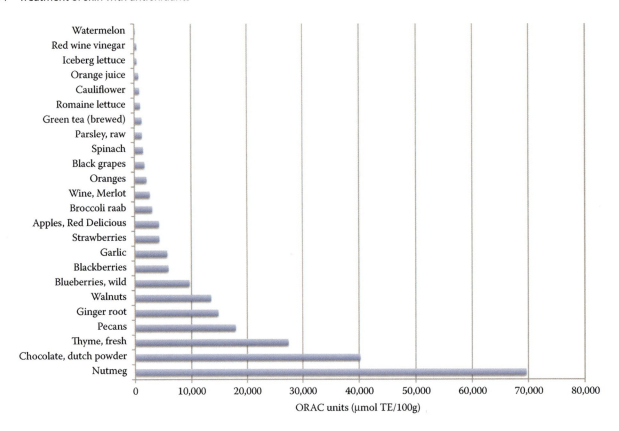

Figure 8.28 ORAC values expressed in micromolar of Trolox equivalents per 100 grams of sample. Data from the USDA website (www.ars.usda.gov).

to yield the lowest ORAC values. This data was obtained from the USDA website[286] but was later withdrawn by the USDA's Nutrient Data Laboratory due to increasing evidence that ORAC values do not correlate with bioactivity of phytonutrients. Nevertheless, the information illustrates the antioxidant capacity of different plant species. One should bear in mind that regardless of a molecule's potential antioxidant properties, bioavailability will ultimately determine if a nutritional supplement is efficacious.

TOPICAL APPLICATION OF ANTIOXIDANTS

Throughout this chapter most of the antioxidant studies summarized focus on topical application unless otherwise noted. Table 8.10 provides a summary of additional studies involving topical application of antioxidants. As compared to dietary intake of antioxidants, in many cases topical application allows: (1) greater concentrations to reach tissues, (2) greater tissue specificity, and (3) reduced side effects to other organs.[95] In some cases, topical application, if high enough concentration is employed, is more efficacious than oral administration. These were the findings of a review researching the combined effects of vitamins C and E by Karen Burke.[287] Unfortunately, not all antioxidants (e.g., from extracts) easily cross the stratum corneum barrier. The fact that some antioxidants are not able to penetrate the skin could be considered a positive benefit in terms of toxicology.[288] Nevertheless, antioxidants deposited on the surface or at the upper layers of the stratum corneum could provide surface protection to the skin analogous to what was discussed in Chapter 1 regarding the delivery of endogenous antioxidants by sebum. In any event, skin permeation and antioxidant stability can be enhanced by utilizing state-of-the-art delivery systems.

FORMULATION CHALLENGES

Chapter 7 discusses lipid peroxidation and its relevance to cosmetic formulations, mainly in the context of prevention of lipid peroxidation by addition of antioxidants. Again, the concept of formulation strategies with antioxidants stems from the need to prevent oxidation within the formulation and also to deliver to the skin an active antioxidant that is bioavailable. In many cases, formulations are based on carrier systems in which oxidation can occur in the oil phase, water phase, or at the interface. More often than not, oxidation occurs at the interface. Some of the hurdles facing formulators in the antioxidant arena are a result of stability issues with antioxidants that are intended to be delivered to skin. Vitamins C and E are two of the most studied ingredients in this area. It is not surprising that so many ester forms of these molecules are available on the commercial specialty chemicals market. As discussed in other sections of this chapter, modified forms of the original antioxidant have oftentimes less efficacy than the parent form. This is the case with vitamin E derivatives, especially

Table 8.10 Additional studies demonstrating benefits of antioxidants in topical formulations.

Antioxidant	Clinical end points studied
Vitamin C (ascorbyl palmitate, magnesium ascorbyl palmitate)	Photoimmunosuppression,[44] Photoaging,[289] Photocarcinogenesis[290]
Vitamin E (alpha-tocopherol acetate, alpha-tocopherol succinate)	Erythema,[291] Photoaging,[14,290] Photoimmunosuppression,[15,16] Photocarcinogenesis[16]
Vitamin A (retinols, carotenoids)	Photoaging[292]
Selenium	Erythema,[78,79] Photocarcinogenesis[79,293]
Silymarin	Photocarcinogenesis,[294,295] Photoimmunosuppression[296]
Green tea polyphenols (epicatechin, epicatechin-3-gallate, epigallocatechin, epigallocatechin-3-gallate)	Erythema, Photoimmunosuppression,[297,298] Photoaging,[299] Photocarcinogenesis[300]
Soy isoflavones (genistein, daidzein, equol)	Erythema,[301,302] Photoaging,[301] Photoimmunosuppression,[303] Photocarcinogenesis[301,303]
Caffeic acid (ferulic acid, caffeic acid, phenethyl ester)	Erythema,[122] Photoimmunosuppression[304]
Apigenin	Photocarcinogenesis[305]
Polypodium leucotomos extract	Erythema,[306] Photoaging,[307] Photocarcinogenesis[307]
Pycnogenol	Inflammation,[308] Photoimmunosuppression,[308] Photocarcinogenesis[308]
Resveratrol	Erythema,[190] Photocarcinogenesis[190]

Source: Chen, L. et al., *J. Am. Acad. Dermatol.*, 67, 1013–1024, 2012.

vitamin E acetate, whose efficacy has been a recurring theme in the literature for the last two decades.

The use of carrier systems represents a real asset for the delivery of antioxidants to skin and can include various types of emulsion, vesicular, or lipid particle systems.[309] Emulsion systems—the first classification of carrier—are dispersions of oil and water and can refer to microemulsions, nanoemulsions, and Pickering emulsions. Microemulsions and nanoemulsions are characterized by the dispersion size of the emulsified phase, while Pickering emulsions refer to a type of emulsion that is stabilized by solid particles (e.g., titanium dioxide, clays, silica).

The second classification of carrier is vesicular systems: liposomes, phytosomes, transfersomes, ethosomes, and niosomes. Liposomes are the most popular vesicular system used in personal care applications and are composed of concentric layers of phospholipid bilayers spherically shaped with a hollow center for the active ingredient. Phytosomes are vesicles of phospholipids that have high affinity for phytocompounds, such as polyphenols. Transfersomes are lipid vesicles that consist of fatty acids and a small amount of ethanol. They are more elastic than liposomes, which improves their deposition characteristics. Ethosomes are lipid vesicles that contain even greater amounts of ethanol, yielding a more flexible vesicle. Niosomes are lamellar vesicles based on nonionic surfactants. Due to the nature of the surfactants in niosomes, crossing the stratum corneum is more facile than in the case with other vesicles.

The third group of carriers is lipid particle systems and consists of lipid microparticles and lipid nanoparticles. Lipid microparticles are created by a process known as microencapsulation where a small solid or liquid droplet is surrounded with a thin layer of shell. Lipid nanoparticles are further categorized as solid lipid nanoparticles and nanostructured carriers. Solid lipid nanoparticles consist of a lipid system in the solid state at room temperature with a thin surfactant coating on the outside as a stabilizer. Nanostructured lipid carriers, on the other hand, are more complex and contain lipids both in the solid and fluid phase. Table 8.11 contains a list of potential carrier systems for antioxidant delivery to skin with a summary of studies and observed effects. Typically, such systems can increase the stability of antioxidants and their permeation efficacy to skin as well as reduce irritation. The reader is referred to the review by Pol and Patravale for a nice introduction to the subject.[310]

ANTIOXIDANT COMBINATIONS

By definition, synergism refers to a process in which two agents used together are greater than the sum of their parts. The term *synergism* is thrown around a lot, even used for outcomes that are in fact additive. In any event, recent years have seen a flurry of antioxidant research toward possible combinations of various antioxidants. More than likely, such ideas evolved from a better understanding of the body's endogenous antioxidant system, which, instead of relying on the activity of a single antioxidant, exploits the multiplicity of an assembly. As discussed in Chapter 3, endogenous glutathione replenishes ascorbic acid, which in turn restores the activity of oxidized alpha-tocopherol. Before bringing a product to market based on multiple antioxidants, knowledge of the interactions and activities of such systems both in vitro and in vivo is imperative.

As shown in Table 8.12, vitamins C and E are probably the most commonly studied antioxidant combinations.

Table 8.11 Lipid-based carrier systems for antioxidants with potential use for delivery to skin.

Carrier	Active ingredients	Effects observed	Year	References
Emulsions				
Microemulsions	Quercetin, vitamin E	Increased skin permeation and diminished irritation	2007	336
Microemulsions	Curcumin	Increased solubility; improved protection against degradation	2009	337
Liquid crystals	Vitamin A palmitate	Sustained release	2003 2008	338,339
Multiple emulsions	Ascorbic acid, vitamin A	Stabilizing effect and improved release profile	2001	340
Vesicular systems				
Liposomes	(−)-Epigallocatechin-3-gallate, retinoic acid	Increased drug deposition	2007	336
Transfersomes	Alpha-tocopherol	Improved skin deposition and photostability	2007	336,341
Niosomes	Tretinoin	Protection against photodegradation	2007	336
Nanotopes	Vitamin E acetate	Increased skin permeation of active	2005	342
Elastic vesicles	Curcumin	Inhibition of UV-induced photoaging	2010	343
Nanotransfersomes	*Punica granatum* extract	Inhibits destruction of endogenous antioxidants and formation of malondialdehyde levels	2011	344
Lipid particulate systems				
Lipid nanoparticles	Retinol, coQ, alpha-lipoic acid, beta-carotene, alpha-tocopherol	Enhanced chemical stability	2007 2009 2009	345–347
Solid lipid nanoparticles	Tretinoin, curcuminoids	Diminished skin irritation; enhanced physical and chemical stability	2007	348–349
Nanostructured lipid carriers	Resveratrol	Greater penetration	2012	350

Source: Pol, A. and Patravale, V., *Household and Personal Care TODAY*, 5–8, 2009.

Two articles appeared by Karen Burke emphasizing the importance of formulating vitamins C and E together, rather than alone, in order to obtain a clinically relevant degree of efficacy.[287,311] Burke recommends a vitamin C (ascorbic acid form) concentration of 15%–20% be used in conjunction with 2%–5% vitamin E (alpha-tocopherol form). Overall, the combination of these two antioxidants has been found to protect skin from sunburn, pigment darkening, photoaging, and photocarcinogenesis.

In another case involving beta-carotene, it was found that delivery of beta-carotene (by dietary supplementation) to skin was slightly more efficacious than a mixture of three carotenoids (beta-carotene, lycopene, and lutein). However, the carotenoid mixture was equally effective as beta-carotene alone at reducing UV-induced erythema in humans.[61] Thus, in this case it may be argued that little synergy exists between carotenoids; however, treatment with smaller doses of each carotenoid (rather than one high beta-carotene supplementation) for patients susceptible to lung cancer (mentioned in the Retinoids section earlier) might be a safer treatment alternative. In yet another study, it was found that dietary supplementation with beta-carotene in combination with vitamin E is more efficacious against UV-induced erythema than beta-carotene alone.[312]

Cell culture studies generated interest in possible synergistic activity of antioxidant combination treatments containing vitamin E and selenium.[313,314] It was reported that vitamin E and selenium operated by distinct protective mechanisms and provided an overall additive antioxidant effect. In contrast, when combinations of the two antioxidants were tested on mouse skin, no synergism or additive effects were found for the mixture.[293]

Table 8.12 In vivo studies investigating combinations of antioxidants.

Antioxidants	Endpoints	Outcome	Year	References
Vitamin E linoleate, magnesium ascorbyl phosphate, butylated hydroxytoluene, nordihydroguaradinic acid	Erythema, immediate pigment darkening (human)	Protective after single topical application	1999	351
Vitamin C, vitamin E, carotenoids, selenium, and proanthocyanidins	Erythema, MMP-1 (mouse)	Oral administration had no effect on erythema, but inhibited MMP-1 expression	2002	352
Lycopene, beta-carotene, alpha-tocopherol, selenium	Erythema, p53 expression, sunburn cells, lipoperoxide (human)	Oral intake resulted in improvement	2003	353
Vitamin C, vitamin E	Erythema, sunburn cells, thymine dimers (pig)	Topical treatment improved all factors	2003	354
Associated bioflavonoids, retinyl palmitate, tocopheryl acetate, and ascorbyl tetraisopalmitate	TEWL, erythema, sunburn cells (mouse)	No effect on TEWL and erythema, but inhibited sunburn cell formation (topical application)	2006	355
Vitamin C, ferulic acid, phloretin	Erythema, thymine dimers, MMP-9, p53, Langerhans cells (human)	Topical treatment effective; proposed that phloretin increases bioavailability of vitamin C and ferulic acid	2008	356
Vitamin C, vitamin E, ferulic acid	Erythema, sunburn cells, thymine dimers, p53, cytokine expression (human)	Topical treatment inhibited all measured factors	2008	357

Finally, it was found that ferulic acid stabilizes vitamins C and E and doubles their photoprotection of skin.[315] The optimal system contained 0.5% ferulic acid, 1% alpha-tocopherol, and 15% L-ascorbic acid. Long-term stability was conducted for 1 month at 45°C. In vivo (porcine skin) efficacy was determined by erythema measurements, histological studies to quantify the number of sunburn cells formed, activity of apoptotic signaling molecules (caspases), and formation of thymine dimers. An increase from fourfold to eightfold protection was observed in the presence of ferulic acid in terms of erythema and the number of sunburn cells. (Minimal erythemal dose, or MED, is the minimum dose required to cause skin reddening 24 hours after UVB exposure.) The number of thymine dimers decreased and a reduction of caspase 3 and caspase 7 was observed, indicating less apoptotic activity.

Overall, there can be many benefits to utilizing combinations of antioxidants. This strategy can improve formulation and delivery of antioxidants, ensuring that the highest concentrations possible come into contact with the skin. Once at the surface of the skin, some antioxidants may permeate better than others (e.g., lipophilic versus hydrophilic). It is possible that one type of antioxidant may make skin more permeable for another. However, many of the mechanisms associated with such processes are still unknown. Also, we should keep in mind that most of the studies in the literature examine combinations of the antioxidants, but do not make a fair comparison of each separately in order to determine if they are simply additive effects, or if true synergism is at play.

USE OF ANTIOXIDANTS IN SUNSCREEN FORMULATIONS

A variety of antioxidants are used in commercial sunscreen formulations to help combat the detrimental effects of UV-induced ROS in skin (Table 8.13). A number of years ago, several studies appeared in the literature with the aim to elucidate the benefits of adding antioxidants to sunscreen formulations.[316-318]

In one study using a human skin equivalent model (MatTek) with two-photon fluorescence microscopy, ROS were monitored in different lamina of skin.[316,317] While sunscreens are very effective at protecting against UV-induced erythema, their findings clearly illustrate a protective benefit of adding antioxidants (vitamin E and diethylhexylsyringlidene malonate) to the sunscreen formulation in terms of reducing the overall number of ROS relative to a placebo containing only the sunscreen filters.[317] This effect (difference between placebo and antioxidant-containing sunscreen) is greater at low SPF values, but it should be noted that the overall amount of ROS decreases with increasing SPF value. Furthermore, some antioxidants behave as prooxidants when exposed to UV radiation. Specifically, Hanson et al. found increases in the number of ROS when chardonnay grape extract, rose extract, and fennel seed

Table 8.13 Commercially available sunscreen formulations containing antioxidants.

Brand name	Supplier	SPF	Sunscreens	Antioxidants
Neutrogena® Clear Face Liquid-Lotion Sunscreen	Johnson & Johnson	55	Avobenzone Homosalate Octisalate Octocrylene Oxybenzone	BHT *Cedrus atlantica* bark extract *Cinnamon zeylanicum* bark extract *Portulaca oleracea* extract
Botanical Sunscreen SPF 50 Tinted Face Mineral Lotion	Australian Gold®	50	Titanium dioxide Zinc oxide	*Butyrospermum parkii* (shea) butter *Eucalyptus globulus* leaf extract *Porphyra umbilicalis* (red algae) extract *Terminalia ferdinandiana* (Kakadu plum) fruit extract Tocopheryl acetate Vitamin E
CeraVe® Suncare Sunscreen Face	CeraVe®	50	Titanium dioxide Zinc oxide	Ascorbic acid *Avena sativa* (oat) kernel extract Tocopheryl acetate BHT
Banana Boat® Sport Performance® Continuous Spray Sunscreen	Edgewell™ Personal Care	30	Avobenzone Homosalate Octisalate Octocrylene Oxybenzone	Aloe vera (*Aloe barbadensis*) extract Ascorbic acid Tocopheryl acetate
Coppertone® Oil Free Sunscreen Lotion for Faces	Bayer	50+	Avobenzone Homosalate Octisalate Octocrylene Oxybenzone	Tocopherol (vitamin E) Sodium ascorbyl phosphate
Hawaiian Tropic® Lotion Sunscreen	Edgewell™ Personal Care	8	Octocrylene Oxybenzone	*Aloe barbadensis* (Aloe vera) leaf juice Tocopheryl acetate (vitamin E) Ascorbic acid (vitamin C) Retinyl palmitate (vitamin A) *Plumeria acutifolia* (plumeria) flower extract *Mangifera indica* (mango) fruit extract *Psidium guajava* (guava) fruit extract *Carica papaya* (papaya) fruit extract *Passiflora incarnata* (passionflower) fruit extract *Colocasia antiquorum* root extract
DermaE® Antioxidant Natural Sunscreen Body	DermaE®	30	Zinc oxide	Organic *Camellia sinensis* (green tea) leaf extract Sodium ascorbyl phosphate (vitamin C) Tocopheryl acetate (vitamin E) *Carthamus tinctorius* (safflower) seed oil

extract were used in combination with the sunscreen filters. In contrast, in an analysis of lipid hydroperoxides present in the stratum corneum—formed as a result of UV exposure—they found that vitamin C, vitamin E, green tea extract, tetrahydrocurcuminoids, and Emblica fruit extract afforded greater protection than the placebo system containing only the UV filters.[317] Other antioxidants had pro-oxidant activity, while some combinations of antioxidants ameliorated prooxidant effects. Overall, it appears that the addition of antioxidants to sun protection formulas can provide superior benefits if there are no pro-oxidant effects, as evidenced by scientific literature and the number of commercial formulations containing antioxidants.

In recent years, a number of studies have evaluated natural materials from plant sources as photoprotectants.[319] Motivation for such development stems from photosensitization and contact dermatitis issues with synthetic sunscreens.[320] While a large quantity of herbal extracts show much promise in the pre- and post-treatment of solar exposed skin, synthetic and mineral sunscreens provide superior protection.[321] To date, there is still no natural sunscreen that is approved by any of the major regulatory agencies. Therefore, it is not surprising that many sunscreen formulations contain natural ingredients, which supplement the activity of synthetic and mineral sunscreens.

ANTIOXIDANT RATING SYSTEMS

Until relatively recently, no antioxidant rating system existed for antioxidant efficacy when topically applied to skin. A number of years ago, a Skin Antioxidative Protection (SAP) system was proposed by Jung et al., utilizing a measurement technique involving electron spin resonance to monitor free radicals in ex vivo sections of skin. SAP describes the ability of skin, relying on its endogenous antioxidant system or fortified with antioxidants, to remove free radicals/ROS.[322] The electron spin resonance measurement technique monitors the reduction of a test radical (probe) in skin, in which case untreated skin would have a baseline of 100%. The results from this study demonstrate the ability of topically applied antioxidants, such as green tea extract, coQ, and an antioxidant mixture (retinol, ascorbyl palmitate, and alpha-tocopherol), to increase the SAP of skin.

The measurement of food antioxidant capacity is commonly carried out using the oxygen radical absorbance capacity (ORAC) assay (Chapter 6) or analysis by emitted light-relative antioxidant capacity (ABEL-RAC). The use of these procedures for measuring antioxidant capacity of skin care formulations was recently proposed.[323] They are both standardized techniques intended to provide uniform results regardless of the testing laboratory. While these techniques were offered as a possible metric for skin care applications, there has not been any type of universal adaptation in their implementation. Furthermore, we must also keep in mind that formulation vehicle and chemical properties of the antioxidant will ultimately determine if it can be delivered to either the stratum corneum or the viable layers of the epidermis. If an antioxidant remains on the surface of skin, its antioxidant capacity may indicate something very different than if it penetrates to lower layers. For example, at the surface it may be more susceptible to oxidation and may not confer protection against free radical damage to viable cells in the lower layers. On the other hand, it could confer more protection to intercellular lipids of the stratum corneum. In any event, an antioxidant rating could be misleading to the general public if it does not factor proper tissue delivery.

CONCLUDING REMARKS

Numerous opportunities exist for the effective treatment of skin with antioxidants. A wealth of research, mostly conducted within the last two decades, demonstrates the value of topical application of skin with antioxidants to diminish a variety of conditions caused by solar exposure, including erythema, photoaging, photoimmunosuppression, and photocarcinogenesis. Equally intriguing, the molecular mechanisms of antioxidant protection behind many of these events are just now starting to be understood, alongside the immunomodulating properties of many of the phyto-antioxidants. Increasingly, natural ingredients are making inroads into personal care formulations. Botanical extracts represent an important aspect of this movement and their use in a myriad of cosmetic formulations demonstrates their utility and versatility. They are loaded with natural polyphenols that protect the plant from harsh environmental and solar effects. Today, most sunscreen formulations contain antioxidants to offer supplemental protection to that supplied by solar filters. With the development of many novel carrier systems, antioxidants can be delivered more efficiently to skin and without irritation. An understanding of combinations of antioxidants is in its infancy but, based on initial studies, offers many prospectives.

REFERENCES

1. Beckman K, Ames B. *Physiol Rev.* 1998;78:547–581.
2. Stahl W, Sies H. Protection against solar radiation—Protective properties of antioxidants. In: Giacomoni P, (Ed.). *Sun Protection in Man.* Amsterdam, the Netherlands: Elsevier; 2001.
3. Kamimura M, Matsuzawa T. *J Vitaminol (Kyoto).* 1968;14:150–159.
4. Norkus E et al. *Photochem Photobiol.* 1993;57:613–615.
5. Trevithick J, Mitton K. *Biochem Mol Biol Int.* 1993;31:869–878.
6. Nabi Z et al. *Curr Probl Dermatol.* 2001;29:175–186.
7. Rangarajan M, Zatz J. *J Cosmet Sci.* 2001;52:35–50.
8. Baschong W et al. *J Cosmet Sci.* 2001;52:155–161.
9. van Henegouwen GB et al. *J Photochem Photobiol B.* 1995;29:45–51.
10. Kramer-Stickland K, Liebler D. *J Invest Dermatol.* 1998;111:302–307.
11. Burke K. Topical nutritional antioxidants. In: Draelos Z, Thaman L, (Eds.) *Cosmetic Formulation of Skin Care Products.* New York: Taylor & Francis; 2006. pp. 377–402.
12. Chen L et al. The role of antioxidants in photoprotection: A critical review. *J Am Acad Dermatol.* 2012. doi: 10.1016/j.jaad.2012.02.009.

13. Lopez-Torres M et al. *Br J Dermatol.* 1998;138:207–215.
14. Jurkiewicz B et al. *J Invest Dermatol.* 1995;104:484–488.
15. Steenvoorden D, Beijersbergen van Henegouwen G. *Int J Radiat Biol.* 1999;75:747–755.
16. Gensler H, Magdaleno M. *Nutr Cancer.* 1991;15:97–106.
17. Thiele J, Dreher F. Antioxidant defense systems in skin. In: Elsner P, Maibach H, (Eds.). *Cosmeceuticals and Active Cosmetics: Drugs Versus Cosmetics.* Boca Raton, FL: Taylor & Francis; 2005. pp. 37–87.
18. Ricciarelli R et al. *Free Radic Biol Med.* 1999;27:729–737.
19. Gerrish K, Gensler H. *Nutr Cancer.* 1993;19:125–133.
20. Tsoureli-Nikita E et al. *Int J Dermatol.* 2002;41:146–150.
21. Malafa M et al. *Surgery.* 2002;131:85–91.
22. Malafa et al. *Ann Surg Oncol.* 2002;9:1023–1032.
23. Chen W et al. *Nutr Cancer.* 1997;29:205–211.
24. McVean M, Liebler D et al. *Mol Carcinog.* 1999;24:169–176.
25. Burke K, Keen, CL et al. *Nutr Cancer.* 2000;38:87–97.
26. Potapenko A et al. *Arch Dermatol Res.* 1984;276:12–16.
27. Berton T et al. *Mol Carcinog.* 1998;23:175–184.
28. Record I et al. *Nutr Cancer.* 1991;16:219–225.
29. Trevithick J et al. *Arch Biochem Biophys.* 1992;296:575–582.
30. Potokar M et al. *Eur J Lipid Sci.* 2006;92:406–410.
31. Gensler H et al. *Nutr Cancer.* 1996;26:183–191.
32. Azzi A et al. *Arch Biochem Biophys* 2016;595:100–108.
33. Hart M. *Schoch Lett.* 1990;40:48.
34. Saperstein H et al. *Arch Dermatol.* 1984;120:906–908.
35. Baumann L, Spencer J. *Dermatol Surg.* 1999;25:311–315.
36. Jenkins M et al. *J Burn Care Rehabil.* 1986;7:309–312.
37. Khoosal D et al. *Can Fam Physician.* 2006;52:855–856.
38. Rangarajan M, Zatz J. *J Cosmet Sci.* 2001;52:225–236.
39. Phillips C et al. *J Invest Dermatol.* 1994;103:228–232.
40. Pinnell S et al. *Arch Dermatol.* 1987;123:1684–1686.
41. Peterkofsky B. *Am J Clin Nutr.* 1991;54:1135S–1140S.
42. Parvez S et al. *Phytother Res.* 2006;20:921–934.
43. Darr D et al. *Br J Dermatol.* 1992;127:247–253.
44. Nakamura T et al. *J Invest Dermatol.* 1997;109:20–24.
45. Nayama S et al. *Biol Pharm Bull.* 1999;22:1301–1305.
46. Pinnell S et al. *Dermatol Surg.* 2001;27:137–142.
47. Davidson J et al. *J Biol Chem.* 1997;272:345–352.
48. Golubitskii G et al. *J Anal Chem.* 2007;62:742–747.
49. Gallarate M et al. *Int J Pharm.* 1999;188:233–241.
50. Ross A. Vitamin A and carotenoids. In: Shils M, Shike M, Ross A, Caballero B, Cousins R, (Eds.). *Modern Nutrition in Health and Disease.* 10th ed. Baltimore, MD: Lippincott Williams & Wilkins; 2006. pp. 351–375.
51. Bissett D. Anti-aging skin care formulations. In: Draelos Z, Thaman L, (Eds.). *Cosmetic Formulation of Skin Care Products.* New York: Taylor & Francis; 2006. pp. 167–186.
52. Fisher G, Voorhees J. *FASEB J.* 1996;10:1002–1013.
53. Bauer E et al. *J Invest Dermatol.* 1983;81:162–169.
54. Darvin M et al. *J Dermatol Sci.* 2011;64:53–58.
55. Darvin M et al. *Exp Dermatol.* 2011;20:125–129.
56. Mathews-Roth M et al. *J Invest Dermatol.* 1972;59:349–383.
57. Garmyn M et al. *Exp Dermatol.* 1995;4:104–111.
58. Wolf C et al. *J Invest Dermatol.* 1988;90:55–57.
59. Noonan F et al. *Clin Exp Immunol.* 1996;103:54–60.
60. Fuller C et al. *Am J Clin Nutr.* 1992;56:684–690.
61. Heinrich U et al. *J Nutr.* 2003;133:98–101.
62. Lee J et al. *Proc Soc Exp Biol Med.* 2000;223:170–174.
63. Krinsky N. *J Nutr.* 1989;119:123–126.
64. Greenberg E et al. *N Engl J Med.* 1990;323:789–795.
65. Green A et al. *Lancet.* 1999;354:723–729.
66. Bayerl C. *Acta Dermatoven APA.* 2008;17:160–166.
67. Kar H. *Indian J Dermatol Venereol Leprol.* 2003;69:92–94.
68. The ATBC Study Group, *N Engl J Med.* 1994;330:1029–1035.
69. Omenn G et al. *J Natl Cancer Inst.* 1996;88:1550–1559.
70. Food and Nutrition Board & Institute of Medicine, *Dietary Reference Intakes for Vitamin C, Vitamin E, Selenium, and Carotenoids.* Washington, DC: National Academy Press; 2000.
71. Biesalski H, Obermueller-Jevic U. *Arch Biochem Biophys.* 2001;389:1–6.
72. Brown K, Arthur, J. *Public Health Nutr.* 2001;4:593–599.
73. Rayman M. *Proc Nutr Soc.* 2005;64:527–542.
74. Clark L et al. *Nutr Cancer.* 1984;6:13–21.
75. Foster H. *J Orthomol Med.* 1998;13:8–10.
76. Clark L et al. *JAMA.* 1996;276:1957–1963.
77. Duffield-Lillico A et al. *J Natl Cancer Inst.* 2003;95:1477–1481.
78. Burke K et al. *Photodermatol Photoimmunol Photomed.* 1992;9:52–57.
79. Burke K et al. *Nutr Cancer.* 1992;17:123–137.
80. Cummins L, Kimuka E. *Toxicol Appl Pharmacol.* 1971;20:189–196.
81. Bereston E. *J Am Med Assoc.* 1954;157:1246–1247.
82. Lin C et al. *Acta Pharmacol Sin.* 2011;32:1181–1190.
83. Vinson J, Anamandla S. *IFSCC Mag.* 2005;8(4):1–6.
84. Prahl S et al. *Biofactors.* 2008;32:245–255.
85. Zhang M et al. *Int J Cosmet Sci.* 2012;34:273–279.
86. Fuller B et al. *J Cosmet Dermatol.* 2006;5:30–38.
87. Blatt T, Littarru G. *Biofactors.* 2011;37:381–385.
88. Inui M et al. *Biofactors.* 2008;32:237–243.
89. Muta-Takada K et al. *Biofactors.* 2009;35:435–441.
90. Hoppe U et al. *Biofactors.* 1999;9:371–378.
91. López L et al. *PLoS One.* 2010;5:e11897.
92. Westerhof W, Kooyers T. *Cosmet Dermatol.* 2005;4:55–59.
93. Deneke S. *Curr Top Cell Regul.* 2000;36:151–180.
94. Munday R. *Free Radic Biol Med.* 1989;7:659–673.
95. Podda M et al. Activity of alpha-lipoic acid in the protection against oxidative stress in skin. In: Thiele J, Elsner P, (Eds.). *Oxidants and Antioxidants in Cutaneous Biology. Curr Probl Dermatol.* 29. Basel, Switzerland: Karger; 2001.

96. Podda M et al. *Biochem Pharmacol.* 1996;52:627–633.
97. Tsuji-Naito K et al. *Connect Tissue Res.* 2010;51:378–387.
98. Beitner H et al. *Br J Dermatol.* 2003;149:841–849.
99. Segall A et al. *J Cosmet Sci.* 2004;55:449–461.
100. Emonet N et al. *J Photochem Photobiol B.* 1997;40:84–90.
101. Morley N et al. *J Photochem Photobiol B.* 2003;72:55–60.
102. Villarama C, Maibach H. *Int J Cosmet Sci.* 2005;27:147–153.
103. Ammar N et al. *JASMR.* 2010;5:141–152.
104. André P, Villain F. *Int J Cosmet Sci.* 2017;39:355–360.
105. Bosch R et al. *Antioxidants (Basel).* 2015;4:248–268.
106. Działo M et al. *Int J Mol Sci.* 2016;17:160. doi: 10.3390/ijms17020160.
107. Jung K et al. *Int J Cosmet Sci.* 2017;39:217–223.
108. Montes de Oca M et al. *Photochem Photobiol.* 2017;93:956–974.
109. Saric S, Sivamani R. *Int J Mol Sci.* 2016;17:1521. doi: 10.3390/ijms17091521.
110. Singh M et al. *Biomed Res Int.* 2014:Article ID 243452. doi: 10.1155/2014/.
111. Lambert J et al. *Am J Clin Nutr.* 2005;81(suppl):284S–291S.
112. Afaq F, Mukhtar H. *Exp Dermatol.* 2006;15:678–684.
113. Hsu H. *J Am Acad Dermatol.* 2005;52:1049–1059.
114. Katiyar S. *Int J Oncol.* 2005;26:169–176.
115. Pinnell S. *J Am Acad Dermatol.* 2003;48:1–19.
116. Sies H, Stahl W. *Annu Rev Nutr.* 2004;24:173–200.
117. Svobodová A et al. *Biomed Papers.* 2003;147:137–145.
118. Yusuf N et al. *Photodermatol Photoimmunol Photomed.* 2007;23:48–56.
119. Bourne L, Rice-Evans C. *Biochem Biophys Res Comm.* 1998;253:222–227.
120. Zhang L et al. *Int J Pharm.* 2010;399:44–51.
121. Saija A et al. *J Sci Food Agric.* 1999;79:476–480.
122. Saija A et al. *Int J Pharm.* 2000;199:39–47.
123. Song H et al. *Korean J Physiol Pharmacol.* 2008;12:343–347.
124. Wang Q et al. *J Cosmet Sci.* 2011;62:483–503.
125. Perchellet et al. *Basic Life Sci.* 1992;59:783–801.
126. Lo C et al. *Melanoma Res.* 2011;21:267–273.
127. Manosroi A et al. *Pharm Biol.* 2011;49:553–562.
128. Manosroi A et al. *Pharm Biol.* 2011;49:1190–1203.
129. Kim Y. *Biol Pharm Bull.* 2007;30:1052–1055.
130. OyetakinWhite P et al. *Oxid Med Cell Longev.* 2012:Article ID 560682. doi: 10.1155/2012/.
131. Meeran S et al. *Clin Cancer Res.* 2006;12:2272–2280.
132. Katiyar S et al. *Cancer Prev Res (Phila).* 2010;3:179–189.
133. Vayalil P et al. *Carcinogenesis.* 2003;24:927–936.
134. Isbrucker R et al. *Food Chem Toxicol.* 2006;44:636–650.
135. Saric S et al. *Antioxidants (Basel).* 2016;6:pii: E2. doi: 10.3390/antiox6010002.
136. Rahman Mazumder M, Hongsprabhas P. *Biomed Pharmacother* 2016;82:379–392.
137. Chevallier A. *The Encyclopedia of Medicinal Plants.* London, UK: Dorling Kindersley; 1996.
138. Vaid M, Katiyar S. *Int J Oncol.* 2010;36:1053–1060.
139. Maheshwari R et al. *Life Sci.* 2006;78:2081–2087.
140. Goel A et al. *Biochem Pharmacol.* 2007;75:787–809.
141. Kilfoyle B et al. The use of quercetin and curcumin in skin care consumer products. In: Dayan N, Kromidas L, (Eds.). *Formulating, Packaging, and Marketing of Natural Cosmetic Products.* Hoboken, NJ: John Wiley & Sons; 2011.
142. Thangapazham R et al. *Adv Exp Med Biol.* 2007;595:343–357.
143. Huang M et al. *J Cell Biochem Suppl.* 1997;27:26–34.
144. Conney A et al. *Adv Enzyme Regul.* 1991;31:385–396.
145. Huang M et al. *Cancer Res.* 1988;48:5941–5946.
146. Marín Y et al. *Melanoma Res.* 2007;17:274–283.
147. Phan T et al. *J Trauma.* 2001;51:927–931.
148. Gopinath D et al. *Biomaterials.* 2004;25:1911–1917.
149. Kumar V et al. *Indian J Physiol Pharmacol.* 2002;46:209–217.
150. Ma Z et al. *J Biomed Mater Res A.* 2008;86:300–310.
151. Bisht S et al. *J Nanobiotechnol.* 2007;5. doi:10.1186/477-3155-5-3.
152. Patel N et al. *Drug Dev Ind Pharm.* 2009;35:234–242.
153. Patel N et al. *Pharm Dev Technol.* 2009;14:80–89.
154. Hussain Z et al. *Colloids Surf B Biointerfaces.* 2017;150:223–241.
155. Vaughn A et al. *Phytother Res.* 2016;30:1243–1264.
156. Baghel S et al. *World J Pharm Pharmaceut Sci.* 2012;1:146–160.
157. Karuppagounder V et al. *Drug Discov Today.* 2016;21:632–639.
158. Afanas'ev I et al. *Biochem Pharmacol.* 1989;38:1763–1769.
159. Bors W et al. *Methods Enzymol.* 1990;186:343–355.
160. Bors W et al. *Methods Enzymol.* 1994;234:420–429.
161. Casagrande R et al. *J Photochem Photobiol B: Biol.* 2006;84:21–27.
162. Erden Inal M et al. *Toxicology.* 2000;154:21–29.
163. Erden Inal M et al. *Clin Exp Dermatol.* 2001;26:536–539.
164. Sim G et al. *Arch Pharm Res.* 2007;30:290–298.
165. Hatahet T et al. *Eur J Pharm Biopharm.* 2016;108:41–53.
166. Casagrande R et al. *Int J Pharm.* 2006;328:183–190.
167. Bonina F et al. *Int J Pharm.* 1996;145:87–94.
168. Kim H et al. *Arch Pharm Res.* 2004;27:763–768.
169. Olivella M et al. *Pharm Dev Technol.* 2007;12:481–484.
170. Kitagawa S et al. *J Pharm Pharmacol.* 2009;61:855–860.
171. Vicentini F et al. *Eur J Pharm Biopharm.* 2008;69:948–957.
172. Scalia S, Mezzena M. *J Pharm Biomed Anal.* 2009;49:90–94.
173. Casagrande R et al. *AAPS PharmSci.* 2006;7:E64–E71.
174. Smith G et al. *J Photochem Photobiol A: Chem.* 2000;136:87–91.
175. Choquenet B et al. *J Nat Prod.* 2008;71:1117–1118.

176. Frutos P et al. *Span J Agric Res.* 2004;2:191–202.
177. Bele A et al. *Asian J Plant Sci.* 2010;9:209–214.
178. Gali-Muhtasib H et al. *Photochem Photobiol.* 1998;67:663–668.
179. Gali-Muhtasib H et al. *Oncol Rep.* 1999;6:847–853.
180. Gali-Muhtasib H et al. *Nutr Cancer.* 2000;37:73–77.
181. Chaudhuri R. *Sunscreens: Regulations and Commercial Development.* Boca Raton, FL: Taylor & Francis; 2005.
182. Chaudhuri R et al. *Cosmet & Toil.* 2004;119:59–68.
183. Smoliga J et al. *Mol Nutr Food Res.* 2011;55:1129–1141.
184. Renaud S, de Lorgeril M. *Lancet.* 1992;339:1523–1526.
185. Wu J et al. *Int J Mol Med.* 2001;8:3–17.
186. Jang M et al. *Science.* 1997;275:218–220.
187. Ndiaye M et al. *Arch Biochem Biophys.* 2011;508:164–170.
188. Aziz M et al. *FASEB J.* 2005;19:1193–1195.
189. Aziz M et al. *Photochem Photobiol.* 2005;81:25–31.
190. Afaq F et al. *Toxicol Appl Pharmacol.* 2003;186:28–37.
191. Kundu J et al. *Carcinogenesis.* 2006;27:1465–1474.
192. Baxter R. *J Cosmet Dermatol.* 2008;7:2–77.
193. Adhami V et al. *Neoplasia.* 2003;5:74–82.
194. Chen M et al. *Zhong Nan Da Xue Xue Bao Yi Xue Ban.* 2006;31:635–639.
195. Reagan-Shaw S et al. *Oncogene.* 2004;23:5151–5160.
196. Reagan-Shaw S et al. *Photochem Photobiol.* 2008;84:415–421.
197. Roy P et al. *Pharm Res.* 2009;26:211–217.
198. Liu Y et al. *Eur J Pharmacol.* 2011;650:130–137.
199. Hung C et al. *Biol Pharm Bull.* 2008;31:955–962.
200. Emer J et al. *Semin Cutan Med Surg.* 2011;30:148–155.
201. Syed D, Mukhtar H. *Pigment Cell Melanoma Res.* 2011;24:688–702.
202. Mukherjee P et al. *Phytomedicine.* 2011;19:64–73.
203. Katiyar S. *Cancer Lett.* 2007;18:1–11.
204. Bonina F et al. *J Cosmet Sci.* 2002;53:321–335.
205. Trombetta D et al. *Phytother Res.* 2005;19:29–33.
206. Aquino R et al. *J Ethnopharmacol.* 2002;79:183–191.
207. Saliou C et al. *Free Radic Biol Med.* 2001;30:154–160.
208. Afaq F et al. *Photochem Photobiol.* 2005;81:38–45.
209. Syed D et al. *Photochem Photobiol.* 2006;82:398–405.
210. Afaq F et al. *Int J Cancer.* 2005;113:423–433.
211. Saija A et al. *Int J Cosmet Sci.* 1998;20:331–342.
212. Tsukahara K et al. *Biol Pharm Bull.* 2001;24:998–1003.
213. Bonina F et al. *J Pharm Pharmacol.* 2000;52:1279–1285.
214. Michel P. *Presse Med.* 1986;15:1450–1454.
215. Chan P et al. *J Environ Sci Health C Environ Carcinog Ecotoxicol Rev.* 2007;25:211–244.
216. Zimmermann M et al. *Cell Mol Biol (Noisy-le-grand).* 2002;48:613–623.
217. Dubber M, Kanfer I. *J Pharm Pharmaceut Sci.* 2004;7:303–309.
218. Strømgaard K, Nakanishi K. *Angew Chem Int Ed.* 2004;43:1640–1658.
219. dal Belo S et al. *Skin Pharmacol Physiol.* 2009;22:299–304.
220. Chuarienthong P et al. *Int J Cosmet Sci.* 2010;32:99–106.
221. Szczurko O et al. *BMC Complement Altern Med.* 2011;15:11:21.
222. dal Belo S et al. *Phytother Res.* 2011;25:1854–1860.
223. Bomser J et al. *Cancer Lett.* 1999;135:151–157.
224. Bomser J et al. *Chem Biol Interact.* 2000;127:45–59.
225. Katiyar S. *Mol Nutr Food Res.* 2008;52:S71–S76.
226. Mittal A et al. *Carcinogenesis.* 2003;24:1379–1388.
227. Zhao J et al. *Carcinogenesis.* 1999;20:1737–1745.
228. Sharma S et al. *Mol Cancer Ther.* 2007;6:995–1005.
229. Mantena S, Katiyar S. et al. *Free Radic Biol Med.* 2006;40:1603–1614.
230. Kim Y et al. *Arch Pharm Res.* 2000;23:396–400.
231. Heo M et al. *Mutat Res.* 2001;496:47–59.
232. Kim Y et al. *J Cosmet Sci.* 2002;53:27–34.
233. Kroto H et al. *Nature.* 1985;318:162–163.
234. Markovic Z, Trajkovic V. *Biomaterials.* 2008;29:3561–3573.
235. Xiao L et al. *Biomed Pharmacother.* 2005;59:351–358.
236. Saitoh Y et al. *J Photochem Photobiol B.* 2011;102:69–76.
237. Kato S et al. *J Nanosci Nanotechnol.* 2011;11:3814–3823.
238. Rouse J et al. *Nano Lett.* 2007;7:155–160.
239. Nelson M et al. *Toxicol Ind Health.* 1993;9:623–630.
240. Huczko A et al. *Fullerene Sci Techn.* 1999;7:935–939.
241. Kato S et al. *Basic Clin Pharmacol Toxicol.* 2009;104:483–487.
242. Halford B. *Chem Eng News.* 2006;84:47.
243. Inui S et al. *Nanotechnol.* 2011;7:238–241.
244. Fujimoto T et al. *Lasers Surg Med.* 2012;44:685–694.
245. Lens M. *Recent Pat Biotechnol.* 2009;3:118–123.
246. Lens M. *Recent Pat Biotechnol.* 2011;5:67–73.
247. World Health Organization (www.who.int). 2012.
248. United States Department of Agriculture (www.ers.usda.gov). 2012.
249. Black H, Rhodes L. Systemic photoprotection: Dietary intervention and therapy. In: Giacomoni P (Ed.). *Sun Protection in Man.* Amsterdam, Netherlands: Elsevier; 2001.
250. Black H et al. *Cancer Res.* 1978;38:1384–1387.
251. De Rios G et al. *J Invest Dermatol.* 1978;70:123–125.
252. Peterson A et al. *J Invest Dermatol.* 1980;75:408–410.
253. Black H et al. *Photochem Photobiol.* 1984;40:69–75.
254. Koone M, Black H. *J Invest Dermatol.* 1986;87:343–347.
255. J. Cordy, Butylated hydroxytoluene, www.TheCosmeticChemist.com, March 15, 2017.
256. Williams G et al. *Food Chem Toxicol.* 1999;37:1027–1038.
257. Epstein J. *Photochem Photobiol.* 1977;25:211–213.
258. Mathews-Roth M, Krinsky N. *Photochem Photobiol.* 1985;42:35–38.
259. Stahl W. *Arch Biochem Biophys.* 2016;595:125–131.
260. Kune G et al. *Nutr Cancer.* 1992;18:237–244.
261. IARC Working Group on the Evaluation of Cancer-Preventive Agents. Carotenoids. *Handbooks of Cancer Prevention;* 1998. Vol 2, Lyon, France.
262. Levy J, Sharoni Y. The inside-out concept as complement to the use of topical sunscreen: The case for endogenous photoprotection from sunlight by natural dietary actives such as tomato carotenoids. In: Dayan

N, Kromidas L, (Eds.). *Formulating, Packaging, and Marketing of Natural Cosmetic Products*. Hoboken, NJ: John Wiley & Sons; 2011. pp. 313–327.
263. Stahl W et al. *J Nutr*. 2001;131:1449–1451.
264. Aust O et al. *Int J Vitam Nutr Res*. 2005;75:54–60.
265. Heinrich U et al. *Skin Pharmacol Physiol*. 2006;19:224–231.
266. Darvin M et al. *Eur J Pharm Biopharm*. 2008;69:943–947.
267. Dunham W et al. *Proc Natl Acad Sci USA*. 1982;79:7532–7536.
268. Werninghaus K et al. *Arch Dermatol*. 1994;130:1257–1261.
269. Kagan V et al. *Free Radic Res Commun*. 1992;16:51–64.
270. Eberlein-König B et al. *J Am Acad Dermatol*. 1998;38:45–48.
271. Fuchs J, Kern H. *Free Radic Biol Med*. 1998;25:1006–1012.
272. Afaq F, Katiyar S. *Mini-Rev Med Chem*. 2011;11:1200–1215.
273. Benzie I et al. *Nutr Cancer*. 1999;34:83–87.
274. Kinden L et al. *Br J Cancer*. 1988;58:397–401.
275. La Vecchia C et al. *Nutr Cancer*. 1992;17:27–31.
276. Goldbohm R et al. *J Natl Cancer Inst*. 1996;88:93–100.
277. Jeon H et al. *Skin Pharmacol Physiol*. 2009;22:137–141.
278. Heinrich U et al. *J Nutr*. 2006;136:1565–1569.
279. Black H et al. *Nutr Cancer*. 1983;5:59–68.
280. Black H et al. *Cancer Res*. 1985;45:6254–6259.
281. Black H et al. *Photochem Photobiol*. 1992;56:195–199.
282. Reeve V et al. *Cancer Lett*. 1996;29:271–279.
283. Black H et al. *Photochem Photobiol*. 1995;62:964–969.
284. Orengo I et al. *Photochem Photobiol*. 1989;49:71–77.
285. McArdle F et al. *Am J Clin Nutr*. 2004;80:1270–1275.
286. USDA Database for the Oxygen Radical Absorbance Capacity (ORAC) of Selected Foods, Release 2—Prepared by Nutrient Data Laboratory, Beltsville Human Nutrition Research Center (BHNRC), Agricultural Research Service (ARS), U.S. Department of Agriculture (USDA). 2010.
287. Burke K. Photoprotection of the skin with vitamins C and E: Antioxidants and synergies. In: Pappas A, (Ed.). *Nutrition and Skin: Lessons for Anti-Aging, Beauty and Healthy Skin. Part 1*. New York: Springer; 2011. pp. 43–58.
288. Pouillot A, Polla L, Tacchini P, Neequaye A, Polla A, Polla B. Natural antioxidants and their effects on the skin. In: Dayan N, Kromidas L, (Eds.). *Formulating, Packaging, and Marketing of Natural Cosmetic Products*. Hoboken, NJ: John Wiley & Sons; 2011.
289. Traikovich S. *Arch Otolaryngol Head Neck Surg*. 1999;125:1091–1098.
290. Bissett D et al. *Photodermatol Photoimmunol Photomed*. 1990;7:56–62.
291. Dreher F et al. *Dermatol*. 1999;198:52–55.
292. Olsen E et al. *J Am Acad Dermatol*. 1997;37:217–226.
293. Burke K et al. *J Am Acad Dermatol*. 2003;49:458–472.
294. Katiyar S et al. *J Natl Cancer Inst*. 1997;89:556–566.
295. Lahiri-Chatterjee M et al. *Cancer Res*. 1999;21:1213–1222.
296. Katiyar S et al. *Int J Oncol*. 2002;21:1213–1222.
297. Katiyar S et al. *Photochem Photobiol*. 1999;69:148–153.
298. Camouse M et al. *Exp Dermatol*. 2009;18:522–526.
299. Kim J et al. *Skin Pharmacol Appl Skin Physiol*. 2001;14:11–19.
300. Lu Y et al. *Proc Natl Acad Sci USA*. 2002;99:12455–12460.
301. Wei H et al. *J Nutr*. 2003;133:3811S–3819S.
302. Lin J et al. *Photodermatol Photoimmunol Photomed*. 2008;24:61–66.
303. Widyarini S et al. *Photochem Photobiol*. 2001;74:465–470.
304. Staniforth V et al. *Carcinogenesis*. 2006;27:1803–1181.
305. Birt D et al. *Anticancer Res*. 1997;17:85–91.
306. Gonzalez S et al. *Photodermatol Photoimmunol Photomed*. 1997;13:50–60.
307. Alcaraz M et al. *Photodermatol Photoimmunol Photomed*. 1999;15:120–126.
308. Sime S, Reeve V. *Photochem Photobiol*. 2004;79:193–198.
309. Saroj S et al. *Asian J Pharm Clin Res*. 2012;5 (Suppl 3):4–9.
310. Pol A, Patravale V. *Household and Personal Care TODAY*. 2009; (4):5–8.
311. Burke K. *Dermatol Ther*. 2007;20:314–321.
312. Stahl W et al. *Am J Clin Nutr*. 2000;71:795–798.
313. Borek C et al. *Proc Natl Acad Sci USA*. 1986;83:1490–1494.
314. Noaman E et al. *Biol Trace Elem Res*. 2002;86:55–64.
315. Lin F et al. *J Invest Dermatol*. 2005;125:826–832.
316. Hanson K, Clegg R. *J Cosmet Sci*. 2003;54:589–598.
317. Hanson K et al. *Cosmet & Toil*. 2011;126(11):710–717.
318. Maia Campos P, Gaspar L. *Int J Pharm*. 2007;343:181–189.
319. Saewan N, Jimtaisong A. *J Cosmet Dermatol*. 2015;14:47–63.
320. Cefali L et al. *Int J Cosmet Sci*. 2016;38:346–353.
321. Radice M et al. *Filoterapia*. 2016;114:144–162.
322. Jung K et al. *SÖFW J*. 2006;132:38–44.
323. Palmer D, Kitchin J. *J Drug Dermatol*. 2010;9:11–15.
324. Roshchupkin D et al. *Arch Dermatol Res*. 1979;266:91–94.
325. Khettab N et al. *Biochimie*. 1988;70:1709–1713.
326. Montenegro L et al. *Int J Cosmet Sci*. 1995;17:91–103.
327. Bissett D et al. *J Soc Cosmet Chem*. 1992;43:85–92.
328. Darr D et al. *Acta Derm Venereol*. 1996;76:264–268.
329. Dreher F et al. *Br J Dermatol*. 1998;139:332–339.
330. Khan W et al. *Cancer Lett*. 1988;42:7–12.
331. Wang Z et al. *Carcinogenesis*. 1991;12:1527–1530.
332. Wang Z et al. *Carcinogenesis*. 1989;10:411–415.
333. Elmets C et al. *J Am Acad Dermatol*. 2001;44:425–432.
334. Soleas G et al. *Clin Biochem*. 2002;35:119–124.
335. Boily G et al. *Oncogene*. 2009;28:2882–2893.
336. Kaur I et al. *Ageing Res Rev*. 2007;6:271–288.
337. Lin C et al. *Food Chem*. 2009;116:923–928.

338. Massaro R et al. *Boll Chim Farm.* 2003;142:264–270.
339. Patravale V et al. *Int J Cosmet Sci.* 2008;30:19–33.
340. Yanaki T. *Stud Surf Sci Catal.* 2001;132:1009–1014.
341. Kumar R, Philip A. *Trop J Pharm Res.* 2007;6:633–644.
342. Baschong W et al. Nanotopes: A novel ultra-small unilamellar carrier system for cosmetic actives. In: Rosen M (Ed.). *Delivery System Handbook for Personal Care and Cosmetic Products.* Norwich, CT: William Andrew; 2005.
343. Agrawal R, Kaur I. *Rejuvenation Res.* 2010;13:397–410.
344. Kaur C, Saraf S. *Int J Drug Delivery.* 2011;3:699–711.
345. Souto E, Müller R. Lipid nanoparticles (solid lipid nanoparticles and nanostructured lipid carriers) for cosmetic, dermal, and transdermal applications. In: Thassu D, Deleers M, Pathak Y (Eds.). *Nanoparticulate Drug Delivery Systems.* New York: Informa Healthcare; 2007, pp. 213–234.
346. Trombino S et al. *Colloids Surf B Biointerfaces.* 2009;72:181–187.
347. Ruktanonchai U et al. *AAPS PharmSciTech.* 2009;10:227–234.
348. Shah K et al. *Int J Pharm.* 2007;345:163–171.
349. Tiyaboonchai W et al. *Int J Pharm.* 2007;337:299–306.
350. Gokce E et al. *Int J Nanomedicine.* 2012;7:1841–1850.
351. Muizzuddin N et al. *Skin Res Tech.* 1999;5:260–265.
352. Greul A et al. *Skin Pharmacol Appl Skin Physiol.* 2002;15:307–315.
353. Césarini J et al. *Photodermatol Photoimmunol Photomed.* 2003;19:182–189.
354. Lin J et al. *J Am Acad Dermatol.* 2003;48:866–874.
355. Maia Campos P et al. *Photochem Photobiol.* 2006;82:683–688.
356. Oresajo C et al. *J Cosmet Dermatol.* 2008;7:290–297.
357. Murray J et al. *J Am Acad Dermatol.* 2008;59:418–425.

Antioxidant properties and application information

Life expectancy has risen continuously in developed societies, yet the mystery of aging remains largely unresolved.

—Barbara Gilchrest and Jean Krutmann, *Skin Aging*

Often when investigating new molecules, we need quick access to fundamental chemical and physical property data in order to anticipate a compound's behavior under a given set of conditions. The intent of this chapter is to be that resource for researchers working with antioxidants. Common antioxidants employed in personal care formulations are presented individually. General information such as a molecule's *empirical formula*, molecular weight, nomenclature, chemical abstract service (CAS) registry number, European commission (EC) number, and simplified molecular-input line-entry system (SMILES) formula is given for each antioxidant. These are useful identifiers that are often needed when conducting research on a particular compound. SMILES is a simple way to input the two-dimensional layout of molecular structure into many computer databases using a simple ASCII formula. Additional chemical and physical data is provided when available, consisting of *melting point*, solubility, dissociation constants, pH, partition coefficient (Log P and *ALOGPs*), Henry's law constant, and hydroxyl radical reaction rate constant. Partition coefficient (Log P) is experimentally determined from the ratio of concentrations of a solute in two immiscible phases (typically water and octanol), which provides the difference in solubility between the aqueous and oil phases. *ALOGPS* is a computer-based prediction of Log P that was developed for the pharmaceutical industry to predict properties of hypothetical molecules not yet synthesized. Henry's law constant can provide similar information as Log P, especially when one of the solvent phases is gas and the other is liquid. The hydroxyl radical reaction rate constant is provided as a reference to differences between each of the antioxidants. Bear in mind, however, that in vivo the hydroxyl radical reacts so quickly that its target is often determined by its rate of diffusion. In addition, stability information is provided when available along with references to analytical methods, electron spin resonance studies, general interest articles, and skin studies.

N-ACETYL CYSTEINE

- *Empirical formula*: $C_5H_9NO_3S$
- *MW*: 163.19
- *Synonyms*: N-acetyl-L-cysteine; acetyl cysteine; mercapturic acid
- *CAS*: 616-91-1
- *EC number*: 210-498-3
- *SMILES*: C(C(O)=O)(NC(C)=O)CS

Description

N-acetylcysteine is a pharmaceutical active used as a mucolytic agent, which breaks down mucous into a less viscous substance by cleaving disulfide bonds. It is also a nutritional supplement for its antioxidant properties. N-acetylcysteine is also used to treat overdoses of paracetamol (acetaminophen)—an OTC pharmaceutical to treat pain and fever that is often taken to induce self-poisoning. In addition, it is utilized as an antidote for cysteine/glutathione deficiency.

The activity of proinflammatory cytokines and growth factors often leads to the production of free radical species. N-acetylcysteine mediates cell signaling pathways by inhibiting the activation of c-Jun N-terminal kinase, p38 MAP kinase, activating protein-1, and nuclear factor-kappa B transcription factor. It also inhibits apoptosis.[1]

Chemical/physical properties

- *Melting point*[2]: 109.5°C
- *Solubilities*[3,4]: H_2O (100 mg/mL with heating); 1 g/4 mL of EtOH; Insoluble in chloroform and ether
- *Dissociation constants*[4,5]: pKa = 3.24 (carboxylic acid moiety); pKa = 9.52 (SH group)
- *pH*[6]: 2–2.75 (1 mg in 100 mL)
- *ALOGPs*[6]: −0.03
- *Henry's law constant*[7]: 1.7×10^{-13} atm · m^3/mol
- *Hydroxyl radical reaction rate constant*[7]: 5.5×10^{-11} cm^3/molec · s
- *Specific optical rotation*[8]: +5° at 20°C (3 g/100 mL)

Stability/shelf life

It is stable in ordinary light, nonhygroscopic (oxidizes in moist air), and stable at temperatures up to 120°C.[9]

Analytical methods

- Toussaint B, Pitti C, Streel B, Ceccato A, Hubert P, Crommen J. Quantitative analysis of N-acetylcysteine and its pharmacopeial impurities in a pharmaceutical formulation by liquid chromatography-UV detection-mass spectrometry. *J Chromatogr A*. 2000;896:191–199.

ESR studies

- Hadley J, Gordy W. Nuclear coupling of 33S and the nature of free radicals in irradiated crystals of N-acetyl-L-cysteine. *Proc Natl Acad Sci USA*. 1977;74:216–220.
- Matsuki K, Hadley J, Nelson W, Yang C. ESR studies of monosulfide radicals in irradiated N-acetyl-L-cysteine single crystals. *J Magnet Res A*. 1993;103:196–202.
- Saxebøl G, Herskedal Ø. Electron spin resonance studies of electron-irradiated peptides. A single crystal of N-acetyl-L-cysteine at 77 K. *Radiat Res*. 1975;62:395–405.

General interest articles

- Agnihotri N, Mishra PC. Mechanism of scavenging action of N-acetylcysteine for the OH radical: A quantum computational study. *J Phys Chem B*. 2009;113:12096–12104.
- Aruoma OI, B. H, Hoey BM, Butler J. The antioxidant action of N-acetylcysteine: Its reaction with hydrogen peroxide, hydroxyl radical, superoxide, and hypochlorous acid. *Free Rad Biol Med*. 1989;6:593–597.
- Atkuri K, Mantovani J, Herzenberg L, Herzenberg L. N-Acetylcysteine—A safe antidote for cysteine/glutathione deficiency. *Curr Opin Pharmacol*. 2007;7:355–359.
- Zafarullah M, Li W, Sylvester J, Ahmad M. Molecular mechanisms of N-acetylcysteine actions. *Cell Mol Life Sci*. 2003;60:6–20.

Skin studies

- Bush JA, Ho VC, Mitchell DL, Tron VA, Li G. Effect of N-acetylcysteine on UVB-induced apoptosis and DNA repair in human and mouse keratinocytes. *Photochem Photobiol*. 1999;70:329–333.
- D'Agostini F, Balansky RM, Camoirano A, De Flora S. Modulation of light-induced skin tumors by N-acetylcysteine and/or ascorbic acid in hairless mice. *Carcinogenesis*. 2005;26:657–664.
- Kang S, Chung JH, Lee JH, Fisher GJ, Wan YS, Duell EA et al. Topical N-acetyl cysteine and genistein prevent ultraviolet-light-induced signaling that leads to photoaging in human skin in vivo. *J Invest Dermatol*. 2003;120:835–841.
- Kowalczyk MC, Walaszek Z, Kowalczyk P, Kinjo T, Hanausek M, Slaga TJ. Differential effects of several phytochemicals and their derivatives on murine keratinocytes in vitro and in vivo: Implications for skin cancer prevention. *Carcinogenesis*. 2009;30:1008–1015.
- Steenvoorden DPT, Hasselbaink DM, van Henegouwen GMJB. Protection against UV-induced reactive intermediates in human cells and mouse skin by glutathione precursors: A comparison of N-acetylcysteine and glutathione ethylester. *Photochem Photobiol*. 1998;67:651–656.
- Sarici, SU, Şahin M, Yurdakök M. Topical N-acetylcysteine treatment in neonatal ichthyosis. *Turk J Pediat*. 2003;45:245–247.
- van den Broeke L, van Henegouwen GB. The effect of N-acetylcysteine on the UVB-induced inhibition of epidermal DNA synthesis in rat skin. *J Photochem Photobiol B: Biol*. 1994;26:271–276.
- Yener G, Öke TI. Development of a w/o/w-emulsion containing N-acetylcysteine for cosmetic use. *Sci Pharm*. 2009;77:639–649.

APIGENIN

- *Empirical formula*: $C_{15}H_{10}O_5$
- *MW*: 270.24
- *Synonyms*: 4′,5,7-trihydroxyflavone; 5,7-dihydroxy-2-(4-hydroxyphenyl)-4H-1-benzopyran-4-one
- *CAS*: 520-36-5
- *EC number*: 208-292-3
- *SMILES*: O=C1c2c(OC(c3ccc(O)cc3)=C1)cc(O)cc2O

Description

Apigenin is a plant-derived flavone (a class of flavonoids) that has antioxidant, anti-inflammatory, and anticancer properties. It is found in many common fruits and vegetables.

Chemical/physical properties

- *Melting point*[2]: 347.5°C
- *Solubilities*[2,3]: water (insoluble); EtOH (soluble); dilute alkali very soluble; DMSO (27 mg/mL); 1M KOH 50 mg/mL
- *LogP (exp)*[10]: 3.02
- *ALOGPs*[6]: 3.07
- *Henry's law constant*[7]: 5.12×10^{-17} atm · m^3/mol
- *Hydroxyl radical reaction rate constant*[7]: 2.31×10^{-10} cm^3/molec · s

Stability/shelf life

Suggested long-term storage: −20°C (stable for two years).[11]

Analytical methods

- Avallone R, Zanoli P, Puia G, Kleinschnitz M, Schreier P, Baraldi M. Pharmacological profile of apigenin, a flavonoid isolated from *Matricaria chamomilla*. *Biochem Pharmacol*. 2000;59:1387–1394.
- Engelmann C, Blot E, Panis Y, Bauer S, Trochon V, Nagy H et al. Apigenin—strong cytostatic and anti-angiogenic action in vitro contrasted by lack of efficacy in vivo. *Phytomedicine*. 2002;9:489–495.
- Li B, Robinson D, Birtx D. Evaluation of properties of apigenin and [G-3H]apigenin and analytic method development. *J Pharm Sci*. 1997;86:721–725.

ESR studies

- Birey M, Sayin Ü, editors. ESR study of quercetin, morin and apigenin single crystals of antioxidant polyphenols. *4th International Conference on Polyphenol Applications*; 2007.

General review articles

- Patel D, Shukla S, Gupta S. Apigenin and cancer chemoprevention: Progress, potential and promise (Review). *Int J Oncol*. 2007;30:233–245.
- Shukla S, Gupta S. Apigenin: A promising molecule for cancer prevention. *Pharm Res*. 2010;27:962–978.

Skin studies

- Balasubramanian S, Eckert RL. Keratinocyte proliferation, differentiation, and apoptosis-Differential mechanisms of regulation by curcumin, EGCG and apigenin. *Toxicol Appl Pharmacol*. 2007;224:214–219.
- Birt DF, Mitchell D, Gold B, Pour P, Pinch HC. Inhibition of ultraviolet light induced skin carcinogenesis in SKH-1 mice by apigenin, a plant flavonoid. *Anticancer Res*. 1997;17:85–91.
- Li BY, Birt DF. In vivo and in vitro percutaneous absorption of cancer preventive flavonoid apigenin in different vehicles in mouse skin. *Pharm Res*. 1996;13:1710–1715.
- Li BY, Pinch H, Birt DF. Influence of vehicle, distant topical delivery, and biotransformation on the chemopreventive activity of apigenin, a plant flavonoid, in mouse skin. *Pharm Res*. 1996;13:1530–1534.
- Segaert S, Courtois, Garmyn M, Degreef H, Bouillon R. The flavonoid apigenin suppresses vitamin D receptor expression and vitamin D responsiveness in normal human keratinocytes. *Biochem Biophys Res Comm*. 2000;268:237–241.
- Yano S, Umeda D, Yamashita S, Yamada K, Tachibana H. Dietary apigenin attenuates the development of atopic dermatitis-like skin lesions in NC/Nga mice. *J Nutr Biochem*. 2009;20:876–881.
- Wei HC, Tye L, Bresnick E, Birt DF. Inhibitory effect of apigenin, a plant flavonoid, on epidermal ornithine decarboxylase and skin tumor promotion in mice. *Canc Res*. 1990;50:499–502.

ARBUTIN

- *Empirical formula*: $C_{12}H_{16}O_7$
- *MW*: 272.25
- *Synonyms*: 4-hydroxyphenyl-beta-D-glucopyranoside; hydroquinone beta-D-glucopyranoside
- *CAS*: 497-76-7
- *EC number*: 207-850-3
- *SMILES*: OC(C(O)C2O)C(OC2CO)OC1=CC=C(O)C=C1

Description

Arbutin is a glycosylated hydroquinone that is found in the leaves of several plant species including the bearberry plant, *Arctostaphylos uva-ursi*. It is used extensively as a skin-whitening agent, which functions as an inhibitor of tyrosinase—resulting in less melanin production by melanocytes.

Chemical/physical properties

- *Melting point*[2]: 199.5°C
- *Solubilities*[2]: water (very soluble); EtOH (soluble)
- *LogP (exp)*[12]: −1.35
- *ALOGPs*[6]: −1.36
- *Henry's law constant*[7]: 1.20×10^{-19} atm · m^3/mol
- *Hydroxyl radical reaction rate constant*: 9.10×10^{-11} cm^3/molec · s
- *Specific optical rotation*[13]: −60.3° at 20°C/D (in H_2O)

Stability/shelf life

Recommended storage: low humidity, away from sunlight at 10°C –30°C (can remain stable for three years).[14]

Analytical methods

- Barsooma B, Abdelsama A, Adib N. Indirect spectrophotometric determination of arbutin, whitening agent through oxidation by periodate and complexation with ferric chloride. *Spectrochim Acta Part A*. 2006;64:844–852.
- Chang M, Chang C. Simultaneous HPLC determination of hydrophilic whitening agents in cosmetic products. *J Pharm Biomed Anal*. 2003;33:617–626.
- Cui T, Nakamura K, Ma L, Li J, Kayahara H. Analyses of arbutin and chlorogenic acid, the major phenolic constituents in oriental pear. *J Agric Food Chem*. 2005;53:3882–3887.
- Huang SC, Lin CC, Huang MC, Wen KC. Simultaneous determination of magnesium ascorbyl phosphate, ascorbyl glucoside, kojic acid, arbutin and hydroquinone in skin whitening cosmetics by HPLC. *J Food Drug Anal*. 2004;12:13–18.
- Kittipongpatana N, Chaiwan A, Pusod U, Kittipongpatana O. High-performance liquid chromatographic method for separation and quantitative analysis of arbutin in plant tissue cultures. *CMU J Nat Sci*. 2007;6:65–74.
- Nycz JE, Malecki G, Morag M, Nowak G, Ponikiewski L, Kusz J et al. Arbutin: Isolation, X-ray structure and computational studies. *J Molec Struct*. 2010;980:13–17.
- Thongchai W, Liawruangrath B, Liawruangrath S. High-performance liquid chromatographic determination of arbutin in skin-whitening creams and medicinal plant extracts. *J Cosmet Sci*. 2007;58:35–44.
- Thongchai W, Liawruangrath B, Liawruangrath S. Arbutin determination in medicinal plants and creams. *Int J Cosmet Sci*. 2009;31:87–96.

ESR studies

- Berkaoui M, Souchard JP, Massol M, Nepveu F. Hydroxyl radical scavenging activity of compounds with pharmaceutical interest–A quantitative analysis by ESR spectroscopy. *J Chim Phys PCB.* 1994;91:1799–1808.

General interest articles

- Takebayashi J, Ishii R, Chen JB, Matsumoto T, Ishimi Y, Tai A. Reassessment of antioxidant activity of arbutin: Multifaceted evaluation using five antioxidant assay systems. *Free Rad Res.* 2010;44:473–478.

Skin studies

- Bang S, Han S, Kim D. Hydrolysis of arbutin to hydroquinone by human skin bacteria and its effect on antioxidant activity. *J Cosmet Dermatol.* 2008;7:189–193.
- O'Donoghue JL. Hydroquinone and its analogues in dermatology–A risk-benefit viewpoint. *J Cosmet Dermatol.* 2006;5:196–203.
- Wen AH, Choi MK, Kim DD. Formulation of liposome for topical delivery of arbutin. *Arch Pharm Res.* 2006;29:1187–1192.

L-ASCORBIC ACID

- *Empirical formula*: $C_6H_8O_6$
- *MW*: 176.12
- *Synonyms*: ascorbic acid; vitamin C; ascorbate; antiscorbutic factor; L-threoascorbic acid
- *CAS*: 50-81-7
- *EC number*: 200-066-2
- *SMILES*: O=C1C(O)=C(O)[CH]([CH](O)CO)O1

Description

L-ascorbic acid, or vitamin C, is a natural antioxidant found in many fruits and vegetables. It is also available from synthetic sources. It is an essential nutrient, which is necessary for proper bone and connective tissue health. Humans, and other primates, lost the ability to synthesize L-ascorbic acid. Therefore, it must be obtained in the diet. L-ascorbic acid is a potent, water-soluble antioxidant against many free radical species, and can even recycle lipid soluble alpha-tocopherol to its active form after it has exerted its antioxidant action.

Chemical/physical properties

- *Melting point*[2]: 191°C (decomposes)
- *Solubilities*[2,13,15]: H_2O (very soluble); EtOH (soluble); insoluble in ether, chloroform, benzene, petroleum ether, oils, fats, and fat solvents; the solubility in g/mL is 0.33 in water, 0.033 in 95 wt% ethanol, 0.02 in absolute ethanol, 0.01 in glycerol USP, 0.05 in propylene glycol.
- *Dissociation constants*[13]: pK1 = 4.17; pK2 = 11.57
- *pH*[13]: pH = 3 (5 mg/mL); pH = 2 (50 mg/mL)
- *LogP (exp)*[16]: −1.85
- *ALOGPs*[6]: −1.58
- *Henry's law constant*[7]: 4.07×10^{-8} atm · m³/mol
- *Hydroxyl radical reaction rate constant*[7]: 5.58×10^{-11} cm³/molec · s
- *Specific optical rotation*[17]: +24° at 20°C/D (in water, 1%)
- *UV max absorption at pH 2*[13]: 245 nm (ε = 695, 1%, 1 cm); at pH 6.4: 265 nm (ε = 940, 1%, 1 cm)

Stability/shelf life

Stable to air when dry; impure preparation and in many natural products vitamin oxidizes on exposure to air and light. Aqueous solutions are rapidly oxidized by air, accelerated by alkalies, iron, and copper.[18]

Analytical methods

- Arya S, Mahajan M, Jain P. Non-spectrophotometric methods for the determination of vitamin C. *Anal Chim Acta.* 2000;417:1–14.
- Pachla L, Reynolds D, Kissinger P. Analytical methods for determining ascorbic acid in biological samples, food products, and pharmaceuticals. *J Assoc Off Anal Chem.* 1985;68:1–12.
- Shukla M, Mishra P. Electronic structures and spectra of two antioxidants: Uric acid and ascorbic acid. *J Molec Struct.* 1996;377:247–259.
- Washko P, Welch R, Dhariwal K, Wang Y, Levine M. Ascorbic acid and dehydroascorbic acid analyses in biological samples. *Anal Biochem.* 1992;204:1–14.

ESR studies

- Bai L, Wang JY, Cui NJ, Zhang Y. The ESR and UV-VIS studies on the reaction between ascorbic acid and iron ion. *Acta Biochim Biophys Sinica.* 1997;29:527–532.
- Buettner G, Jurkiewicz B. Ascorbate free radical as a marker of oxidative stress: An EPR study. *Free Rad Biol Med.* 1993;14:49–55.
- Cossins E, Lee R, Packer L. ESR studies of vitamin C regeneration, order of reactivity of natural source phytochemical preparations. *Biochem Biol Int.* 1998;45:583–597.
- Kalus W, Filby W. The effect of additives on the free radical formation in aqueous solutions of ascorbic acid. *Int J Vitam Nutr Res.* 1977;47:258–264.
- Lohmann W, Holz D. Structure of ascorbic acid and its biological function. I. ESR determination of the ascorbyl radical in biological samples and in model systems. *Biophys Struct Mech.* 1984;10:197–204.
- McAlpine R, Ocivera M, Chen H. Photooxidation and reduction of ascorbic acid studied by E.S.R. *Can J Chem.* 1973;51:1682–1686.
- McDearmon G, Moulton G. Radiation-induced free radicals in L-ascorbic acid: An ESR study. *Rad Res.* 1982;89:468–480.
- Satoh K, Ao Y, Asano K, Sakagami H. Rapid determination of ascorbate by ESR spectroscopy. *Anticancer Res.* 1997;17:3479–3483.
- Van Duijn M, Van der Zee J, Van den Broek P. Electron spin resonance study on the formation of ascorbate free radical from ascorbate: The effect of dehydroascorbic acid and ferricyanide. *Protoplasma.* 1998;205:122–128.

General review articles

- Arrigoni O, DeTullio M. Ascorbic acid: Much more than just an antioxidant. *Biochim Biophys Acta.* 2002;1569:1–9.
- Iqbal K, Khan A, Khattak M. Biological significance of ascorbic acid (vitamin C) in human health—A review. *Pak J Nutr.* 2004;3:5–13.
- Lodge J. Molecular actions of ascorbic acid. *Curr Top Nutr Res.* 2008;6:1–13.
- Zümreoglu-Karan B. The coordination chemistry of Vitamin C: An overview. *Coord Chem Rev.* 2006;250:2295–2307.

Skin studies

- Buettner GR. The pecking order of free radicals and antioxidants: Lipid peroxidation, alpha-tocopherol, and ascorbate. *Arch Biochem Biophys.* 1993;300:535–543.
- Burke KE. Interaction of vitamins C and E as better cosmeceuticals. *Dermatol Ther.* 2007;20:314–321.
- Elmore A. Final report of the safety assessment of L-ascorbic acid, calcium ascorbate, magnesium ascorbate, magnesium ascorbyl phosphate, sodium ascorbate, and sodium ascorbyl phosphate as used in cosmetics. *Int J Toxicol.* 2005;24(Suppl. 2):51–111.
- Fuchs J. Potentials and limitations of the natural antioxidants RRR-alpha-tocopherol, L-ascorbic acid, and β-carotene in cutaneous photoprotection. *Free Rad Biol Med.* 1998;25:848–873.
- Oresajo C, Stephens T, Hino PD, Law RM, Yatskayer M, Foltis P et al. Protective effects of a topical antioxidant mixture containing vitamin C, ferulic acid, and phloretin against ultraviolet-induced photodamage in human skin. *J Cosmet Dermatol.* 2008;7:290–297.
- Murray JC, Burch JA, Streilein RD, Iannacchione MA, Hall RP, Pinnell SR. A topical antioxidant solution containing vitamins C and E stabilized by ferulic acid provides protection for human skin against damage caused by ultraviolet irradiation. *J Am Acad Dermatol.* 2008;59:418–425.
- Saraf S, Kaur CD. Phytoconstituents as photoprotective novel cosmetic formulations. *Pharmacogn Rev.* 2010;4:1–11.

TERT-BUTYLHYDROQUINONE

- *Empirical formula*: $C_{10}H_{14}O_2$
- *MW*: 166.22
- *Synonyms*: 2-(1,1-dimethylethyl)-1,4-benzenediol; TBHQ; tert-butyl-1,4-benzenediol
- *CAS*: 1948-33-0
- *EC number*: 217-752-2
- *SMILES*: c1(C(C)(C)C)c(O)ccc(O)c1

Description

tert-Butylhydroquinone (TBHQ) is a synthetic antioxidant that is used to prevent oxidation and stabilize formulations. In addition to its utility in cosmetics, it is a common ingredient in foods, which is added to prevent lipid peroxidation of fats and oils.

Chemical/physical properties

- *Melting point*[3]: 127°C–129°C
- *Solubilities*[19]: 60% (EtOH), 60% (ethyl acetate), 30% (propylene glycol), 10% (glyceryl monooleate), 10% (cottonseed oil), 10% (corn oil), 10% (soybean oil), 5% (safflower oil), and <1% (H_2O) (all at 25°C)
- *ALOGPs*[6]: 2.61

Analytical methods

- Cortés A, Armisen P, Ruiz M, Yáñez-Sedeño P, Pingarrón J. Electroanalytical study of the antioxidant tert-butylhydroquinone (TBHQ) in an oil-in-water emulsified medium. *Electroanalysis.* 1994;6:1014–1019.
- Cortés A, García A, Yáñez-Sedeño P, Pingarrón J. Polarographic determination of tert-butylhydroquinone in micellar and emulsified media. *Anal Chim Acta.* 1993;273:545–551.
- de la Fuente C, Acuna J, Vazquez M, Tascon M, Batanero P. Voltammetric determination of the phenolic antioxidants 3-tert-butyl-4-hydroxyanisole and tert-butylhydroquinone at a polypyrrole electrode modified with a nickel phthalocyanine complex. *Talanta.* 1999;49:441–452.
- González M, Ballesteros E, Gallego M, Valcárce M. Continuous-flow determination of natural and synthetic antioxidants in foods by gas chromatography. *Anal Chim Acta.* 1998;359:47–55.
- Guan Y, Chu Q, Fu L, Ye J. Determination of antioxidants in cosmetics by micellar electrokinetic capillary chromatography with electrochemical detection. *J Chromatogr A.* 2005;1074:201–204.
- Guan Y, Chu Q, Fu L, Wu T, Ye J. Determination of phenolic antioxidants by micellar electrokinetic capillary chromatography with electrochemical detection. *Food Chem.* 2006;94:157–162.
- Ni Y, Wang L, Kokot S. Voltammetric determination of butylated hydroxyanisole, butylated hydroxytoluene, propyl gallate and tert-butylhydroquinone by use of chemometric approaches. *Anal Chim Acta.* 2000;412:185–193.
- Rababah T, Hettiarachchy N, Horax R. Total phenolics and antioxidant activities of fenugreek, green tea, black tea, grape seed, ginger, rosemary, gotu kola, gingko extracts, vitamin E, and tert-butylhydroquinone. *J Agr Food Chem.* 2004;52:5183–5186.
- Raymundo M, Paula M, Franco C, Fett R. Quantitative determination of the phenolic antioxidants using voltammetric techniques. *LWT.* 2007;40:1133–1139.
- Ruiz M, García-Moreno E, Barbas C, Pingarrón J. Determination of phenolic antioxidants by HPLC

with amperometric detection at a nickel phthalocyanine polymer modified electrode. *Electroanalysis.* 1999;11:470–474.

ESR studies

- Kim J, Lee J, Choi D, Won B, Jung M, Park J. Kinetic study of the quenching reaction of singlet oxygen by common synthetic antioxidants (tert-butylhydroxyanisol, tert-di-butylhydroxytoluene, and tert-butylhydroquinone) as compared with α-tocopherol. *J Food Sci.* 2009;74: C362–C369.
- Okubo T, Nagai F, Ushiyama K, Kano I. Contribution of oxygen radicals to DNA cleavage by quinone compounds derived from phenolic antioxidants, tert-butylhydroquinone and 2,5-di-tert-butylhydroquinone. *Toxicol Lett.* 1997;90:11–18.
- Stolze K, Nohl H. Free radical formation and erythrocyte membrane alterations during MetHb formation induced by the BHA metabolite, tert-butylhydroquinone. *Free Rad Res.* 1999;30:295–303.

General interest articles

- Gharavi N, Haggarty S, El-Kadi A. Chemoprotective and carcinogenic effects of tert-butylhydroquinone and its metabolites. *Curr Drug Metab.* 2007;8:1–7.
- Yu R, Tan T, Kong A. Butylated hydroxyanisole and its metabolite tert-butylhydroquinone differentially regulate mitogen-activated protein kinases. The role of oxidative stress in the activation of mitogen-activated protein kinases by phenolic antioxidants. *J Biol Chem.* 1997;272:28962–28970.

Skin studies

- Patrick E, Juberg D, O'Donoghue J, Maibach H. Depigmentation with tert-butyl hydroquinone using black guinea pigs. *Food Chem Toxicol.* 1999;37:169–175.

2-*TERT*-BUTYL-4-HYDROXYANISOLE AND 3-*TERT*-BUTYL-4-HYDROXYANISOLE

- *Empirical formula*: $C_{11}H_{16}O_2$
- *MW*: 180.24
- *Synonyms*: 2-*t*-butyl-4-hydroxyanisole; (2-*tert*-butyl-4-methoxyphenol); BHA
- *CAS*: 25013-16-5 (121-00-6)
- *EC number*: 246-563-8 (204-442-7)
- *SMILES*: c1(C(C)(C)C)c(O)ccc(OC)c1

Description

Butylated hydroxyanisole (BHA) is an isomeric mixture of 2-*tert*-butyl-4-hydroxyanisole and 3-*tert*-butyl-4-hydroxyanisole. It acts by a free radical scavenging mechanism and is used for the preservation of rubber, petroleum, food, and cosmetic products. Please note that 3-*tert*-butyl-4-hydroxyanisole is catalogued with distinct CAS (121-00-6) and EC (204-442-7) numbers. Normally the use of the term BHA infers that both isomers are present in the product.

Chemical/physical properties

- *Melting point*[3]: 58°C–60°C
- *Boiling point*[20]: 264°C–270°C (733 mm Hg)
- *Solubilities*[20]: Soluble in 50% EtOH (or higher), petroleum ether, propylene glycol, fats, and oils; insoluble in H_2O
- *ALOGPs*[6]: 3.25

Stability

Note: There are reports indicating that BHA is ineffective in vegetable oils.[21]

Analytical studies

- Aguilar-Caballos MP, Gómez-Hens A, Pérez-Bendito D. Simultaneous kinetic determination of butylated hydroxyanisole and propyl gallate by coupling stopped-flow mixing technique and diode-array detection. *Anal Chim Acta.* 1997;354:173–179.
- de la Fuente C, Acuna J, Vazquez M, Tascon M, Batanero P. Voltammetric determination of the phenolic antioxidants 3-tert-butyl-4-hydroxyanisole and tert-butylhydroquinone at a polypyrrole electrode modified with a nickel phthalocyanine complex. *Talanta.* 1999;49:441–452.
- García-Jiménez J, Valencia M, Capitán-Vallvey L. Simultaneous determination of antioxidants, preservatives and sweetener additives in food and cosmetics by flow injection analysis coupled to a monolithic column. *Anal Chim Acta.* 2007;594:226–233.
- González M, Ballesteros E, Gallego M, Valcárce M. Continuous-flow determination of natural and synthetic antioxidants in foods by gas chromatography. *Anal Chim Acta.* 1998;359:47–55.
- González A, Ruiz M, Yáñez-Sedeño P, Pingarrón J. Voltammetric determination of tert-butylhydroxyanisole in micellar and emulsified media. *Anal Chim Acta.* 1994;285:63–71.
- Guan Y, Chu Q, Fu L, Ye J. Determination of antioxidants in cosmetics by micellar electrokinetic capillary chromatography with electrochemical detection. *J Chromatogr A.* 2005;1074:201–204.
- Guan Y, Chu Q, Fu L, Wu T, Ye J. Determination of phenolic antioxidants by micellar electrokinetic capillary chromatography with electrochemical detection. *Food Chem.* 2006;94:157–162.
- Ni Y, Wang L, Kokot S. Voltammetric determination of butylated hydroxyanisole, butylated hydroxytoluene, propyl gallate and tert-butylhydroquinone by use of chemometric approaches. *Anal Chim Acta.* 2000;412:185–193.

- Raymundo M, Paula M, Franco C, Fett R. Quantitative determination of the phenolic antioxidants using voltammetric techniques. *LWT*. 2007;40:1133–1139.
- Ruiz M, García-Moreno E, Barbas C, Pingarrón J. Determination of phenolic antioxidants by HPLC with amperometric detection at a nickel phthalocyanine polymer modified electrode. *Electroanalysis*. 1999;11:470–474.
- Zhang W, Wu C, Wang C, Yang Z, Liu L. Determination of antioxidants butylated hydroxyanisole (BHA) and butylated hydroxytoluene (BHT) in cosmetics by gas chromatography-mass spectrometry selected ion method. *Se Pu*. 2002;20:178–181.

ESR studies

- Satoh K, Atsumi T, Sakagami H, Kashiwagi Y, Ida Y, Ueha T et al. Radical intensity and cytotoxicity of butylated hydroxyanisole and its orthobisphenol dimer. *Anticancer Res*. 1999;19:3947–3952.

General interest articles

- Kraybill H, Dugan L, Beadle B, Vibrans F, Swartz V, Rezabek H. Butylated hydroxyanisole as an antioxidant for animal fats. *J Am Oil Chem Soc*. 1949;26:449–453.
- Yu R, Tan T, Kong A. Butylated hydroxyanisole and its metabolite tert-butylhydroquinone differentially regulate mitogen-activated protein kinases. The role of oxidative stress in the activation of mitogen-activated protein kinases by phenolic antioxidants. *J Biol Chem*. 1997;272:28962–28970.

Skin studies

- Kono T, Taniguchi S, Mizuno N, Fukuda M, Maekawa N, Hisa T et al. Effects of butylated hydroxyanisole on ornithine decarboxylase activity induced by ultraviolet-B and PUVA in mouse skin. *J Dermatol*. 1992;19:389–392.
- Pino M, Billack B. Reduction of vesicant toxicity by butylated hydroxyanisole in A-431 skin cells. *Cutan Ocul Toxicol*. 2008;27:161–172.
- Taniguchi S, Furukawa M, Kono T, Hisa T, Ishii M, Hamada T. Butylated hydroxyanisole blocks the inhibitory effects of tumor necrosis factor-alpha on collagen production in human dermal fibroblasts. *J Dermatol Sci*. 1996;12:44–49.
- Timmins G, Davies M. Free radical formation in isolated murine keratinocytes treated with organic peroxides and its modulation by antioxidants. *Carcinogenesis*. 1993;14:1615–1620.

BUTYLATED HYDROXYTOLUENE

- *Empirical formula*: $C_{15}H_{24}O$
- *MW*: 220.35
- *Synonyms*: 2,6-di-*tert*-butyl-4-methylphenol; 2,6-di-*tert*-butyl-*p*-cresol
- *CAS*: 128-37-0
- *EC number*: 204-881-4
- *SMILES*: c1(O)c(C(C)(C)C)cc(C)cc1C(C)(C)C

Description

Butylated hydroxytoluene (BHT) is a lipid/fat-soluble antioxidant, which acts by free radical scavenging mechanisms. It is used extensively in food and cosmetic products for its preservation properties.

Chemical/physical properties

- *Boiling point*[2]: 265°C
- *Melting point*[2]: 71°C
- *Solubilities*[3,20]: Insoluble in H_2O. Soluble in EtOH (100 mg/mL). Soluble in vegetable oils; Freely soluble in toluene; soluble in methanol, isopropanol, methyl ethyl ketone, acetone, cellosolve, benzene, most hydrocarbon solvents, petroleum ether, liquid petrolatum, and linseed oil (0.5% w/w); more soluble in food oils and fats than BHA.
- *LogP (exp)*: 5.10
- *ALOGPs*[6]: 5.25
- *Max absorption (isopropanol)*[22]: 227 nm (log ε = 3.75), 277 nm (log ε = 3.34), 283 nm (log ε = 3.34)
- *Intense mass spectral peaks*[23]: 205 m/z (100%), 220 m/z (27%), 57 m/z (27%), 206 m/z (15%)

Stability/shelf life

Stable in light and air.[9] Note that BHT has been reported to be ineffective in vegetable oils.[21]

Analytical studies

- Capitan-Vallvey L, Valencia M, Nicolas E. Flow-through sensor for determination of butylated hydroxytoluene in cosmetics. *Anal Lett*. 2002;35:65–81.
- González M, Ballesteros E, Gallego M, Valcárce M. Continuous-flow determination of natural and synthetic antioxidants in foods by gas chromatography. *Anal Chim Acta*. 1998;359:47–55.
- Guan Y, Chu Q, Fu L, Ye J. Determination of antioxidants in cosmetics by micellar electrokinetic capillary chromatography with electrochemical detection. *J Chromatogr A*. 2005;1074:201–204.
- Guan Y, Chu Q, Fu L, Wu T, Ye J. Determination of phenolic antioxidants by micellar electrokinetic capillary chromatography with electrochemical detection. *Food Chem*. 2006;94:157–162.
- Irache J, Vega F, Ezpeleta I. Antioxidants in some pharmaceuticals, cosmetics and food from the European market. *Pharm Acta Helv*. 1992;67:152–155.
- Ni Y, Wang L, Kokot S. Voltammetric determination of butylated hydroxyanisole, butylated hydroxytoluene, propyl gallate and tert-butylhydroquinone by use of chemometric approaches. *Anal Chim Acta*. 2000;412:185–193.
- Raymundo M, Paula M, Franco C, Fett R. Quantitative determination of the phenolic antioxidants using voltammetric techniques. *LWT*. 2007;40:1133–1139.

- Ruiz M, García-Moreno E, Barbas C, Pingarrón J. Determination of phenolic antioxidants by HPLC with amperometric detection at a nickel phthalocyanine polymer modified electrode. *Electroanalysis*. 1999;11:470–474.
- Zhang W, Wu C, Wang C, Yang Z, Liu L. Determination of antioxidants butylated hydroxyanisole (BHA) and butylated hydroxytoluene (BHT) in cosmetics by gas chromatography-mass spectrometry selected ion method. *Se Pu*. 2002;20:178–181.

ESR studies

- Kim J, Lee J, Choi D, Won B, Jung M, Park J. Kinetic study of the quenching reaction of singlet oxygen by common synthetic antioxidants (tert-butylhydroxyanisol, tert-di-butylhydroxytoluene, and tert-butylhydroquinone) as compared with α-tocopherol. *J Food Sci*. 2009;74:C362–C369.

General interest articles

- Babich H. Butylated hydroxytoluene (BHT): A review. *Environ Res*. 1982;29:1–29.
- Jori A. Toxico-kinetic aspects of butylated hydroxytoluene (BHT): A review. *Ann 1st Super Sanita*. 1983;19:271–286.
- Lanigan R, Yamarik T. Final report on the safety assessment of BHT(1). *Int J Toxicol*. 2002;21(Suppl. 2):19–94.

Skin studies

- Black H. Pro-oxidant and anti-oxidant mechanism(s) of BHT and beta-carotene in photocarcinogenesis. *Front Biosci*. 2002;7:d1044–d1055.
- Black H, Mathews-Roth M. Protective role of butylated hydroxytoluene and certain carotenoids in photocarcinogenesis. *Photochem Photobiol*. 1991;53:707–716.
- Koone M, Black H. A mode of action for butylated hydroxytoluene-mediated photoprotection. *J Invest Dermatol*. 1986;87:343–347.
- Potapenko A, Kyagova A. The application of antioxidants in investigations and optimization of photochemotherapy. *Membr Cell Biol*. 1998;12:269–278.
- Schoonderwoerd S, van Henegouwen GB, Persons K. Effect of alpha-tocopherol and di-butyl-hydroxytoluene (BHT) on UV-A-induced photobinding of 8-methoxy-psoralen to Wistar rat epidermal biomacromolecules in vivo. *Arch Toxicol*. 1991;65:490–494.
- Väänänen A, Hannuksela M. UVB erythema inhibited by topically applied substances. *Acta Derm Venereol*. 1989;69:12–17.
- Vile G, Tanew-Ilitschew A, Tyrrell R. Activation of NF-kappa B in human skin fibroblasts by the oxidative stress generated by UVA radiation. *Photochem Photobiol*. 1995;62:463–468.

CAFFEIC ACID

- *Empirical formula*: $C_9H_8O_4$
- *MW*: 180.16
- *Synonyms*: 3,4-dihydroxy-cinnamic acid; 3-(3,4-dihydroxyphenyl)-2-propenoic acid
- *CAS*: 331-39-5
- *EC number*: 206-361-2
- *SMILES*: C(C=Cc1cc(O)c(O)cc1)(O)=O

Description

Caffeic acid is a phenolic acid commonly found in fruits and grains. Despite its name, the only relation with caffeine is that they are both found in coffee. In addition to its antioxidant properties, caffeic acid is an anti-inflammatory, immunomodulatory, and anticancer agent.

Chemical/physical properties

- *Melting point*[13]: 223°C–225°C (decomposes). Softens at 194°C
- *Solubilities*[13]: Sparingly soluble in cold water. Freely soluble in hot water and cold alcohol
- *LogP (exp)*[24]: 1.15
- *ALOGPs*[6]: 1.67
- Observed light absorption wavelengths[25] = 265 nm, 325 nm, and 442 nm

Analytical studies

- Cao Y, Wang Y, Yuan Q. Analysis of flavonoids and phenolic acid in propolis by capillary electrophoresis. *Chromatographia*. 2004;59:135–140.
- Rivelli D, da Silva V, Ropke C, Miranda D, Almeida R, Sawada T et al. Simultaneous determination of chlorogenic acid, caffeic acid and caffeine in hydroalcoholic and aqueous extracts of *Ilex paraguariensis* by HPLC and correlation with antioxidant capacity of the extracts by DPPH reduction. *Braz J Pharm Sci*. 2007;43:215–222.

ESR studies

- Atherton N, Willder J. EPR and ENDOR of free-radicals formed during the aerobic oxidation of chlorogenic acid and of caffeic acid in strongly alkaline-solution. *Res Chem Intermed*. 1993;19:787–795.
- Maegawa Y, Sugino K, Sakurai H. Identification of free radical species derived from caffeic acid and related polyphenols. *Free Rad Res*. 2007;41:110–119.

General interest articles

- al-Sereiti M, Abu-Amer K, Sen P. Pharmacology of rosemary (*Rosmarinus officinalis* Linn.) and its therapeutic potentials. *Ind J Exp Biol*. 1999;37:124–130.
- Bors W, Michel C, Stettmaier K, Lu Y, Yeap Foo L. Antioxidant mechanisms of polyphenolic caffeic acid oligomers, constituents of *Salvia officinalis*. *Biol Res*. 2004;37:301–311.
- Jiang R-W, Lau K-M, Hon P-M, Mak TCW, Woo K-S, Fung K-P. Chemistry and biological activities of caffeic acid derivatives from *Salvia miltiorrhiza*. *Curr Med Chem*. 2005;12:237–246.

- Laranjinha J. Redox cycles of caffeic acid with alpha-tocopherol and ascorbate. *Methods Enzymol.* 2001;335:282–295.
- Mateos J, Rivera M, Arrizon J, Canales A, Sandoval G. Enzymes useful in the synthesis of bioactive caffeic acid derivatives: Practical screening and structure-function relationships. In: Pandev A et al. (Eds.). *New Horizons in Biotechnology 2007.* New Delhi, India: Asiatech Publishers; 2008.

Skin studies

- Bonina F, Puglia C, Ventura D, Aquino R, Tortora S, Sacchi A et al. In vitro antioxidant and in vivo photoprotective effects of a lyophilized extract of *Capparis spinosa* L. buds. *J Cosmet Sci.* 2002;53:321–335.
- Huang MT, Ma W, Yen P, Xie J-G, Han J, Frenkel K et al. Inhibitory effects of caffeic acid phenethyl ester (CAPE) on 12-0-tetradecanoylphorbol-13-acetate-induced tumor promotion in mouse skin and the synthesis of DNA, RNA and protein in HeLa cells. *Carcinogenesis.* 1996;17:761–765.
- Huang M, Smart R, Wong C, Conney A. Inhibitory effect of curcumin, chlorogenic acid, caffeic acid, and ferulic acid on tumor promotion in mouse skin by 12-O-tetradecanoylphorbol-13-acetate. *Cancer Res.* 1988;48:5941–5946.
- Kang NJ, Lee KW, Shin BJ, Jung SK, Hwang MK, Bode AM et al. Caffeic acid, a phenolic phytochemical in coffee, directly inhibits Fyn kinase activity and UVB-induced COX-2 expression. *Carcinogenesis.* 2009;30:321–330.
- Marti-Mestres G, Mestres J, Bres J, Martin S, Ramosc J, Vian L. The "in vitro" percutaneous penetration of three antioxidant compounds. *Int J Pharm.* 2007;331:139–144.
- Neradil J, Veselska R, Slanina J. UVC-protective effect of caffeic acid on normal and transformed human skin cells in vitro. *Folia Biol.* 2003;49:197–202.
- Saija A, Tomaino A, Trombetta D, De Pasquale A, Uccella N, Barbuzzi T et al. In vitro and in vivo evaluation of caffeic and ferulic acids as topical photoprotective agents. *Int J Pharm.* 2000;199:39–47.
- Staniforth V, Chiu L, Yang N. Caffeic acid suppresses UVB radiation-induced expression of interleukin-10 and activation of mitogen-activated protein kinases in mouse. *Carcinogenesis.* 2006;27:1803–1811.
- Yamada Y, Yasui H, Sakurai H. Suppressive effect of caffeic acid and its derivatives on the generation of UVA-induced reactive oxygen species in the skin of hairless mice and pharmacokinetic analysis on organ distribution of caffeic acid in ddY mice. *Photochem Photobiol.* 2006;82:1668–1676.

BETA-CAROTENE

- *Empirical formula*: $C_{40}H_{56}$
- *MW*: 536.87
- *Synonyms*: 1,1′-(3,7,12,16-tetramethyl-1,3,5,7,9,11,13, 15,17-octadecanonaene-1,18-diyl)bis[2,6,6-trimethyl-cyclohexene]; beta, beta-carotene; provitamin A
- *CAS*: 7235-40-7
- *EC number*: 230-636-6
- *SMILES*: C(=CC(=C(C)2)C(C)(C)CCC2)C(C)=CC= CC(=CC=CC=C(C)C=CC=C(C=CC(=C(C)1)C(C)(C)CCC1)C)C

Description

Beta-carotene is an orange-yellow pigment found in many vegetables including carrots, sweet potatoes, pumpkin, green kale, and spinach. In terms of antioxidant behavior, it is most well known for its quenching of $^1O_2$, but it can also quench $O_2^{-\cdot}$ and $HO^\cdot$. It is also used for the treatment of a number of ailments of the skin including erythropoetic protoporphyria—a skin disease characterized by photosensitivity.

Chemical/physical properties

- *Melting point*[13]: 183°C
- *Solubilities*[13]: Soluble in benzene, chloroform, and carbon disulfide; moderately soluble in ether, petroleum ether, and oils; 100 mL hexane dissolves 109 mg at 0°C; very sparingly soluble in methanol and ethanol; practically insoluble in water, acids, and alkalies
- *Henry's law constant*[7]: 1.10×10^2 atm · m³/mol
- *Hydroxyl radical reaction rate constant*[7]: 7.40×10^{-10} cm³/molec · s
- *Max absorption (chloroform)*[13]: 466, 497 nm
- *Max absorption (benzene)*[26]: 278 nm (log ε = 4.30), 364 nm (log ε = 4.62), 463 nm (log ε = 5.10), 494 nm (log ε = 4.77)

Stability/shelf life

Absorbs oxygen from air resulting in the formation of inactive, colorless oxidation products.[20]

ESR studies

- Iannone A, Rota C, Bergamini S, Tomasi A, Canfield L. Antioxidant activity of carotenoids: An electron-spin resonance study on beta-carotene and lutein interaction with free radicals generated in a chemical system. *J Biochem Mol Toxicol.* 1998;12:299–304.
- Konovalova T, Kispert L. EPR and ENDOR studies of carotenoid-solid Lewis acid interactions. *J Chem Soc Faraday Trans.* 1998;94:1465–1468.
- Piekara-Sady L, Kispert L. Carotenoid action radical: An EPR and ENDOR study. *Mol Phys Rep.* 1994;6:220–223.
- Tkáč A, Scott G. The β-carotene dilemma: ESR study with coordinated peroxyl radicals. *Chem Pap.* 2006;60:179–185.

General interest articles

- Burton G, Ingold K. β-Carotene: An unusual type of lipid antioxidant. *Science.* 1984;224:569–573.

- Edge R, McGarvey DJ, Truscott TG. The carotenoids as anti-oxidants—A review. *J Photochem Photobiol B: Biol.* 1997;41:189–200.
- Goodwin T. Metabolism, nutrition, and function of carotenoids. *Annu Rev Nutr.* 1986;6:273–297.
- Liebler D. Antioxidant reactions of carotenoids. *Ann New York Acad Sci.* 1993;691:20–31.
- Namitha KK, Negi PS. Chemistry and biotechnology of carotenoids. *Crit Rev Food Sci Nutr.* 2010;50:728–760.
- Omaye S, Krinsky N, Kagan V, Mayne S, Liebler D, Bidlack W. β-Carotene: Friend or Foe? *Fundam Appl Toxicol.* 1997;40:163–174.
- Ozhogina O, Kasaikina O. Beta-carotene as an interceptor of free radicals. *Free Rad Biol Med.* 1995;19:575–581.
- Palozza P, Serini S, Calviello G. Carotenoids as modulators of intracellular signaling pathways. *Curr Signal Transduct Ther.* 2006;1:325–335.
- Wood A, Britton G, Jackson M. Carotenoids and protection of phospholipids in solution or in liposomes against oxidation by peroxyl radicals: Relationship between carotenoid structure and protective ability. *Biochem Biophys Acta.* 1997;1336:575–586.
- Woutersen R, Wolterbeek A, Appel M, van den Berg H, Goldbohm R, Feron V. Safety evaluation of synthetic beta-carotene. *Crit Rev Toxicol.* 1999;29:515–542.
- www.carotenoidsociety.org

Skin studies

- Alaluf S, Heinrich U, Stahl W, Tronnier H, Wiseman S. Dietary carotenoids contribute to normal human skin color and UV photosensitivity. *J Nutr.* 2002;132:399–403.
- Bayerl C. Beta-carotene in dermatology: Does it help? *Acta Dermatoven APA.* 2008;17:160–166.
- Biesalski H, Obermueller-Jevic U. UV light, beta-carotene and human skin - Beneficial and potentially harmful effects. *Arch Biochem Biophys.* 2001;389:1–6.
- Black H. Pro-oxidant and anti-oxidant mechanism(s) of BHT and beta-carotene in photocarcinogenesis. *Front Biosci.* 2002;7:d1044–d1055.
- Darvin M, Gerzonde I, Ey S, Brandt N, Albrecht H, Gonchukov S et al. Noninvasive detection of beta-Carotene and lycopene in human skin using Raman spectroscopy. *Laser Phys.* 2004;14:231–233.
- Garmyn M, Ribaya-Mercado J, Russel R, Bhawan J, Gilchrest B. Effect of beta-carotene supplementation on the human sunburn reaction. *Exper Derm.* 1995;4:104–111.
- Heinrich U, Gärtner C, Wiebusch M, Eichler O, Sies H, Tronnier H et al. Supplementation with β-carotene or a similar amount of mixed carotenoids protects humans from UV-induced erythema. *J Nutr.* 2003;133:98–101.
- Huang Z, Lin Y, Fang J. Biological and pharmacological activities of squalene and related compounds: Potential uses in cosmetic dermatology. *Molecules.* 2009;14:540–554.
- Maharshak N, Shapiro J, Trau H. Carotenoderma—A review of the current literature. *Int J Derm.* 2003;42:178–181.
- McArdle F, Rhodes L, Parslew R, Close G, Jack C, Friedmann P et al. Effects of oral vitamin E and {beta}-carotene supplementation on ultraviolet radiation-induced oxidative stress in human skin. *Am J Clin Nutr.* 2004;80:1270–1275.
- Ribaya-Mercado J, Garmyn M, Gilchrest B, Russell R. Skin lycopene is destroyed preferentially over beta-carotene during UV irradiation in humans. *J Nutr.* 1995;125:1854–1859.
- Richelle M, Sabatier M, Steiling H, Williamson G. Skin bioavailability of dietary vitamin E, carotenoids, polyphenols, vitamin C, zinc and selenium. *Br J Nutr.* 2005;96:801–808.
- Rosen C. Topical and systemic photoprotection. *Dermatol Ther.* 2003;16:8–15.
- Stahl W, Heinrich U, Jungmann H, Tronnier H, Sies H. Carotenoids in human skin: Noninvasive measurement and identification of dermal carotenoids and carotenol esters. *Methods Enzymol.* 2000;319:494–502.
- Wertz K, Seifert N, Buchwald P, Hunziker P, Riss G, Wyss A et al. Beta-carotene inhibits UVA-induced matrix metalloprotease 1 and 10 expression in keratinocytes by a singlet oxygen-dependent mechanism. *Free Rad Biol Med.* 2004;37:654–670.
- Stahl W, Sies H. Carotenoids and protection against solar UV radiation. *Skin Pharmacol Appl Skin Physiol.* 2002;15:291–296.

CURCUMIN

- *Empirical formula*: $C_{21}H_{20}O_6$
- *MW*: 368.39
- *Synonyms*: diferuloylmethane, diferulylmethane, natural yellow 3
- IUPAC name: (1E,6E)-1,7-bis(4-hydroxy-3-methoxyphenyl) hepta-1,6-diene-3,5-dione
- *CAS*: 458-37-7
- *EC number*: 207-280-5
- *SMILES*: COC1=C(C=CC(=C1)C=CC(=O)CC(=O)C=CC2=CC(=C(C=C2)O)OC)O

Description

Curcumin is the principal component of the spice turmeric (*Curcuma longa*), which gives it a characteristic yellow color. In recent years, a great deal of research has elucidated a number of pharmacological properties including antioxidant, anti-inflammatory, and anti-tumor activity. In skin care, a significant amount of work has demonstrated curcumin's utility in wound healing as well as its possible role in ameliorating skin conditions, such as psoriasis, scleroderma, and cancer.

Chemical/physical properties

- *Melting point*[13]: 183°C
- *Solubilities*[13]: Insoluble in water. Soluble in alcohol

- *ALOGPs[6]*: 3.62
- *Max absorption[27]*: 265 nm (log ε = 4.18); 420 nm (log ε = 4.77)

Stability/shelf life

Kharat M, Du Z, Zhang G, McClements D. Physical and chemical stability of curcumin in aqueous solutions and emulsions: Impact of pH, temperature, and molecular environment. *J Agric Food Chem.* 2017;65:1525–1532.

Analytical studies

- Lestari M, Indrayanto G. Curcumin. *Profiles Drug Subst Excip Relat Methodol.* 2014;39:113–204.

ESR studies

- Morales N, Sirijaroonwong S, Yamanont P, Phisalaphong C. Electron paramagnetic resonance study of the free radical scavenging capacity of curcumin and its demethoxy and hydrogenated derivatives. *Biol Pharm Bull.* 2015;38:1478–1483.

General interest articles

- Hewlings S, Kalman D. Curcumin: A review of its effects on human health. *Foods.* 2017;6(10):E92.
- Stanić Z. Curcumin, a compound from natural sources, a true scientific challenge—A review. *Plant Foods Hum Nutr.* 2017;72:1–12.

Skin studies

- Hussain Z, Thu H, Ng S, Khan S, Katas H. Nanoencapsulation, an efficient and promising approach to maximize wound healing efficacy of curcumin: A review of new trends and state-of-the-art. *Colloids Surf B Biointerfaces.* 2017;150:223–241.
- Mohanty C, Sahoo S. Curcumin and its topical formulations for wound healing applications. *Drug Discov Today.* 2017;22:1582–1592.
- Vaughn A, Branum A, Sivamani R. Effects of turmeric (*Curcuma longa*) on skin health: A systematic review of the clinical evidence. *Phytother Res.* 2016;30:1243–1264.
- Vaughn A, Haas K, Burney W, Andersen E, Clark A, Crawford R et al. Potential role of curcumin against biofilm-producing organisms on the skin: A review. *Phytother Res.* 2017. doi:10.1002/ptr.5912.

ELLAGIC ACID

- *Empirical formula*: $C_{14}H_6O_8$
- *MW*: 302.19
- *Synonyms*: 4,4′,5,5′,6,6′-hexahydroxydiphenic acid 2,6,2′,6′-dilactone
- *CAS*: 476-66-4
- *EC number*: 207-508-3
- *SMILES*: c12c3c(O)c(O)cc2C(Oc4c1c(C(O3)=O)cc(O)c4O)=O

Description

Ellagic acid is primarily used as a skin whitening agent, but also is an antioxidant. It is a phytochemical found in cranberries, raspberries, strawberries, pomegranate, walnuts, and pecans. Although studies have demonstrated anticarcinogenic activity of ellagic acid, there is considerable controversy surrounding its use as an anticancer agent. In fact, the FDA identified it on its list of *Fake Cancer Cures.*[28] In in vitro and animal model studies, promising results with ellagic acid acting as an anticancer agent were found. However, such observations have never been made in humans. Thus, several organizations, including the American Cancer Society, have recommended ellagic acid's category of use as antioxidant and not as an anticancer agent.

Chemical/physical properties

- *Melting point[13]*: >360°C
- *Solubilities[13]*: Slightly soluble in alcohol; soluble in alkalies and in pyridine; practically insoluble in ether
- *ALOGPs[6]*: 1.59
- *Hydroxyl radical reaction rate constant[7]*: 1.48×10^{-11} cm^3/molec · s
- *UV max (ethanol)[13]*: 366, 255 nm (log ε = 3.93, 4.60)

General interest articles

- Bell C, Hawthorne S. Ellagic acid, pomegranate and prostate cancer—A mini review. *J Pharm Pharmacol.* 2008;60:139–144.
- Jurenka JS. Therapeutic applications of pomegranate (*Punica granatum* L.): A review. *Altern Med Rev.* 2008;13:128–144.

Skin studies

- Almeida IF, Valentão P, Andrade PB, Seabra RM, Pereira TM, Amaral MH et al. In vivo skin irritation potential of a *Castanea sativa* (Chestnut) leaf extract, a putative natural antioxidant for topical application. *Basic Clin Pharmacol Toxicol.* 2008;103:461–467.
- Almeida IF, Valentão P, Andrade PB, Seabra RM, Pereira TM, Amaral MH et al. Oak leaf extract as topical antioxidant: Free radical scavenging and iron chelating activities and in vivo skin irritation potential. *Biofactors.* 2008;33:267–279.
- Bae JY, Choi JS, Kang SW, Lee YJ, Park J, Kang YH. Dietary compound ellagic acid alleviates skin wrinkle and inflammation induced by UV-B irradiation. *Exper Derm.* 2010;19:182–190.
- Kim YH, Kim KH, Han CS, Yang HC, Park SH, Jang HI et al. Anti-wrinkle activity of *Platycarya strobilacea* extract and its application as a cosmeceutical ingredient. *J Cosmet Sci.* 2010;61:211–224.
- Kim S, Liu Y, Gaber *MW*, Bumgardner JD, Haggard WO, Yang Y. Development of chitosan-ellagic acid

films as a local drug delivery system to induce apoptotic death of human melanoma cells. *J Biomed Mater Res B Appl Biomater*. 2009;90:145–155.
- Kowalczyk MC, Kowalczyk P, Tolstykh O, Hanausek M, Walaszek Z, Slaga TJ. Synergistic effects of combined phytochemicals and skin cancer prevention in SENCAR mice. *Cancer Prev Res (Phila)* 2010;3:170–178.
- Kowalczyk MC, Walaszek Z, Kowalczyk P, Kinjo T, Hanausek M, Slaga TJ. Differential effects of several phytochemicals and their derivatives on murine keratinocytes in vitro and in vivo: Implications for skin cancer prevention. *Carcinogenesis*. 2009;30:1008–1015.
- Shimogaki H, Tanaka Y, Tamai H, Masuda M. In vitro and in vivo evaluation of ellagic acid on melanogenesis inhibition. *Int J Cosmet Sci*. 2000;22:291–303.

(−)-EPICATECHIN

- *Empirical formula*: $C_{15}H_{14}O_6$
- *MW*: 290.27
- *Synonyms*: (−)-*cis*-3,3′,4′,5,7-pentahydroxyflavane; (2R,3R)-2-(3,4-dihydroxyphenyl)-3,4-dihydro-1(2H)-benzopyran-3,5,7-triol
- *CAS*: 490-46-0
- *EC number*: 207-710-1
- *SMILES*: O1c2c(CC(O)C1c3cc(O)c(O)cc3)c(O)cc(O)c2

Description

Epicatechin belongs to a class of flavonoids known as flavanols. The *cis* form, (−)-epicatechin, is shown above, while its common epimer, (+)-catechin (154-23-4), is not shown. (−)-Epicatechin and (+)-catechin are the most common epimers found for this molecule. Often, epicatechin and similar compounds are also referred to as catechins. They are found in green tea (*Camellia sinensis*), cocoa, wine, and other fruits and vegetables. The catechins also consist of (−)-epicatechin gallate, (−)-epigallocatechin, and (−)-epigallocatechin gallate, which are also tabulated in this chapter. In addition to their antioxidant activity, research also suggests that they have anticarcinogenic and immunomodulating properties.

Chemical/physical properties

- *Melting point*[3]: 240 °C
- *LogP (exp)*[10]: 0.51
- *ALOGPs*[6]: 1.02

Stability/shelf life

Lun Su Y, Leung LK, Huang Y, Chen Z-Y. Stability of tea theaflavins and catechins. *Food Chem*. 2003;83:189–195.

Analytical studies

- Frauen M, Rode T, Rapp C, Steinhart H. Determination of green-tea catechins in cosmetic formulations and in in-vitro skin extracts by high-performance liquid chromatography coupled with electrospray ionization mass spectrometry. *Chromatographia*. 2002;55:43–48.
- Guanqun S, Jinming L, Feng Q, Huie CW. Extraction of catechins and caffeine from different tea leaves and comparison with micellar electrokinetic chromatography. *Chin Sci Bull*. 2003;48:2438–2443.
- Kofink M, Papagiannopoulos M, Galensa R. Enantioseparation of catechin and epicatechin in plant food by chiral capillary electrophoresis. *Eur Food Res Tech*. 2007;225:569–577.
- Teshima N, Ogawa K, Yamashita M, Sakai T. Separation and determination of catechins and caffeine in Japanese teas by capillary zone electrophoresis. *Anal Sci*. 2001;17(suppl):a125–a127.
- Vuong QV, Golding JB, Nguyen M, Roach PD. Extraction and isolation of catechins from tea. *J Separ Sci*. 2010;33:3415–3428.

ESR studies

- Guo Q, Zhao B, Shen S, Hou J, Hu J, Xin W. ESR study on the structure–antioxidant activity relationship of tea catechins and their epimers. *Biochim Biophys Acta*. 1999;1427:13–23.
- Jensen ON, Pedersen JA. The oxidative transformations of (+)catechin and (−)epicatechin as studied by ESR: Formation of hydroxycatechinic acids. *Tetrahedron*. 1983;39:1609–1615.
- Martin TS, Kikuzaki H, Hisamoto M, Nakatani N. Constituents of *Amomum tsao-ko* and their radical scavenging and antioxidant activities. *J Am Oil Chem Soc*. 2000;77:667–673.
- Oniki T, Takahama U. Free radicals produced by the oxidation of gallic acid and catechin derivatives. *J Wood Sci*. 2004;50:545–547.
- Pedrielli P, Skibsted LH. Antioxidant synergy and regeneration effect of quercetin, (−)-epicatechin, and (+)-catechin on α-tocopherol in homogeneous solutions of peroxidating methyl linoleate. *J Agric Food Chem*. 2002;50:7138–7144.

General interest articles

- Frei B, Higdon JV. Proceedings of the third international scientific symposium on tea and human health: Role of flavonoids in the diet. *J Nutr*. 2003;133:3275S–3284S.
- Kuroda Y, Hara Y. Antimutagenic and anticarcinogenic activity of tea polyphenols. *Mutat Res*. 1999;436:69–97.
- Lambert JD, Elias RJ. The antioxidant and pro-oxidant activities of green tea polyphenols: A role in cancer prevention. *Arch Biochem Biophys*. 2010;501:65–72.
- Mukhtar H, Ahmad M. Tea polyphenols: Prevention of cancer and optimizing health. *Am J Clin Nutr*. 2000;71(suppl):1698S–16702S.

Skin studies

- Elmets CA, Singh D, Tubesing K, Matsui M, Katiyar S, Mukhtar H. Cutaneous photoprotection from ultraviolet injury by green tea polyphenols. *J Am Acad Dermatol*. 2001;44:425–432.

- Hsu S. Green tea and the skin. *J Am Acad Dermatol.* 2005;52:1049–1059.
- Katiyar SK, Perez A, Mukhtar H. Green tea polyphenol treatment to human skin prevents formation of ultraviolet light B-induced pyrimidine dimers in DNA. *Clin Canc Res.* 2000;6:3864–3869.
- Katiyar SK, Bergamo BM, Vyalil PK, Elmets CA. Green tea polyphenols: DNA photodamage and photoimmunology. *J Photochem Photobiol B: Biol.* 2001;65:109–114.
- Katiyara S, Elmetsa CA, Katiyar SK. Green tea and skin cancer: Photoimmunology, angiogenesis and DNA repair. *J Nutr Biochem.* 2007;18:287–296.
- Mahmood T, Akhtar N, Khan BA, Ahmad M, Khan HMS, Zaman SU. Applications of a stable green tea extract cream on human cheeks. *J Acad Res.* 2010;2:121–126.
- Mantena SK, Meeran SM, Elmets CA, Katiyar SK. Orally administered green tea polyphenols prevent ultraviolet radiation-induced skin cancer in mice through activation of cytotoxic T cells and inhibition of angiogenesis in tumors. *J Nutr.* 2005;135:2871–2877.
- Saraf S, Kaur CD. Phytoconstituents as photoprotective novel cosmetic formulations. *Pharmacogn Rev.* 2010;4:1–11.
- Saric S, Notay M, Sivamani R. Green tea and other tea polyphenols: Effects on sebum production and acne vulgaris. *Antioxidants (Basel).* 2016;6:pii: E2. doi:10.3390/antiox6010002.
- Yusuf N, Irby C, Katiyar SK, Elmets CA. Photoprotective effects of green tea polyphenols. *Photochem Photoimmunol Photomed.* 2007;23:48–56.
- Zhao JF, Zhang YJ, Jin XH, Athar M, Santella RM, Bickers DR et al. Green tea protects against psoralen plus ultraviolet A-induced photochemical damage to skin. *J Invest Dermatol.* 1999;113:1070–1075.

(−)-EPICATECHIN GALLATE*

- *Empirical formula*: $C_{22}H_{18}O_{10}$
- *MW*: 442.37
- *Synonyms*: (−)-cis-2-(3,4-dihydroxyphenyl)-3,4-dihydro-1(2H)-benzopyran-3,5,7-triol 3-gallate; (−)-cis-3,3′,4′,5,7-pentahydroxyflavane 3-gallate
- *CAS*: 1257-08-5

Description

Epicatechin gallate belongs to a class of flavonoids known as flavanols. Structurally, it is similar to epicatechin, but has the additional gallate functionality. Often, epicatechin gallate and similar compounds are also referred to as catechins. They are found in green tea (*Camellia sinensis*), cocoa, wine, and other fruits and vegetables. The catechins also consist of (−)-epicatechin, (−)-epigallocatechin, and (−)-epigallocatechin gallate, which are also tabulated in this chapter. In addition to their antioxidant activity, research also suggests that they have anticarcinogenic properties.

ESR studies

- Shi X, Ye J, Leonard SS, Ding M, Vallyathan V, Castranova V et al. Antioxidant properties of (−)-epicatechin-3-gallate and its inhibition of Cr (VI)-induced DNA damage and Cr (IV)- or TPA-stimulated NF-κB activation. *Mol Cell Biochem.* 2000;206:125–132.

(−)-EPIGALLOCATECHIN*

- *Empirical formula*: $C_{15}H_{14}O_7$
- *MW*: 306.27
- *Synonyms*: (−)-cis-2-(3,4,5-trihydroxyphenyl)-3,4-dihydro-1(2H)-benzopyran-3,5,7-triol; (−)-cis-3,3′,4′,5,5′,7-hexahydroxyflavane
- *CAS*: 970-74-1

Description

Epigallocatechin belongs to a class of flavonoids known as flavanols. Structurally, it differs from epicatechin by an additional hydroxyl group on one of its aromatic rings. Often, epigallocatechin and similar compounds are also referred to as catechins. They are found in green tea (*Camellia sinensis*), cocoa, wine, and other fruits and vegetables. The catechins also consist of (−)-epicatechin, (−)-epicatechin gallate, and (−)-epigallocatechin gallate, which are also tabulated in this chapter. In addition to their antioxidant activity, research also suggests that they have anticarcinogenic properties.

(−)-EPIGALLOCATECHIN GALLATE*

- *Empirical formula*: $C_{22}H_{18}O_{11}$
- *MW*: 458.37

---

* For related studies see section on Epicatechin.

- *Synonyms*: (−)-cis-2-(3,4,5-trihydroxyphenyl)-3,4-dihydro-1(2H)-benzopyran-3,5,7-triol 3-gallate; (−)-cis-3,3′,4′,5,5′,7-hexahydroxy-flavane-3-gallate
- CAS: 989-51-5

Description

Epigallocatechin gallate belongs to a class of flavonoids known as flavanols. Structurally, it differs from epicatechin gallate by an additional hydroxyl group on one of its aromatic rings. In comparison with epicatechin gallate, epigallocatechin gallate contains a gallate moiety. Often, epigallocatechin gallate and similar compounds are also referred to as catechins. They are found in green tea (Camellia sinensis), cocoa, wine, and other fruits and vegetables. The catechins also consist of (−)-epicatechin, (−)-epicatechin gallate, and (−)-epigallocatechin, which are also tabulated in this chapter. In addition to their antioxidant activity, research also suggests that they have anticarcinogenic properties. Epigallocatechin gallate is the most abundant catechin found in green tea (Camellia sinensis).

General interest articles

- Fujiki H, Suganuma M, Okabe S, Sueoka E, Suga K, Imai K et al. A new concept of tumor promotion by tumor necrosis factor-alpha, and cancer preventive agents (−)-epigallocatechin gallate and green tea—a review. *Canc Det Prev*. 2000;24:91–99.

Skin studies

- Balasubramanian S, Eckert RL. Keratinocyte proliferation, differentiation, and apoptosis—differential mechanisms of regulation by curcumin, EGCG and apigenin. *Toxicol Appl Pharmacol*. 2007;224:214–219.
- Nomura M, Akira K, He Z, Ma W-Y, Miyamoto K, Yang CS et al. Inhibitory mechanisms of tea polyphenols on the ultraviolet B-activated phosphatidylinositol 3-kinase-dependent pathway. *J Biol Chem*. 2001;276:46624–46631.

EQUOL

- *Empirical formula*: $C_{15}H_{14}O_3$
- MW: 242.30
- *Synonyms*: 4′,7-isoflavandiol; 4′,7-dihydroxyisoflavan
- IUPAC name: (3S)-3-(4-hydroxyphenyl)-7-chromanol
- CAS: 531-95-3
- EC number: 208-522-2

Description

Equol is an isoflavonoid that has antioxidant, extracellular matrix enhancing, and phytoestrogenic properties. A considerable amount of research has gone into understanding its anti-aging properties in human skin. Equol is a metabolic product of daidzein—an isoflavone found in soybeans—which is metabolized by intestinal bacteria. Equol is also found in beans, cabbage, lettuce, and other plant species.

It should be noted that isoflavonoids are often referred to as phytoestrogens—meaning that they can exert biological effects by interacting with estrogen receptors. Interestingly, equol interacts with estrogen receptor beta, found in keratinocytes and fibroblasts, although the resulting biological outcome has not yet been elucidated.

Chemical/physical properties

- *Melting point*[29]: 192°C–193°C
- *Solubilities*: Soluble in ethanol and other organic solvents
- *Specific optical rotation*[29]: −23.5° (in ethanol)

Analytical studies

- Kašparovská J, Dadáková K, Lochman J, Hadrová S, Křížová L, Kašparovský T. Changes in equol and major soybean isoflavone contents during processing and storage of yogurts made from control or isoflavone-enriched bovine milk determined using LC–MS (TOF) analysis. *Food Chem*. 2017;222:67–73.
- Kim Y, Pyo H, Chung B, Moon M, Lee J. GC-MS Analysis of various phytoestrogens in health functional foods. *Bull Kor Chem Soc*. 2017;38:448–458.
- Rodriguez-Morato J, Farre M, Perez-Mana C, Papaseit E, Martinez-Riera R, de la Torre R et al. Pharmacokinetic comparison of soy isoflavone extracts in human plasma. *J Agric Food Chem*. 2015;63:6946–6953.
- Yerramsetty V, Roe M, Cohen J, Hegeman A, Ismail B. Development of a simple, fast, and accurate method for the direct quantification of selective estrogen receptor modulators using stable isotope dilution mass spectrometry. *J Agric Food Chem*. 2013;61:7028–7037.

General interest articles

- Lund T, Munson D, Haldy M, Setchell K, Lephart E, Handa R. Equol is a novel anti-androgen that inhibits prostate growth and hormone feedback. *Biol Reprod*. 2004;70:1188–1195.
- Setchell K, Brown N, Lydeking-Olsen E. The clinical importance of the metabolite equol—a clue to the effectiveness of soy and its isoflavones. *J Nutr*. 2002;132:3577–3584.
- Setchell K, Clerici C, Lephart E, Cole S, Heenan C, Castellani D et al. S-equol, a potent ligand for estrogen receptor beta, is the exclusive enantiomeric form of the soy isoflavone metabolite produced by human intestinal bacterial flora. *Am J Clin Nutr*. 2005;81:1072–1079.
- Setchell K, Clerici C. Equol: History, chemistry, and formation. *J Nutr*. 2010;140:1355S–1362S.
- Setchell K, Clerici C. Equol: Pharmacokinetics and biological actions. *J Nutr*. 2010;140:1363S–1368S.

Skin studies

- Gopaul R, Knaggs H, Lephart E. Biochemical investigation and gene analysis of equol: A plant and soy-derived

isoflavonoid with antiaging and antioxidant properties with potential human skin applications. *Biofactors*. 2012;38:44–52.
- Jackson R, Greiwe J, Schwen R. S-equol, an antioxidant metabolite of soy daidzein, and oxidative stress in aging: A focus on skin and on the cardiovascular system. In: Preedy V (Ed.). *Aging: Oxidative Stress and Dietary Antioxidants*. Amsterdam, Netherlands: Elsevier; 2014.
- Lephart E. Skin aging and oxidative stress: Equol's antiaging effects via biochemical and molecular mechanisms. *Ageing Res Rev*. 2016;31:36–54.
- Widyarini S, Allanson M, Gallagher N, Pedley J, Boyle G, Parsons P et al. Isoflavonoid photoprotection in mouse and human skin is dependent on metallothionein. *J Invest Dermatol*. 2006;126:198–204.

FERULIC ACID

- *Empirical formula*: $C_{10}H_{10}O_4$
- *MW*: 194.18
- *Synonyms*: (E)-3-(4-hydroxy-3-methoxy-phenyl)prop-2-enoic acid; cinnamic acid; *trans*-4-hydroxy-3-methoxycinnamic acid
- *CAS*: 537-98-4
- *EC number*: 208-679-7

Description

Ferulic acid, like caffeic acid, is a hydroxycinnamic acid that is found in grains, fruits, and vegetables. Normally, it is present in the cell wall of plants where it is covalently attached to the polysaccharide scaffold. In addition to its antioxidant properties, ferulic acid is also a UV absorber and it has anticarcinogenic properties.

Chemical/physical properties

- *Melting point*[13]: 174°C
- *Solubilities*[13]: Soluble in hot water, alcohol, and ethyl acetate; moderately soluble in ether; sparingly soluble in petroleum ether and benzene; forms a sodium salt (*trans*-form)
- *Dissociation constants*[5]: pKa = 4.58
- *Henry's law constant*[7]: 7.96×10^{-14} atm · m^3/mol
- *Hydroxyl radical reaction rate constant*[7]: 4.83×10^{-11} cm^3/molec ·s
- *UV max (EtOH)*[13]: 236, 322 nm

Analytical studies

- Abd-Alla HI, Shaaban M, Shaaban KA, Abu-Gabal NS, Shalaby NM, Laatsch H. New bioactive compounds from *Aloe hijazensis*. *Nat Prod Res*. 2009;23:1035–1049.
- Liu YF, Yang XW. HPLC fingerprint of chemical constituents of Flos Farfarae. *Yao Xue Bao*. 2009;44:510–514.
- Luo L, Wang X, Li Q, Ding Y, Jia J, Deng D. Voltammetric determination of ferulic acid by didodecyldimethylammonium bromide/nafion composite film-modified carbon paste electrode. *Anal Sci*. 2010;26:907–911.

ESR studies

- Ogiwara T, Satoh K, Kadoma Y, Murakami Y, Unten S, Atsumi T et al. Radical scavenging activity and cytotoxicity of ferulic acid. *Anticancer Res*. 2002;22:2711–2717.
- Sun YP, Yates B, Abbot J, Chen CL. ESR study of lignin model compounds irradiated by UV (254 nm photons) in the presence of hydrogen peroxide. *Holzforschung*. 1996;50:233–236.
- Zhou KQ, Yin JJ, Yu LL. ESR determination of the reactions between selected phenolic acids and free radicals or transition metals. *Food Chem*. 2006;95:446–457.

General interest articles

- Graf E. Antioxidant potential of ferulic acid. *Free Rad Biol Med*. 1992;13:435–448.
- Kikuzaki H, Hisamoto M, Hirose K, Akiyama K, Taniguchi H. Antioxidant properties of ferulic acid and its related compounds. *Agr Food Chem*. 2002;50:2161–2168.
- Ogiwara T, Satoh K, Kadoma Y, Murakami Y, Unten S, Atsumi T et al. Radical scavenging activity and cytotoxicity of ferulic acid. *Anticancer Res*. 2002;22:2711–2717.
- Ou S, Kwok K. Ferulic acid: Pharmaceutical functions, preparation and applications in foods. *J Sci Food Agric*. 2004;84:1261–1269.
- Scott B, Butler J, Halliwell B, Aruoma O. Evaluation of the antioxidant actions of ferulic acid and catechins. *Free Radic Res Commun*. 1993;19:241–253.
- Srinivasan M, Sudheer A, Menon V. Ferulic acid: Therapeutic potential through its antioxidant property. *J Clin Biochem Nutr*. 2007;40:92–100.
- Voisin-Chiret AS, Bazin M-A, Lancelot J-C, Rault S. Synthesis of new L-ascorbic ferulic acid hybrids. *Molecules*. 2007;12:2533–2545.

Skin studies

- Asanoma M, Takahashi K, Miyabe M, Yamamoto K, Yosbimi N, Mori H et al. Inhibitory effect of topical application of polymerized ferulic acid, a synthetic lignin, on tumor promotion in mouse skin two-stage tumorigenesis. *Carcinogenesis*. 1994;15:2069–2071.
- Bonina F, Puglia C, Ventura D, Aquino R, Tortora S, Sacchi A et al. In vitro antioxidant and in vivo photoprotective effects of a lyophilized extract of *Capparis spinosa* L. buds. *J Cosmet Sci*. 2002;53:321–335.
- Calabrese V, Calafato S, Puleo E, Cornelius C, Sapienza M, Morganti P et al. Redox regulation of cellular stress response by ferulic acid ethyl ester in human dermal fibroblasts: Role of vitagenes. *Clin Dermatol*. 2008;26:358–363.
- Huang M, Smart R, Wong C, Conney A. Inhibitory effect of curcumin, chlorogenic acid, caffeic acid, and ferulic acid on tumor promotion in mouse skin by

12-O-tetradecanoylphorbol-13-acetate. *Cancer Res.* 1988;48:5941–5946.
- Lesca P. Protective effects of ellagic acid and other plant phenols on benzo[a]pyrene-induced neoplasia in mice. *Carcinogenesis.* 1983;4:1651–1653.
- Lin F-H, Lin J-Y, Gupta RD, Tournas JA, Burch JA, Selim MA et al. Ferulic acid stabilizes a solution of vitamins C and E and doubles its photoprotection of skin. *J Invest Dermatol.* 2005;125:826–832.
- Lin X-F, Min W, Luo D. Anticarcinogenic effect of ferulic acid on ultraviolet-B irradiated human keratinocyte HaCaT cells. *J Med Plants Res.* 2010;4:1686–1694.
- Murray JC, Burch JA, Streilein RD, Iannacchione MA, Hall RP, Pinnell SR. A topical antioxidant solution containing vitamins C and E stabilized by ferulic acid provides protection for human skin against damage caused by ultraviolet irradiation. *J Am Acad Dermatol.* 2008;59:418–425.
- Neradil J, Veselska R, Slanina J. UVC-protective effect of caffeic acid on normal and transformed human skin cells in vitro. *Folia Biol.* 2003;49:197–202.
- Oresajo C, Stephens T, Hino PD, Law RM, Yatskayer M, Foltis P et al. Protective effects of a topical antioxidant mixture containing vitamin C, ferulic acid, and phloretin against ultraviolet-induced photodamage in human skin. *J Cosmet Dermatol.* 2008;7:290–297.
- Puoci F, Cirillo G, Settino R, Curcio M, Parisi OI, Iemma F et al. UV protecting activity of ferulic acid polymeric derivative. *Chem Today.* 2010;28(2):8–10.
- Saija A, Tomaino A, Trombetta D, De Pasquale A, Uccella N, Barbuzzi T et al. In vitro and in vivo evaluation of caffeic and ferulic acids as topical photoprotective agents. *Int J Pharm.* 2000;199:39–47.
- Zhang LW, Al-Suwayeh SA, Hsieh PW, Fang JY. A comparison of skin delivery of ferulic acid and its derivatives: Evaluation of their efficacy and safety. *Int J Pharm.* 2010;399:44–51.

GENISTEIN

- *Empirical formula*: $C_{15}H_{10}O_5$
- *MW*: 270.24
- *Synonyms*: 4′,5,7-trihydroxyisoflavone; 5,7-dihydroxy-3-(4-hydroxyphenyl)-4H-1-benzopyran-4-one
- *CAS*: 446-72-0
- *EC number*: 207-174-9
- *SMILES*: c3(C1=COc2c(C1=O)c(O)cc(O)c2)ccc(O)cc3

Description

Genistein is an isoflavone that is found in soy beans (*Glycine max*) as well as in several other plant species. In recent years, there has been a great deal of interest in soy, primarily due to its bountiful consumption by Southeastern Asians, who coincidentally, have lower incidences of certain diseases. In addition to its antioxidant activity, genistein interacts with various molecular targets in the body and influences cardiovascular health, reproductive tissue state (breast and prostate cancer), enzyme inhibition, and bone viability. Its molecular structure is similar to estrogen; thus, it competitively binds to estrogen receptors. These receptors have diverse biological functions, sometimes resulting in adverse reactions, and other times more favorable.[30]

Chemical/physical properties

- *Melting point*[13]: 297°C–298°C (slight decomposition)
- *Solubilities*[13]: Soluble in the usual organic solvents; soluble in dilute alkalies with yellow color. Practically insoluble in water.
- *ALOGPs*[6]: 3.04
- *Henry's law constant*[7]: 5.10×10^{-17} atm · m^3/mol
- *Hydroxyl radical reaction rate constant*[7]: 2.3×10^{-10} cm^3/molec · s
- *UV max (EtOH)*[13]: 236, 322 nm

Analytical studies

- Delmonte P, Rader JI. Analysis of isoflavones in foods and dietary supplements. *J AOAC Int.* 2006;89:1138–1146.
- Dentith S, Lockwood B. Development of techniques for the analysis of isoflavones in soy foods and nutraceuticals. *Curr Opin Clin Nutr Metab Care.* 2008;11:242–247.
- Qu LP, Fan GR, Peng JY, Mi HM. Isolation of six isoflavones from *Semen sojae praeparatum* by preparative HPLC. *Fitoterapia.* 2007;78:200–204.
- Thomas BF, Zeisel SH, Busby MG, Hill JM, Mitchell RA, Scheffler NM et al. Quantitative analysis of the principle soy isoflavones genistein, daidzein and glycitein, and their primary conjugated metabolites in human plasma and urine using reversed-phase high-performance liquid chromatography with ultraviolet detection. *J Chromatogr B Biomed Sci Appl.* 2001;760:191–205.
- Wu Q, Wang M, Sciarappa WJ, Simon JE. LC/UV/ESI-MS analysis of isoflavones in Edamame and Tofu soybeans. *J Agric Food Chem.* 2004;19:2763–2769.

ESR studies

- Guo Q, Rimbach G, Moini H, Weber S, Packer L. ESR and cell culture studies on free radical-scavenging and antioxidant activities of isoflavonoids. *Toxicol.* 2002;179:171–180.
- Kruk I, Aboul-Enein HY, Michalska T, Lichszteld K, Kładna A. Scavenging of reactive oxygen species by the plant phenols genistein and oleuropein. *Luminescence.* 2005;20:81–89.
- Shirataki Y, Tani S, Sakagami H, Satoh K, Nakashima H, Gotoh K et al. Relationship between cytotoxic activity and radical intensity of isoflavones from Sophora species. *Anticancer Res.* 2001;21:2643–2648.

General interest articles

- Dang ZC. Dose-dependent effects of soy phyto-oestrogen genistein on adipocytes: Mechanisms of action. *Obes Rev.* 2009;10:342–349.
- Klein CB, King AA. Genistein genotoxicity: Critical considerations of in vitro exposure dose. *Toxicol Appl Pharmacol.* 2007;224:1–11.
- Polkowski K, Mazurek AP. Biological properties of genistein. A review of in vitro and in vivo data. *Acta Pol Pharm.* 2000;57:135–155.
- Reiter E, Beck V, Medjakovic S, Jungbauer A. Isoflavones are safe compounds for therapeutical applications—Evaluation of in vitro data. *Gynecol Endocrinol.* 2009;25:554–580.
- Rusin A, Krawczyk Z, Grynkiewicz G, Gogler A, Zawisza-Puchałka J, Szeja W. Synthetic derivatives of genistein, their properties and possible applications. *Acta Biochim Pol.* 2010;57:23–34.
- Sarkar FH, Adsule S, Padhye S, Kulkarni S, Li Y. The role of genistein and synthetic derivatives of isoflavone in cancer prevention and therapy. *Mini Rev Med Chem.* 2006;6:401–407.
- Sarkar FH, Li Y, Wang Z, Padhye S. Lesson learned from nature for the development of novel anti-cancer agents: Implication of isoflavone, curcumin, and their synthetic analogs. *Curr Pharm Des.* 2010;16:1801–1812.
- Si H, Liu D. Phytochemical genistein in the regulation of vascular function: New insights. *Curr Med Chem.* 2007;14:2581–2589.
- Wegrzyn G, Jakóbkiewicz-Banecka J, Gabig-Cimińska M, Piotrowska E, Narajczyk M, Kloska A et al. Genistein: A natural isoflavone with a potential for treatment of genetic diseases. *Biochem Soc Trans.* 2010;38:695–701.

Skin studies

- Huang ZR, Hung CF, Lin YK, Fang JY. In vitro and in vivo evaluation of topical delivery and potential dermal use of soy isoflavones genistein and daidzein. *Int J Pharm.* 2008;19:36–44.
- Kang S, Chung JH, Lee JH, Fisher GJ, Wan YS, Duell EA et al. Topical N-acetyl cysteine and genistein prevent ultraviolet-light-induced signaling that leads to photoaging in human skin in vivo. *J Invest Dermatol.* 2003;120:835–841.
- Kitagawa S, Inoue K, Teraoka R, Morita SY. Enhanced skin delivery of genistein and other two isoflavones by microemulsion and prevention against UV irradiation-induced erythema formation. *Chem Pharm Bull (Tokyo).* 2010;58:398–401.
- Lin JY, Tournas JA, Burch JA, Monteiro-Riviere NA, Zielinski J. Topical isoflavones provide effective photoprotection to skin. *Photodermatol Photoimmunol Photomed.* 2008;24:61–66.
- Minghetti P, Cilurzo F, Casiraghi A, Montanari L. Evaluation of ex vivo human skin permeation of genistein and daidzein. *Drug Deliv.* 2006;13:411–415.
- Miyazaki K, Hanamizu T, Iizuka R, Chiba K. Genistein and daidzein stimulate hyaluronic acid production in transformed human keratinocyte culture and hairless mouse skin. *Skin Pharmacol Appl Skin Physiol.* 2002;15:175–183.
- Saraf S, Kaur CD. Phytoconstituents as photoprotective novel cosmetic formulations. *Pharmacogn Rev.* 2010;4:1–11.
- Sharma S, Sultana S. Modulatory effect of soy isoflavones on biochemical alterations mediated by TPA in mouse skin model. *Food Chem Toxicol.* 2004;42:1669–1675.
- Silva APC, Nunes BR, de Oliveira MC, Koester LS, Mayorga P, Bassani VL et al. Development of topical nanoemulsions containing the isoflavone genistein. *Pharmazie.* 2009;64:32–35.
- Wang Y, Yaping E, Zhang X, Lebwohl M, DeLeo V, Wei H. Inhibition of ultraviolet (UVB-induced) c-fos and c-jun expression in vivo by protein kinase inhibitor genistein. *Carcinogenesis.* 1998;19:649–654.
- Wei H, Bowen R, Cai Q, Barnes S, Wang Y. Antioxidant and antipromotional effects of the soybean isoflavone genistein. *Proc Soc Exp Biol Med.* 1995;208:124–130.
- Wei H, Cai Q, Rahn RO. Inhibition of UV light- and fenton reaction-induced oxidative DNA damage by the soybean isoflavone genistein. *Carcinogenesis.* 1996;17:73–77.
- Widyarini S, Spinks N, Husband AJ, Reeve VE. Isoflavonoid compounds from red clover (*Trifolium pratense*) protect from inflammation and immune suppression induced by UV radiation. *Photochem Photobiol.* 2001;74:465–470.

GLUTATHIONE

- *Empirical formula*: $C_{10}H_{17}N_3O_6S$
- *MW*: 307.32
- *Synonyms*: Gamma-L-glutamyl-L-cysteinyl-glycine
- *CAS*: 70-18-8
- *EC number*: 200-725-4
- *SMILES*: O=C(N[CH](CS)C(NCC(O)=O)=O)CC[CH](C(O)=O)N

Description

Glutathione (gamma-glutamylcysteinylglycine) is an endogenous aqueous phase antioxidant composed of three amino acid moieties. Its antioxidant activity (strong reducing power) stems from the sulfhydryl group (-SH) of the cysteine residue, which donates electrons. It is found in many life forms, including plants and organisms, usually at higher concentrations than other antioxidants. Glutathione, a cofactor for many enzymes (e.g., glutathione peroxidase), can exist in the reduced form (GSH) or oxidized state (GSSG), where two glutathione molecules are covalently linked together at the sulfur groups.

Chemical/physical properties

- *Melting point*[27]: 195°C
- *Solubilities*[27]: very soluble in H_2O; insoluble in EtOH and ether; soluble in DMF

- *Dissociation constants*[20]: pK1 = 2.12, pK2 = 353, pK3 = 8.66, pK4 = 9.12
- *ALOGPs*[6]: −2.74
- *Specific optical rotation*[20]: −18.9° at 25°C/D (c=4.653); −21° at 27°C/D (c = 2.74)

Analytical studies

- Gotti R, Andrisano V, Cavrini V, Bongini A. Determination of glutathione in pharmaceuticals and cosmetics by HPLC with UV and fluorescence detection. *Chromatographia*. 1994;39:23–28.
- Griffith OW. Biologic and pharmacologic regulation of mammalian glutathione synthesis. *Free Rad Biol Med*. 1999;27:922–935.

ESR studies

- Khramtsov VV, Grigor'ev IA, Foster MA, Lurie DJ. In vitro and in vivo measurement of pH and thiols by EPR-based techniques. *Antioxid Redox Signal*. 2004;6:667–676.

General interest articles

- Anderson ME. Glutathione: An overview of biosynthesis and modulation. *Chem Biol Interact*. 1998;111–112:1–14.
- Circu ML, Aw TY. Glutathione and apoptosis. *Free Rad Res*. 2008;42:689–706.
- Forman HJ, Zhang H, Rinna A. Glutathione: Overview of its protective roles, measurement, and biosynthesis. *Mol Aspects Med*. 2009;30:1–12.
- Kidd PM. Glutathione: Systemic protectant against oxidative and free radical damage. *Altern Med Rev*. 1997;2:155–176.
- Li Y, Wei G, Chen J. Glutathione: A review on biotechnological production. *Appl Microbiol Biotechnol*. 2004;66:233–242.

Skin studies

- Kopal C, Deveci M, Öztürk S, Sengezer M. Effects of topical glutathione treatment in rat ischemic wound model. *Ann Plast Surg*. 2007;58:449–455.
- Sonthalia S, Daulatabad D, Sarkar R. Glutathione as a skin whitening agent: Facts, myths, evidence and controversies. *Indian J Dermatol Venereol Leprol* 2016;82:262–272.

KOJIC ACID

- *Empirical formula*: $C_6H_6O_4$
- *MW*: 142.11
- *Synonyms*: 5-hydroxy-2-(hydroxymethyl)-4h-pyran-4-one
- *CAS*: 501-30-4
- *EC number*: 207-922-4
- *SMILES*: C(C1=CC(C(O)=CO1)=O)O

Description

Kojic acid is a commonly utilized skin whitening agent (also referred to as lightening or depigmentation agent), powerful antioxidant, and antibacterial agent. It is produced by some species of the fungi *Aspergillus* and *Penicillium*. As a skin whitening agent, kojic acid impedes the activity of tyrosinase by chelating with the copper ion of the enzyme. Normally, tyrosine is converted to melanin through a series of steps and tyrosinase is responsible for the first two steps of the reaction sequence. Although less known, kojic acid also has antioxidant activity. It is often employed in foods for preservation.

Chemical/physical properties

- *Melting point*[2]: 153.5°C
- *Solubilities*[2,31]: Soluble in ethanol, ethyl ether, acetone, and DMSO; slightly soluble in benzene; soluble in water, acetone; slightly soluble in ether; insoluble in benzene
- *Dissociation constants*[5]: pKa = 7.66 (25°C)
- *LogP (exp)*[32]: −0.64
- *ALOGPs*[6]: −1.02
- *Henry's law constant*[7]: 2.39×10^{-7} atm · m³/mol
- *Hydroxyl radical reaction rate constant*: 6.44×10^{-11} cm³/molec ·s

Stability/shelf life

Kojic acid has several inherent stability problems. It chelates with metal ions, especially iron, leading to yellow discoloration and may become oxidized. To circumvent these problems, metal chelating agents and other antioxidants are normally added to formulations containing kojic acid.[33]

Analytical studies

- Chisvert A, Sisternes J, Balaguer A, Salvador A. A gas chromatography-mass spectrometric method to determine skin-whitening agents in cosmetic products. *Talanta*. 2010;15:530–536.
- Dobias J, Brtko J, Nemec P. [Quantitative determination of kojic acid in fungal fermentation broth using diffusion in agar plates and spectrophotometry]. *Kvasný Prum*. 1985;31:260–262.
- Huang SC, Lin CC, Huang MC, Wen KC. Simultaneous determination of magnesium ascorbyl phosphate, ascorbyl glucoside, kojic acid, arbutin and hydroquinone in skin whitening cosmetics by HPLC. *J Food Drug Anal*. 2004;12:13–18.
- Ichimoto I, Tatsumi C. Studies on kojic acid derivatives: The acylation of kojic acid. *Bull Univ Osaka Pref Ser B*. 1962;13:53–58.
- Kawate S, Koike M, Fukuo T. Spectrophotometric determination of kojic acid. *Technol Rep Kansai Univ*. 1972;13:67–79.
- Kimura K, Hirokado M, Yasuda K, Nishijima M. [Determination of kojic acid in various commercial foods by HPLC]. *Shokuhin Eiseigaku Zasshi*. 2000;41:70–73.
- Manabe M, Shinshi E, Goto T, Misawa Y, Tanaka K, Matsuura S. [Fluorescent compound in fermented

foods. VI. High-performance liquid chromatographic analysis of kojic acid]. *Nippon Shoyu Kenkyusho Zasshi.* 1984;10:146–150.
- Manabe M, Shinshi E, Goto T, Tanaka K, Misawa Y. [Fluorescent constituents in fermented foods. VIII. Gas–liquid chromatographic analytical system for kojic acid]. *Nippon Shoyu Kenkyusho Zasshi.* 1988;14:183–186.
- Owens RG, Welty RE, Lucas GB. Gas chromatographic analysis of the mycotoxins kojic acid, terreic acid, and terrein. *Anal Biochem.* 1970;35:249–258.
- Shih Y, Zen J-M. Voltammetric determination of kojic acid in cosmetic bleaching products using a disposable screen-printed carbon electrode. *Electroanalysis.* 1999;11:229–233.
- Shih Y, Zen J-M, Ke J-H, Hsu J-C, Chen P-C. Flow injection analysis of kojic acid in cosmetics by a carbon-nanotube modified screen-printed electrode. *J Food Drug Anal.* 2007;15:151–155.
- Tanigaki H, Obata H, Tokuyama T. The determination of kojic acid using the stopped-flow method. *Bull Chem Soc Jpn.* 1980;53:3195–3197.

ESR studies

- Dixon WT, Moghimi M, Murphy D. Electron spin resonance study of radicals obtained from the oxidation of naturally occurring hydroxypyrones. *J Chem Soc Perkin Trans 2.* 1975(2):101–103.

General interest articles

- Bentley R. From miso, saké and shoyu to cosmetics: A century of science for kojic acid. *Nat Prod Rep.* 2006;23:1046–1062.
- Brtko J, Rondahl L, Ficková M, Hudecová D, Eybl V, Uher M. Kojic acid and its derivatives: History and present state of art. *Cent Eur J Public Health.* 2004;12(Suppl):S16–S18.
- Burdock GA, Soni MG, Carabin IG. Evaluation of health aspects of kojic acid in food. *Regulatory Toxicol Pharmacol.* 2001;33:80–101.
- Gomes AJ, Lunardi CN, Gonzalez S, Tedesco AC. The antioxidant action of *Polypodium leucotomos* extract and kojic acid: Reactions with reactive oxygen species. *Braz J Med Biol Res.* 2001;34:1487–1494.
- Mohamad R, Mohamed MS, Suhaili N, Salleh MM, Ariff AB. Kojic acid: Applications and development of fermentation process for production. *Biotechnol Molec Biol Rev.* 2010;5:24–37.

Skin studies

- Burnett CL, Bergfeld WF, Belsito DV, Hill RA, Klaassen CD, Liebler DC et al. Final report of the safety assessment of Kojic acid as used in cosmetics. *Int J Toxicol.* 2009;29(6 Suppl):244S–273S.
- Cabanes J, Chazarra S, Garcia-Carmona F. Kojic acid, a cosmetic skin whitening agent, is a slow-binding inhibitor of catecholase activity of tyrosinase. *J Pharm Pharmacol.* 1994;46:982–985.
- Mitani H, Koshiishi I, Sumita T, Imanari T. Prevention of the photodamage in the hairless mouse dorsal skin by kojic acid as an iron chelator. *Eur J Pharmacol.* 2001;411:169–174.

ALPHA-LIPOIC ACID

- *Empirical formula*: $C_8H_{14}O_2S_2$
- *MW*: 206.33
- *Synonyms*: (±)-1,2-dithiolane-3-pentanoic acid; 6,8-dithiooctanoic acid; DL-alpha-lipoic acid; thioctic acid
- CAS: 1077-28-7
- EC number: 214-071-2
- SMILES: S1SCCC1CCCCC(O)=O

Description

Lipoic acid exists in both the oxidized disulfide form (shown above) and the reduced dithiol form (dihydrolipoic acid). Both forms of the molecule have antioxidant activity. It is a cofactor for several enzymes where it carries out a role in oxidative decarboxylation reactions, such as those that occur with alpha-keto acids. It has been cited as a *universal antioxidant* because it is so versatile in its specificity for radical species and for its ability to function in both lipid and aqueous phases. While lipoic acid is a very strong reducing agent, its endogenous levels in tissues are not very high.

Chemical/physical properties

- *Melting point*[34]: 47.5°C–48°C
- *Solubilities*[34]: Soluble in methanol, ethanol, diethyl ether, and chloroform
- *Dissociation constants*[35]: pKa = 5.10
- White powder, soluble in water, pH of aqueous solutions about 7.4 (sodium salt of lipoic acid)[13]
- *Crystals by vacuum sublimation (at 85°C–90°C and 25 µm). MP*[13]: 46°C–48°C (microblock). pKa = 5.4. Practically insoluble in water. Soluble in fat solvents. (d-form)
- *Yellow needles from cyclohexane. MP*: 60°C–61°C. BP[13]: 160°C–165°C. Practically insoluble in water; soluble in fat solvents. Forms a water-soluble sodium salt. (dl-form)
- *Crystals from cyclohexane. MP*: 45°C–47.5°C (microblock).
- *ALOGPs*[6]: 2.75
- *Henry's law constant*[7]: 1.64×10^{-8} atm · m³/mol
- *Hydroxyl radical reaction rate constant*[7]: 2.52×10^{-10} cm³/molec · s
- Crystals by vacuum sublimation (at 85°C–90°C and 25 µm). Specific optical rotation: + 104° at 23°C/D (c = 0.88 in benzene). UV max (methanol)[13]: 333 nm (ε = 150)
- Crystals from cyclohexane. Specific optical rotation[13]: –113 at 23°C/D (c = 1.88 in benzene). UV max (methanol): 330 nm (ε = 140). (l-form)

Stability/shelf life

Segall A, Sosa M, Alami A, Enero C, Hormaechea F, Pizzorno MT et al. Stability study of lipoic acid in the presence of vitamins A and E in o/w emulsions for cosmetic application. *J Cosmet Sci.* 2004;55:449–461.

Analytical studies

- Han D, Handelman GJ, Packer L. Analysis of reduced and oxidized lipoic acid in biological samples by high-performance liquid chromatography. *Methods Enzymol.* 1995;251:315–325.
- Kataoka H. Chromatographic analysis of lipoic acid and related compounds. *J Chromatogr B: Biomed Sci Appl.* 1998;717:247–262.
- Moyano MA, Broussalis AM, Segall AI. Thermal analysis of lipoic acid and evaluation of the compatibility with excipients. *J Therm Anal Calorim.* 2009;99:631–637.
- Ravanić N, Filipić S, Nikolić K, Popović G, Vovk I, Simonovska B et al. Analysis of α-lipoic acid in drug formulations and dietary supplement preparations. *Acta Chromatographica.* 2009;21:433–441.
- Sen CK, Roy S, Khanna S, Packer L. Determination of oxidized and reduced lipoic acid using high-performance liquid chromatography and coulometric detection. *Methods Enzymol.* 1999;299:239–246.
- Sittona A, Schmid MG, Gübitza G, Aboul-Enein HY. Determination of lipoic acid in dietary supplement preparations by capillary electrophoresis. *J Biochem Biophys Meth.* 2004;61:119–124.

ESR studies

- Smissman EE, Sorenson JRJ. The electron spin resonance spectra of disulfides irradiated with ultraviolet light. *J Org Chem.* 1965;30:4008–4010.

General interest articles

- Bilska A, Włodek L. Lipoic acid—The drug of the future? *Pharmacol Rep.* 2005;57:570–577.
- Kagan VE, Shvedova A, Serbinova E, Khan S, Swanson C, Powell R et al. Dihydrolipoic acid—A universal antioxidant both in the membrane and in the aqueous phase. *Biochem Pharmacol.* 1992;44:1637–1649.
- Navari-Izzo F, Quartacci MF, Sgherri C. Lipoic acid: A unique antioxidant in the detoxification of activated oxygen species. *Plant Physiol Biochem.* 2002;40:463–470.
- Packer L, Witt EH, Tritschler HJ. Alpha-lipoic acid as a biological antioxidant. *Free Rad Biol Med.* 1995;19:227–250.

Skin studies

- Fuchs J, Milbradt R. Antioxidant inhibition of skin inflammation induced by reactive oxidants: Evaluation of the redox couple dihydrolipoate/lipoate. *Skin Pharmacol.* 1994;7:278–284.
- Gelo-Pujic M, Desmurs JR, Kassem T, Delaire S, Adao A, Tawil D. Synthesis of new antioxidant conjugates and their in vitro hydrolysis with stratum corneum enzymes. *Int J Cosmet Sci.* 2008;30:195–204.
- Ho YS, Lai CS, Liu HI, Ho SY, Tai C, Pan MH et al. Dihydrolipoic acid inhibits skin tumor promotion through anti-inflammation and anti-oxidation. *Biochem Pharmacol.* 2007;73:1786–1795.
- Kim GD, Kim TH, Jang AH, Ahn HJ, Park YS, Park CS. α-Lipoic acid suppresses the development of DNFB-induced atopic dermatitis-like symptoms in NC/Nga mice. *Exp Dermatol.* 2011;20:97–101.
- Lin JY, Lin FH, Burch JA, Selim MA, Monteiro-Riviere NA, Grichnik JM et al. α-lipoic acid is ineffective as a topical antioxidant for photoprotection of skin. *J Invest Dermatol.* 2004;123:996–998.
- Podda M, Rallis M, Traber MG, Packer L, Maibach HI. Kinetic study of cutaneous and subcutaneous distribution following topical application of [7,8-14C]rac-alpha-lipoic acid into hairless mice. *Biochem Pharmacol.* 1996;52:627–633.
- Podda M, Zollner TM, Grundmann-Kollmann M, Thiele JJ, Packer L, Kaufmann R. Activity of alpha-lipoic acid in the protection against oxidative stress in skin. *Curr Prob Dermatol.* 2001;29:43–51.
- Richert S, Schrader A, Schrader K. Transdermal delivery of two antioxidants from different cosmetic formulations. *Int J Cosmet Sci.* 2003;25:5–13.
- Tsuji-Naito K, Ishikura S, Akagawa M, Saeki H. α-Lipoic acid induces collagen biosynthesis involving prolyl hydroxylase expression via activation of TGF-β-Smad signaling in human dermal fibroblasts. *Connect Tissue Res.* 2010;51:378–387.
- Venkatraman MS, Chittiboyina A, Meingassner J, Ho CI, Varani J, Ellis CN et al. Alpha-lipoic acid-based PPARgamma agonists for treating inflammatory skin diseases. *Arch Dermatol Res.* 2004;296:97–104.
- Wada N, Wakami H, Konishi T, Matsugo S. The degradation and regeneration of alpha-lipoic acid under the irradiation of UV light in the existence of homocysteine. *J Clin Biochem Nutr.* 2009;44:218–222.
- Wang YJ, Yang MC, Pan MH. Dihydrolipoic acid inhibits tetrachlorohydroquinone-induced tumor promotion through prevention of oxidative damage. *Food Chem Toxicol.* 2008;46:3739–3748.

LYCOPENE

- *Empirical formula*: $C_{40}H_{56}$
- *MW*: 536.87
- *Synonyms*: 2,6,10,14,19,23,27,31-octamethyl-dotriaconta-2,6,8,10,12,14,16,18,20,22,24,26,30-tridecaene; ψ,ψ-carotene
- *CAS*: 502-65-8
- *EC number*: 207-949-1

- *SMILES*: C(C=CC=C(C)CCC=C(C)C)(C)=CC=CC(C)=CC=CC=C(C)C=CC=C(C)C=CC=C(C)CCC=C(C)C

Description

Lycopene is a carotenoid that gives tomatoes their characteristic red color. Like other carotenoids, lycopene's antioxidant properties stem from its highly conjugated backbone structure, which is capable of quenching reactive oxygen species such as $^1O_2$. In skin, lycopene and beta-carotene account for about 70% of the carotenoids.[36]

Chemical/physical properties

- *Melting point*[37]: 172°C–173°C (trans-form), 105°C (15,15′-cis-form)
- *Solubilities*[37]: 1 g dissolves in 50 mL carbon disulfide (0°C); soluble in chloroform and benzene; almost insoluble in MeOH and EtOH
- *ALOGPs*[6]: 9.16
- *UV/vis absorption max*[37]: 446, 472, and 505 nm (trans-form) with the following respective molar absorption coefficients: 2250, 3450, and 3150 (1% and 1 cm)
- *UV/vis absorption max*[37]: 361, 444, 470, and 502 nm (cis-form) with the following respective molar absorption coefficients: 1110, 1280, 1660, and 1280 (1% and 1 cm)
- UV spectrum available in Trevithick-Sutton et al.[38]

Stability/shelf life

Cámara M, Sánchez-Mata MC, Fernández-Ruiz V, Piera G. Stability of lycopene in tomato products and extracts. In: Pitblado R, Routledge J (Eds). ISHS Acta Horticulturae 823: XI International Symposium on the Processing Tomato. Toronto: ISHS; 2009.

Analytical studies

- Ishida BK, Ma J, Chan B. A simple, rapid method for HPLC analysis of lycopene isomers. *Phytochem Anal.* 2001;12:194–198.
- Lin CH, Chen BH. Determination of carotenoids in tomato juice by liquid chromatography. *J Chromatogr A.* 2003;1012:103–109.
- Rajendran V, Pu YS, Chen BH. An improved HPLC method for determination of carotenoids in human serum. *J Chromatogr B Analyt Technol Biomed Life Sci.* 2005;824:99–106.
- Vasta JD, Sherma J. Analysis of lycopene in nutritional supplements by silica gel high-performance thin-layer chromatography with visible-mode densitometry. *Acta Chromatographica.* 2008;20:673–683.

ESR studies

- Haila KM, Nielsen BR, Heinonen MI, Skibsted LH. Carotenoid reaction with free radicals in acetone and toluene at different oxygen partial pressures. An ESR spin-trapping study of structure–activity relationships. *Z Lebensm Unters Forsch A.* 1997;204:81–87.

General interest articles

- Edge R, McGarvey DJ, Truscott TG. The carotenoids as anti-oxidants—A review. *J Photochem Photobiol B: Biol.* 1997;41:189–200.
- Kavanaugh CJ, Trumbo PR, Ellwood KC. The U.S. Food and Drug Administration's evidence-based review for qualified health claims: Tomatoes, lycopene, and cancer. *J Natl Cancer Inst.* 2007;99:1074–1085.
- Namitha KK, Negi PS. Chemistry and biotechnology of carotenoids. *Crit Rev Food Sci Nutr.* 2010;50:728–760.
- Palozza P, Parrone N, Catalano A, Simone R. Tomato lycopene and inflammatory cascade: Basic interactions and clinical implications. *Curr Med Chem.* 2010;17:2547–2563.
- Rao AV, Ray MR, Rao LG. Lycopene. *Adv Food Nutr Res.* 2006;51:99–164.

Skin studies

- Aust O, Stahl W, Sies H, Tronnier H, Heinrich U. Supplementation with tomato based products increases lycopene, phytofluene, and phytoene levels in human serum and protects against UV-induced erythema. *Int J Vitam Nutr Res.* 2003;75:54–60.
- Stahl W, Heinrich U, Aust O, Tronnier H, Sies H. Lycopene-rich products and dietary photoprotection. *Photochem Photobiol Sci.* 2006;5:238–242.
- Stahl W, Heinrich U, Wiseman S, Eichler O, Sies H, Tronnier H. Dietary tomato paste protects against ultraviolet light–induced erythema in humans. *J Nutr.* 2001;131:1449–1451.
- Stahl W, Sies H. Carotenoids and protection against solar UV radiation. *Skin Pharmacol Appl Skin Physiol.* 2002;15:291–296.

NORDIHYDROGUAIARETIC ACID

- *Empirical formula*: $C_{18}H_{22}O_4$
- *MW*: 302.36
- *Synonyms*: 4,4′-(2,3-dimethyltetramethylene)dipyrocatechol; 1,4-bis(3,4-dihydroxyphenyl)-2,3-dimethylbutane
- *CAS*: 500-38-9
- *EC number*: 207-903-0
- *SMILES*: C(c1cc(O)c(O)cc1)C(C)C(C)Cc2cc(O)c(O)cc2

Description

Nordihydroguaiaretic acid occurs naturally in the creosote bush (*Larrea tridentata*), which is native to Mexico and the Southwestern region of the U.S. Nordihydroguaiaretic acid has various pharmacological properties, and for this reason it is often utilized in folk medicine. In addition, it is a potent antioxidant and also inhibits lipoxygenase (enzyme responsible for the formation of lipid hydroperoxide) and cycloxygenase (enzyme responsible for the conversion of arachidonic acid to prostaglandin H2) pathways. Up until the 1960s, it was used extensively as a food preservative until it was withdrawn for toxicity reasons. It was determined that the toxicity was a result of the formation of alpha-quinone during nordihydroguaiaretic acid metabolism. Nowadays, some naturopathic practitioners use chaparral (leaves and flowers from the creosote bush); however, it is not recommended by the FDA. Consumers are warned of possible hepatoxicity and renal complications due to chronic use.

Chemical/physical properties

- *Melting point*[3]: 184°C–186°C
- *ALOGPs*[6]: 3.44

Analytical studies

- Gay ML, Musser SM. Single-laboratory validated method for determination of nordihydroguaiaretic acid in chaparral-containing dietary supplements. *J AOAC Int.* 2008;91:501–505.

General interest articles

- Arteaga S, Andrade-Cetto A, Cárdenas R. *Larrea tridentata* (Creosote bush), an abundant plant of Mexican and US-American deserts and its metabolite nordihydroguaiaretic acid. *J Ethnopharmacol.* 2005;98:231–239.
- Chen Q. Nordihydroguaiaretic acid analogues: Their chemical synthesis and biological activities. *Curr Top Med Chem.* 2009;9:1636–1659.
- Fonyo A. The availability of nordihydroguaiaretic acid antioxidant. *J Am Oil Chem Soc.* 1946;23:75–77.
- Lü JM, Nurko J, Weakley SM, Jiang J, Kougias P, Lin PH et al. Molecular mechanisms and clinical applications of nordihydroguaiaretic acid (NDGA) and its derivatives: An update. *Med Sci Monit.* 2010;16:RA93–RA100.

Skin studies

- Athar M, Raza H, Bickers DR, Mukhtar H. Inhibition of benzoyl peroxide-mediated tumor promotion in 7, 12-dimethylbenz(a)anthracene-initiated skin of Sencar mice by antioxidants nordihydroguaiaretic acid and diallyl sulfide. *J Invest Dermatol.* 1990;94:162–165.
- Gonzales M, Bowden GT. Nordihydroguaiaretic acid-mediated inhibition of ultraviolet B-induced activator protein-1 activation in human keratinocytes. *Mol Carcinog.* 2002;34:102–111.
- Nakadate T, Yamamoto S, Aizu E, Kato R. Inhibition by lipoxygenase inhibitors of 7-bromomethylbenz[a]anthracene-caused epidermal ornithine decarboxylase induction and skin tumor promotion in mice. *Carcinogenesis.* 1989;10:2053–2057.
- Rahman S, Ansari RA, Rehman H, Parvez S, Raisuddin S. Nordihydroguaiaretic acid from creosote Bush (*Larrea tridentata*) mitigates 12-O-tetradecanoylphorbol-13-acetate-induced inflammatory and oxidative stress responses of tumor promotion cascade in mouse skin. *Evid Based Complement Alternat Med.* 2011;734785:1–10.
- Saarinen JV, Harvima RJ, Horsmanheimo M, Harvima IT. Modulation of the immediate allergic wheal reaction in the skin by drugs inhibiting the effects of leukotriene C4 and prostaglandin D2. *Eur J Clin Pharmacol.* 2001;57:1–4.
- Wang ZY, Agarwal R, Zhou ZC, Bickers DR, Mukhtar H. Antimutagenic and antitumorigenic activities of nordihydroguaiaretic acid. *Mutat Res Genet Toxicol.* 1991;261:153–162.

POGOSTONE

- *Empirical formula*: $C_{12}H_{16}O_4$
- *MW*: 224.26
- *Synonyms*: patchouli oil, dhelwangin, 4-hydroxy-6-methyl- 3-(4-methylpentanoyl)pyran-2-one
- *CAS number*: 23800-56-8
- *SMILES*: CC1=CC(=C(C(=O)O1)C(=O)CCC(C)C)O

Description

Pogostone is one of the key components of patchouli oil, which is the essential oil of the aerial part (*Pogostemonis herba*) of the herbaceous plant, *Pogostemon cablin* (Blanco) Benth. In terms of its chemical characterization, pogostone is a pyranone—a pyran ring containing a ketone functional group. It is used in traditional Chinese and Indian (Ayurveda) medicine to treat a variety of ailments and symptoms including dampness, diarrhea, dermatitis, fever, and vomiting as well as to help stimulate appetite.[39] Curiously, pogostone also has insect repellant properties.

Chemical/physical properties

- *Melting point*[39]: 41°C–41.6°C
- *Solubility*[39]: 0.39 g/L
- *ALOGPs*[39]: 1.6

Analytical studies

- Klein E, Rojahn W. Isolation, structure, and synthesis of dhelwangin. *Tetrahedron Lett.* 1969;27:2279–2280.
- Li L, Hu C, Quan Z. Isolation and identification of dhelwangin in *Agastache rugosa*. *Zhongnan Minzu Daxue Xuebao, Ziran Kexueban.* 2005;24:14–16.
- Zhao X, Li C, Cao Y, Yi Y, Shi S, Feng X et al. Structural elucidation of pogostone and its dimers-two novel diastereomers combined with X-ray diffraction and spectroscopy. *J Mol Struct.* 2014;1058:189–196.

General interest articles

- Murugan R, Livingstone C. Origin of the name 'patchouli' and its history. *Curr Sci.* 2010;99:1274–1276.

Skin studies

- Lin R, Feng X, Li C, Zhang X, Yu X, Zhou J et al. Prevention of UV radiation-induced cutaneous photoaging in mice by topical administration of patchouli oil. *J Ethnopharmacol.* 2014;154:408–418.
- Wang X, Huang Y, Wang L, Xu L, Yu X, Liu Y et al. Photoprotective activity of pogostone against UV-induced skin premature aging in mice. *Exp Gerontol.* 2016;77:76–86.

PROPYL GALLATE

- *Empirical formula*: $C_{10}H_{12}O_5$
- *MW*: 212.20
- *Synonyms*: 3,4,5-trihydroxybenzoic acid propyl ester; propyl ester gallic acid; propyl 3,4,5-trihydroxybenzoate
- *CAS*: 121-79-9
- *EC number*: 204-498-2
- *SMILES*: O=C(OCCC)C1=CC(O)=C(O)C(O)=C1

Description

Propyl gallate is a common synthetic antioxidant that has been used for many years to prevent lipid oxidation in foods. It is also utilized in cosmetic preparations.

Chemical/physical properties

- *Melting point*[40]: 130°C
- *Solubilities*[20]: At 25°C in water 0.35 g/100 mL, in alcohol 103 g/100 g, in ether 83 g/100 g, in cottonseed oil at 30°C 1.23 g/100 g, in lard at 45°C 1.14 g/100 g
- *LogP (exp)*[41]: 1.80
- *ALOGPs*[6]: 1.96
- Darkens in presence of iron and iron salts[20]
- Synergistic with acids, BHA, BHT[20]

Stability/shelf life

Due to its solubility profile, propyl gallate will often seek the water phase in systems containing both lipid and aqueous phases. As a result, it can associate with iron in the aqueous phase, resulting in product discoloration.[21]

Analytical studies

- Aguilar-Caballos MP, Gómez-Hens A, Pérez-Bendito D. Simultaneous kinetic determination of butylated hydroxyanisole and propyl gallate by coupling stopped-flow mixing technique and diode-array detection. *Anal Chim Acta.* 1997;354:173–179.
- Ni Y, Wang L, Kokot S. Voltammetric determination of butylated hydroxyanisole, butylated hydroxytoluene, propyl gallate and tert-butylhydroquinone by use of chemometric approaches. *Anal Chim Acta.* 2000;412:185–193.

ESR studies

- Matsunaga Y, McDowell CA. The electron spin resonance absorption spectra of semiquinone ions. Part I. The hyperfine splitting due to alkoxyl groups. *Can J Chem.* 1960;38:1158–1166.

General interest articles

- Becker L. Final report on the amended safety assessment of propyl gallate. *Int J Toxicol.* 2007;26(Suppl. 3):89–118.
- Bors W, Michel C. Antioxidant capacity of flavanols and gallate esters: Pulse radiolysis studies. *Free Rad Biol Med.* 1999;27:1413–1426.
- Deeble DJ, Parsons BJ, Phillips GO, Schuchmann HP, von Sonntag C. Superoxide radical reactions in aqueous solutions of pyrogallol and n-propylgallate: The involvement of phenoxyl radicals. A pulse radiolysis study. *Int J Radiat Biol.* 1988;54:179–193.
- Kim JH, Kang NJ, Lee BK, Lee KW, Lee HJ. Gallic acid, a metabolite of the antioxidant propyl gallate, inhibits gap junctional intercellular communication via phosphorylation of connexin 43 and extracellular-signal-regulated kinase1/2 in rat liver epithelial cells. *Mutat Res Fund Molec Mech Mutagen.* 2008;638:175–183.

Skin studies

- Athavale NV, Srinivas CR. Contact cheilitis from propyl gallate in lipstick. *Contact Dermatitis.* 1994;30:307.
- Baer-Dubowska W, Gnojkowski J, Fenrych W. Effect of tannic acid on benzo[a]pyrene-DNA adduct formation in mouse epidermis: Comparison with synthetic gallic acid esters. *Nutr Cancer.* 1997;29:42–47.
- Cusano F, Capozzi M, Errico G. Safety of propyl gallate in topical products. *J Am Acad Dermatol.* 1987;17:308–309.
- Jacobi H, Hinrichsen M-L, Weß D, Witte I. Induction of lipid peroxidation in human fibroblasts by the antioxidant propyl gallate in combination with copper(II). *Toxicol Lett.* 1999;110:183–190.
- Law E, Lewis AJ. The effect of systemically and topically applied drugs on ultraviolet-induced erythema in the rat. *Br J Pharmacol.* 1977;59:591–597.
- McDonald-Gibson WJ, Saeed SA, Schneider C. The local antinociceptive and topical anti-inflammatory effects of propyl gallate in rodents. *Br J Pharmacol.* 1976;58:573–581.
- Muñoz D, Audicana M, Gastaminza G, Fernández E. Dermatitis de contacto por galatos. *Alergol Inmunol Clin.* 2002;17:173–177.
- van der Meeren HL. Dodecyl gallate, permitted in food, is a strong sensitizer. *Contact Dermatitis.* 1987;16:260–262.

- Wilkinson SM, Beck MH. Allergic contact dermatitis from dibutyl phthalate, propyl gallate and hydrocortisone in Timodine. *Contact Dermatitis*. 1992;27:197.

QUERCETIN

- *Empirical formula*: $C_{15}H_{10}O_7$
- *MW*: 302.24
- *CAS*: 117-39-5
- *EC number*: 204-187-1
- *SMILES*: O=C1c2c(OC(c3cc(O)c(O)cc3)=C1O)cc(O)cc2O

Description

Quercetin is a flavonoid that is found in many common fruits and vegetables such as broccoli, lettuce, Brussel sprouts, onion (high levels), olive, berries, cranberry, and apple (high levels), as well as red wine and tea.[42] Like many polyphenols, it has anti-inflammatory and antioxidant activity.

Chemical/physical properties

- *Melting point*[17]: 316.5°C
- *Boiling point*[17]: sublimes
- *Solubilities*[17]: very soluble in ether and methanol; soluble in ethanol, acetone, pyridine, and acetic acid; soluble in alcohol and glacial acetic acid; insoluble in water
- *LogP (exp)*[6,43,44,45]: 1.82, 1.20, 1.48
- *ALOGPs*: 1.81
- *Henry's law constant*[7]: 6.60×10^{-21} atm·m³/mol
- *Hydroxyl radical reaction rate constant*[7]: 2.39×10^{-10} cm³/molec·s
- *Max absorption (EtOH)*[26]: 256 nm (log ε = 4.32); 301 nm (log ε = 3.89); 373 nm (log ε = 4.32)

Stability/shelf life

Vicentini FTMC, Vaz MOLL, Fonseca YM, Bentley MVLB, Fonseca MJV. Characterization and stability study of a water-in-oil microemulsion incorporating quercetin. *Drug Develop Industr Pharm*. 2011;37:47–55.

Analytical studies

- Ibrahim ESA, Hassan MA, El-Mahdy MM, Mohamed AS. Formulation and evaluation of quercetin in certain dermatological preparations. *J Drug Deliv Sci Tech*. 2007;17:431–436.
- Lee DH, Sim GS, Kim JH, Lee GS, Pyo HB, Lee BC. Preparation and characterization of quercetin-loaded polymethyl methacrylate microcapsules using a polyol-in-oil-in-polyol emulsion solvent evaporation method. *J Pharm Pharmacol*. 2007;59:1611–1620.
- Vicentini FTMC, Casagrande R, Georgetti SR, Bentley MVLB, Fonseca MJV. Influence of vehicle on antioxidant activity of quercetin: A liquid crystalline formulation. *Lat Amer J Pharm*. 2007;26:805–810.
- Vicentini FTMD, Georgetti SR, Bentley MVLB, Fonseca MJV. Assessment of in vitro methodologies to determine topical and transdermal delivery of the flavonoid quercetin. *Braz J Pharm Sci*. 2009;46:357–364.

ESR studies

- Jorgensen LV, Madsen HL, Thomsen MK, Dragsted LO, Skibsted LH. Regeneration of phenolic antioxidants from phenoxyl radicals: An ESR and electrochemical study of antioxidant hierarchy. *Free Rad Res*. 1999;30:207–220.
- Pedrielli P, Skibsted LH. Antioxidant synergy and regeneration effect of quercetin, (−)-epicatechin, and (+)-catechin on α-tocopherol in homogeneous solutions of peroxidating methyl linoleate. *J Agric Food Chem*. 2002;50:7138–7144.

General interest articles

- Boots A, Haenen G, Aalt Bast A. Health effects of quercetin: From antioxidant to nutraceutical. *Eur J Pharmacol*. 2008;585:325–337.
- Chen C, Zhou J, Ji C. Quercetin: A potential drug to reverse multidrug resistance. *Life Sci*. 2010;87:333–338.
- Formica JV, Regelson W. Review of the biology of quercetin and related bioflavonoids. *Food Chem Toxicol*. 1995;33:1061–1080.
- Goniotaki M, Hatziantoniou S, Dimas K, Wagner M, Demetzos C. Encapsulation of naturally occurring flavonoids into liposomes: Physicochemical properties and biological activity against human cancer cell lines. *J Pharm Pharmacol*. 2004;56:1217–1224.
- Jan AT, Kamli MR, Murtaza I, Singh JB, Ali A, Haq QMR. Dietary flavonoid quercetin and associated health benefits. An overview. *Food Rev Int*. 2010;26:302–317.

Skin studies

- Casagrande R, Georgetti SR, Verri WAJ, Dorta DJ, dos Santos AC, Fonseca MJ. Protective effect of topical formulations containing quercetin against UVB-induced oxidative stress in hairless mice. *J Photochem Photobiol B*. 2006;84:21–27.
- Hatahet T, Morille M, Hommoss A, Devoisselle J, Müller R, Bégu S. Quercetin topical application, from conventional dosage forms to nanodosage forms. *Eur J Pharm Biopharm*. 2016;108:41–53.
- Karuppagounder V, Arumugam S, Thandavarayan R, Sreedhar R, Giridharan V, Watanabe K. Molecular targets of quercetin with anti-inflammatory properties in atopic dermatitis. *Drug Discov Today*. 2016;21:632–639.
- Kim H, Gwak H, Chun I. The effect of vehicles and pressure sensitive adhesives on the percutaneous absorption of quercetin through the hairless mouse skin. *Arch Pharm Res*. 2004;27:763–768.

- Kitagawa S, Tanaka Y, Tanaka M, Endo K, Yoshii A. Enhanced skin delivery of quercetin by microemulsion. *J Pharm Pharmacol.* 2009;61:855–860.
- Saraf S, Kaur CD. Phytoconstituents as photoprotective novel cosmetic formulations. *Pharmacogn Rev.* 2010;4:1–11.
- Scalia S, Mezzena M. Photostabilization effect of quercetin on the UV filter combination, butyl methoxydibenzoylmethane-octyl methoxycinnamate. *Photochem Photobiol.* 2010;86:273–278.
- Vicentini FTMC, Fonseca YM, Pitol DL, Iyomasa MM, Bentley MV, Fonseca MJ. Evaluation of protective effect of a water-in-oil microemulsion incorporating quercetin against UVB-induced damage in hairless mice skin. *J Pharm Pharmaceut Sci.* 2010;13:274–285.
- Vicentini FT, Simi TR, Del Ciampo JO, Wolga NO, Pitol DL, Iyomasa MM et al. Quercetin in w/o microemulsion: In vitro and in vivo skin penetration and efficacy against UVB-induced skin damages evaluated in vivo. *Eur J Pharm Biopharm.* 2008;69:948–957.

RESORCINOL

- *Empirical formula*: $C_6H_6O_2$
- *MW*: 110.11
- *Synonyms*: 1,3-benzenediol
- *CAS*: 108-46-3
- *EC number*: 203-585-2
- *SMILES*: OC1=CC(O)=CC=C1

Description

Resorcinol is phenol derivative (*m*-dihydroxybenzene), which has been used as a chemical peeling agent for the last 100 years. It also has antiseptic (1%–3% according to FDA), antifungal, anti-itch (anti-pruritic), and keratolytic (the softening/shedding of the horny layer) properties. In addition to its use as a chemical peeling agent, it is most commonly employed to treat acne vulgaris and pigmentary disorders.[46] In hair care preparations, resorcinol is an important component of hair dyes where it functions as a coupler. Moreover, resorcinol may also be found in shampoos as an anti-dandruff agent.

Chemical/physical properties

- *Melting point*[37]: 109°C–111°C
- *Boiling point*[37]: 280°C
- *Solubilities*[37]: 1 g dissolves in 0.9 mL water at room temperature, 0.2 mL water at 80°C, 0.9 mL alcohol; freely soluble in ether and glycerol; slightly soluble in chloroform
- *Dissociation constants*[5]: pKa = 9.32
- *LogP (exp)*[47]: 0.80
- *ALOGPs*[6]: 0.70
- *Max absorption (EtOH)*[26]: 220 nm (log ε = 3.79); 276 nm (log ε = 3.33)

Stability/shelf life

- Volatizes at a temperature lower than its *boiling point*. Also, slightly volatile with steam.[48]

Analytical studies

- Peñarrieta JM, Alvarado JA, Akesson B, Bergenstahl B. Separation of phenolic compounds from foods by reversed-phase high performance liquid chromatography. *Rev Boliv Quím.* 2007;24:1–4.
- Sakuma K, Ogawa M, Sugibayashi K, Yamada K, Yamamoto K. Relationship between tyrosinase inhibitory action and oxidation-reduction potential of cosmetic whitening ingredients and phenol derivatives. *Arch Pharm Res.* 1999;22:335–339.
- Vincent U, Bordin G, Rodriguez AR. Validation of an analytical procedure for the determination of oxidative hair dyes in cosmetic formulations. *J Cosmet Sci.* 2002;53:43–58.
- Yates RL, Havery DC. Determination of phenol, resorcinol, salicylic acid and α-hydroxy acids in cosmetic products and salon preparations. *J Cosmet Sci.* 1999;50:315–325.

ESR studies

- Campbell D, Symons MCR. Unstable intermediates. Part LXI. Electron spin resonance study of radicals and radical pairs in irradiated resorcinol at 77°K. *J Chem Soc A.* 1969:1494–1498.

General interest articles

- Stasiuk M, Kozubek A. Biological activity of phenolic lipids. *Cell Mol Life Sci.* 2010;67:841–860.
- Yamada F, Nishiyama T, Nakai Y. A study of benzylphenols as antioxidants. *JAOCS.* 1983;60:1651–1652.

Skin studies

- Cassano N, Alessandrini G, Mastrolonardo M, Vena GA. Peeling agents: Toxicological and allergological aspects. *J Eur Acad Dermatol Vener.* 1999;13:14–23.
- Karam PG. 50% Resorcinol peel. *Int J Derm.* 1993;32:569–574.

RESVERATROL

- *Empirical formula*: $C_{14}H_{12}O_3$
- *MW*: 228.24
- *Synonyms*: 5-[(1E)-2-(4-hydroxyphenyl)-ethenyl]-1,3-benzenediol; 3,4′,5-trihydroxy-*trans*-stilbene

- CAS: 501-36-0
- SMILES: C(c1cc(O)cc(O)c1)=Cc2ccc(O)cc2

Description

Resveratrol is a stilbenoid (and a phytoalexin) that is found in the skin of red grapes. It is expressed in plants in response to stress-induced situations caused by foreign bacteria and fungi. Much publicity has centered around resveratrol's potential as a chemopreventive agent as well as its benefits in cardiovascular and neurological health. It is suspected to be one of the key components of red wine that provides it with it therapeutic properties. For example, in regions of the world such as the Mediterranean, where the level of saturated fat intake is concurrently high with red wine consumption, the level of coronary heart disease is low—a phenomenon that has become known as *The French Paradox*. Regardless, many studies have been conducted on skin utilizing this compound as a treatment modality.

Chemical/physical properties

- *Melting point*[13]: 253°C–255°C
- *Solubilities*[17]: very soluble in ethanol
- *ALOGPs*[6]: 2.57
- *Henry's law constant*[7]: 1.39×10^{-16} atm · m^3/mol
- *Hydroxyl radical reaction rate constant*[7]: 2.57×10^{-10} cm^3/molec · s

Stability/shelf life

- Ansari KA, Vavia PR, Trotta F, Cavalli R. Cyclodextrin-based nanosponges for delivery of resveratrol: In vitro characterisation, stability, cytotoxicity and permeation study. *AAPS PharmSciTech*. 2011;Online First:January 15.
- Bertelli AA, Gozzini A, Stradi R, Stella S, Bertelli A. Stability of resveratrol over time and in the various stages of grape transformation. *Drugs Exp Clin Res*. 1998;24:207–211.

Analytical studies

- Brandolini V, Maietti A, Tedeschi P, Durini E, Vertuani S, Manfredini S. Capillary electrophoresis determination, synthesis, and stability of resveratrol and related 3-O-β-d-glucopyranosides. *J Agr Food Chem*. 2002;50:7407–7411.
- Hemar Y, Cheng LJ, Oliver CM, Sanguansri L, Augustin M. Encapsulation of resveratrol using water-in-oil-in-water double emulsions. *Food Biophys*. 2010;5:141–150.

ESR studies

- Jung MY, Choi DS. Electron spin resonance and luminescence spectroscopic observation and kinetic study of chemical and physical singlet oxygen quenching by resveratrol in methanol. *J Agr Food Chem*. 2010;58:11888–11895.

General interest articles

- Brisdelli F, D'Andrea G, Bozzi A. Resveratrol: A natural polyphenol with multiple chemopreventive properties. *Curr Drug Metab*. 2009;10:530–546.
- Fan EG, Zhang K, Zhu MZ, Wang QA. Obtaining resveratrol: From chemical synthesis to biotechnological production. *Mini-Rev Org Chem*. 2010;7:272–281.
- Hsieh TC, Wu JM. Resveratrol: Biological and pharmaceutical properties as anticancer molecule. *Biofactors*. 2010;36:360–369.
- Kalantari H, Das DK. Physiological effects of resveratrol. *Biofactors*. 2010;36:401–406.
- Pervaiz S, Holme AL. Resveratrol: Its biologic targets and functional activity. *Antioxid Redox Signal*. 2009;11:2851–2897.

Skin studies

- Afaq F, Adhami VM, Ahmad N. Prevention of short-term ultraviolet B radiation-mediated damages by resveratrol in SKH-1 hairless mice. *Toxicol Appl Pharmacol*. 2003;186:28–37.
- Aziz MH, Afaq F, Ahmad N. Prevention of ultraviolet-B radiation damage by resveratrol in mouse skin is mediated via modulation in survivin. *Photochem Photobiol*. 2005;81:25–31.
- Aziz MH, Reagan-Shaw S, Wu J, Longley BJ, Ahmad N. Chemoprevention of skin cancer by grape constituent resveratrol: Relevance to human disease? *FASEB J*. 2005;19:1193–5.
- Baxter RA. Anti-aging properties of resveratrol: Review and report of a potent new antioxidant skin care formulation. *J Cosmet Dermatol*. 2008;7:2–7.
- Chann MM. Antimicrobial effect of resveratrol on dermatophytes and bacterial pathogens of the skin. *Biochem Pharmacol*. 2002;63:99–104.
- Gelo-Pujic M, Desmurs JR, Kassem T, Delaire S, Adao A, Tawil D. Synthesis of new antioxidant conjugates and their in vitro hydrolysis with stratum corneum enzymes. *Int J Cosmet Sci*. 2008;30:195–204.
- Hung CF, Lin YK, Huang ZR, Fang JY. Delivery of resveratrol, a red wine polyphenol, from solutions and hydrogels via the skin. *Biol Pharm Bull*. 2008;31:955–962.
- Kowalczyk MC, Walaszek Z, Kowalczyk P, Kinjo T, Hanausek M, Slaga TJ. Differential effects of several phytochemicals and their derivatives on murine keratinocytes in vitro and in vivo: Implications for skin cancer prevention. *Carcinogenesis*. 2009;30:1008–1015.
- Liu Y, Chan F, Sun H, Yan J, Fan D, Zhao D et al. Resveratrol protects human keratinocytes HaCaT cells from UVA-induced oxidative stress damage by downregulating Keap1 expression. *Eur J Pharmacol*. 2011;650:130–137.
- Ndiaye M, Philippe C, Mukhtar H, Ahmad N. The grape antioxidant resveratrol for skin disorders: Promise,

prospects, and challenges. *Arch Biochem Biophys.* 2011;508(2):164–170.
- Reagan-Shaw S, Afaq F, Aziz MH, Ahmad N. Modulations of critical cell cycle regulatory events during chemoprevention of ultraviolet B-mediated responses by resveratrol in SKH-1 hairless mouse skin. *Oncogene.* 2004;23:5151–5160.
- Saraf S, Kaur CD. Phytoconstituents as photoprotective novel cosmetic formulations. *Pharmacogn Rev.* 2010;4:1–11.
- Tomaino A, Cristani M, Cimino F, Speciale A, Trombetta D, Bonina F et al. In vitro protective effect of a Jacquez grapes wine extract on UVB-induced skin damage. *Toxicol In Vitro.* 2006;20:1395–1402.

ROSMARINIC ACID

- *Empirical formula*: $C_{18}H_{16}O_8$
- *MW*: 360.31
- *Synonyms*: (R)-O-(3,4-dihydroxycinnamoyl)-3-(3,4-dihydroxyphenyl)lactic acid; (2R)-2-(2″E″)-3-(3,4-dihydroxyphenyl)-1-oxo-2-propenyloxy]-3-(3,4-dihydroxyphenyl)propanoic acid
- *CAS*: 20283-92-5

Description

Rosmarinic occurs naturally in *Lamiaceae* herbs such as mint, rosemary, sage, oregano, basil, etc. Biologically, it has anti-pathogenic, anti-inflammatory, and antioxidant properties.

Chemical/physical properties

- *Solubilities*: low solubility in H_2O; soluble in many organic solvents.

Stability/shelf life

- Discoloration; chemically unstable.
- Kim H-J, Kim T-H, Kang K-C, Pyo H-B, Jeong H-H. Microencapsulation of rosmarinic acid using polycaprolactone and various surfactants. *Int J Cosmet Sci.* 2010;32:185–191.

Analytical studies

- Almela L, Sánchez-Muñoz B, Fernández-López JA, Roca MJ, Rabe V. Liquid chromatographic-mass spectrometric analysis of phenolics and free radical scavenging activity of rosemary extract from different raw material. *J Chromatogr A.* 2006;1120:221–229.
- Frankel EN, Huang S-W, Aeschbach R, Prior E. Antioxidant activity of a rosemary extract and its constituents, carnosic acid, carnosol, and rosmarinic acid, in bulk oil and oil-in-water emulsion. *J Agr Food Chem.* 1996;44:131–135.
- Ibañez E, Kubátová A, Señoráns FJ, Cavero S, Reglero G, Hawthorne SB. Subcritical water extraction of antioxidant compounds from rosemary plants. *J Agric Food Chem.* 2003;15:375–382.
- Ibarra A, Cases J, Bily A, He K, Bai N, Roller M et al. Importance of extract standardization and in vitro/ex vivo assay selection for the evaluation of antioxidant activity of botanicals: A case study on three *Rosmarinus officinalis* L. extracts. *J Med Food.* 2010;13:1167–1175.

ESR studies

- Maegawa Y, Sugino K, Sakurai H. Identification of free radical species derived from caffeic acid and related polyphenols. *Free Rad Res.* 2007;41:110–119.
- Pedersen JA. Naturally occurring quinols and quinones studied as semiquinones by electron spin resonance. *Phytochem.* 1978;17:775–778.

General interest articles

- al-Sereiti M, Abu-Amer K, Sen P. Pharmacology of rosemary (*Rosmarinus officinalis* Linn.) and its therapeutic potentials. *Ind J Exp Biol.* 1999;37:124–130.
- Luis J, Johnson C. Seasonal variations of rosmarinic and carnosic acids in rosemary extracts. Analysis of their in vitro antiradical activity. *Span J Agr Res.* 2005;3:106–112.
- Moreno S, Scheyer T, Romano CS, Vojnov AA. Antioxidant and antimicrobial activities of rosemary extracts linked to their polyphenol composition. *Free Radic Res.* 2006;40:223–231.
- Park S, Uddin M, Xu H, Kim Y, Lee S. Biotechnological applications for rosmarinic acid production in plant. *Afr J Biotech.* 2008;7:4959–4965.
- Romano CS, Abadi K, Repetto V, Vojnov AA, Moreno S. Synergistic antioxidant and antibacterial activity of rosemary plus butylated derivatives. *Food Chem.* 2009;115:456–461.

Skin studies

- Lee J, Jung E, Koh J, Kim YS, Park D. Effect of rosmarinic acid on atopic dermatitis. *J Dermatol.* 2008;35:768–771.
- Lee J, Kim YS, Park D. Rosmarinic acid induces melanogenesis through protein kinase A activation signaling. *Biochem Pharmacol.* 2007;74:960–968.
- Osakabe N, Yasuda A, Natsume M, Yoshikawa T. Rosmarinic acid inhibits epidermal inflammatory responses: Anticarcinogenic effect of *Perilla frutescens* extract in the murine two-stage skin model. *Carcinogenesis.* 2004;25:549–557.
- Psotova J, Svobodova A, Kolarova H, Walterova D. Photoprotective properties of *Prunella vulgaris* and

rosmarinic acid on human keratinocytes. *J Photochem Photobiol B: Biol.* 2006;84:167–174.
- Ritschel WA, Starzacher A, Sabouni A, Hussain AS, Koch HP. Percutaneous absorption of rosmarinic acid in the rat. *Methods Find Exp Clin Pharmacol.* 1989;11:345–352.
- Sánchez-Campillo M, Gabaldon JA, Castillo J, Benavente-García O, Del Baño MJ, Alcaraz M et al. Rosmarinic acid, a photo-protective agent against UV and other ionizing radiations. *Food Chem Toxicol.* 2009;47:386–392.
- Vostálová J, Zdarilová A, Svobodová A. *Prunella vulgaris* extract and rosmarinic acid prevent UVB-induced DNA damage and oxidative stress in HaCaT keratinocytes. *Arch Dermatol Res.* 2010;302:171–181.

SILIBININ

- *Empirical formula*: $C_{25}H_{22}O_{10}$
- *MW*: 482.44
- *Synonyms*: silybin; 2,3-dihydro-3-(4-hydroxy-3-methoxyphenyl)-2-(hydroxymethyl)-6-(3,5,7-trihydroxy-4-oxobenzopyran-2-yl)benzodioxin
- *CAS*: 22888-70-6

Description

Silbinin is a flavolignan that comes from the milk thistle plant (*Silybum marianum*). Silibinin is a chief component of silymarin. It is renowned for its therapeutic properties against various liver conditions.

Stability/shelf life

- Tang N, Wu D, Lu Y, Chen J, Zhang B, Wu W. A comparative study on the stability of silybin and that in silymarin in buffers and biological fluids. *Drug Metab Lett.* 2009;3:115–119.

Analytical studies

- Liu X, Zhang Y, Tang X, Zhang H. Determination of entrapment efficiency and drug phase distribution of submicron emulsions loaded silybin. *J Microencapsul.* 2009;26:180–186.
- Maheshwari H, Agarwal R, Patil C, Katare OP. Preparation and pharmacological evaluation of silibinin liposomes. *Arzneimittelforschung.* 2003;53:420–427.
- Parveen R, Ahmad S, Baboota S, Ali J, Alka A. Stability-indicating HPTLC method for quantitative estimation of silybin in bulk drug and pharmaceutical dosage form. *Biomed Chromatogr.* 2010;24:639–647.
- Woo JS, Kim TS, Park JH, Chi SC. Formulation and biopharmaceutical evaluation of silymarin using SMEDDS. *Arch Pharm Res.* 2007;30:82–89.
- Wu W, Wang Y, Que L. Enhanced bioavailability of silymarin by self-microemulsifying drug delivery system. *Eur J Pharm Biopharm.* 2006;63:288–294.

ESR studies

- Seršeň F, Vencel T, Annus J. Silymarin and its components scavenge phenylglyoxylic ketyl radicals. *Fitoterapia.* 2006;77:525–529.

General interest articles

- Abenavoli L, Capasso R, Milic N, Capasso F. Milk thistle in liver diseases: Past, present, future. *Phytother Res.* 2010;24:1423–1432.
- Deep G, Agarwal R. Antimetastatic efficacy of silibinin: Molecular mechanisms and therapeutic potential against cancer. *Cancer Metastasis Rev.* 2010;29:447–463.
- Gazák R, Walterová D, Kren V. Silybin and silymarin—New and emerging applications in medicine. *Curr Med Chem.* 2007;14:315–338.
- Ramasamy K, Agarwal R. Multitargeted therapy of cancer by silymarin. *Cancer Lett.* 2008;269:352–362.

Skin studies

- Ahmad N, Gali H, Javed S, Agarwal R. Skin cancer chemopreventive effects of a flavonoid antioxidant silymarin are mediated via impairment of receptor tyrosine kinase signaling and perturbation in cell cycle progression. *Biochem Biophys Res Comm.* 1998;247:294–301.
- Hung CF, Lin YK, Zhang LW, Chang CH, Fang JY. Topical delivery of silymarin constituents via the skin route. *Acta Pharmacol Sin.* 2010;31:118–126.
- Katiyar SK, Korman NJ, Mukhtar H, Agarwal R. Protective effects of silymarin against photocarcinogenesis in a mouse skin model. *J Natl Cancer Inst.* 1997;89:556–566.
- Kitajima S, Yamaguchi K. Silybin from Silybum marianum seeds inhibits confluent-induced keratinocytes differentiation as effectively as retinoic acid without inducing inflammatory cytokine. *J Clin Biochem Nutr.* 2009;45:178–184.
- Onat D, Boscoboinik D, Azzi A, Basaga H. Effect of alpha-tocopherol and silibin dihemisuccinate on the proliferation of human skin fibroblasts. *Biotechnol Appl Biochem.* 1999;29:213–215.
- Saraf S, Kaur CD. Phytoconstituents as photoprotective novel cosmetic formulations. *Pharmacogn Rev.* 2010;4:1–11.
- Singh RP, Agarwal R. Cosmeceuticals and silibinin. *Clin Dermatol.* 2009;27:479–484.
- Singh RP, Agarwal R. Mechanisms and preclinical efficacy of silibinin in preventing skin cancer. *Eur J Cancer.* 2005;41:1969–1979.
- Svobodová A, Zdarilová A, Walterová D, Vostálová J. Flavonolignans from *Silybum marianum* moderate UVA-induced oxidative damage to HaCaT keratinocytes. *J Dermatol Sci.* 2007;48:213–224.

THEAFLAVIN

- *Empirical formula*: $C_{29}H_{24}O_{12}$
- *MW*: 564.49
- *CAS*: 4670-05-7

Description

Theaflavins are found in black tea and have antioxidant, anti-carcinogenic, and anti-pathogenic properties. While epicatechins are associated with green tea, theaflavins are found in black tea. The four principle compounds in the theaflavin class are theaflavin, theaflavin-3-gallate, theaflavin-3′-gallate, and theaflavin-3,3′-digallate. The antioxidant activity of these compounds comes from their free radical scavenging capability (hydroxyl groups) and the ability to chelate metal ions.

Chemical/physical properties

- *Melting point*[37]: Crystals from H_2O, decompose at 237°C–240°C.
- *Crystals from* H_2O[37]: Absorption max (EtOH): 216, 271, 384, 470 (ε = 35500, 19500, 8700, 3600).

Stability/shelf life

- Stable in acidic medium; unstable in alkaline medium.[49]
- Lun Su Y, Leung LK, Huang Y, Chen Z-Y. Stability of tea theaflavins and catechins. *Food Chem.* 2003;83:189–195.

Analytical studies

- Alastair R, Derek SB. Production and HPLC analysis of black tea theaflavins and thearubigins during in vitro oxidation. *Phytochem.* 1983;22:883–887.
- Menet MC, Sang S, Yang CS, Ho CT, Rosen RT. Analysis of theaflavins and thearubigins from black tea extract by MALDI-TOF mass spectrometry. *J Agr Food Chem.* 2004;52:2455–2461.
- Nishimura M, Ishiyama K, Watanabe A, Kawano S, Miyase T, Sano M. Determination of theaflavins including methylated theaflavins in black tea leaves by solid-phase extraction and HPLC analysis. *J Agr Food Chem.* 2007;55:7252–7257.
- Wang K, Liu Z, Huang J, Gong Y. [Determination of theaflavins in black tea by high performance liquid chromatography]. *Se Pu.* 2004;22:151–153.
- Yanagida A, Shoji A, Shibusawa Y, Shindo H, Tagashira M, Ikeda M et al. Analytical separation of tea catechins and food-related polyphenols by high-speed counter-current chromatography. *J Chromatogr A.* 2006;1112:195–201.

General interest articles

- Frei B, Higdon JV. Proceedings of the third international scientific symposium on tea and human health: Role of flavonoids in the diet. *J Nutr.* 2003;133:3275S–3284S.
- Kuroda Y, Hara Y. Antimutagenic and anticarcinogenic activity of tea polyphenols. *Mutat Res.* 1999;436:69–97.
- Mukhtar H, Ahmad M. Tea polyphenols: Prevention of cancer and optimizing health. *Am J Clin Nutr.* 2000;71(suppl):1698S–1702S.
- Leung LK, Su Y, Chen R, Zhang Z, Huang Y, Chen ZY. Theflavins in black tea and catechins in green tea are equally effective antioxidants. *J Nutr.* 2001;131:2248–2251.
- Lin JK. Cancer chemoprevention by tea polyphenols through modulating signal transduction pathways. *Arch Pharm Res.* 2002;25:561–571.
- Łuczaj W, Skrzydlewska E. Antioxidative properties of black tea. *Prev Med.* 2005;40:910–918.
- Masaaki N, Ma WY, Huang C, Yang CS, Bowden GT, Miyamoto K et al. Inhibition of ultraviolet B-induced AP-1 activation by theaflavins from black tea. *Mol Carcinog.* 2000;28:148–155.
- Wang C, Li Y. Research progress on property and application of theaflavins. *Afr J Biotech.* 2006;5:213–218.

Skin studies

- Hakim IA, Harris RB, Weisgerber UM. Tea intake and squamous cell carcinoma of the skin: Influence of type of tea beverages. *Cancer Epidemiol Biomarkers Prev.* 2000;9:727–731.
- Liang YC, Tsai DC, Lin-Shiau SY, Chen CF, Ho CT, Lin JK. Inhibition of 12-O-tetradecanoylphorbol-13-acetate-induced inflammatory skin edema and ornithine decarboxylase activity by theaflavin-3,3′-digallate in mouse. *Nutr Cancer.* 2002;42:217–223.
- Nomura M, Akira K, He Z, Ma W-Y, Miyamoto K, Yang CS et al. Inhibitory mechanisms of tea polyphenols on the ultraviolet B-activated phosphatidylinositol 3-kinase-dependent pathway. *J Biol Chem.* 2001;276:46624–46631.
- Nomura M, Ma WY, Huang C, Yang CS, Bowden GT, Miyamoto K et al. Inhibition of ultraviolet B-induced AP-1 activation by theaflavins from black tea. *Carcinogenesis.* 2000;28:148–155.
- Rees JR, Stukel TA, Perry AE, Zens MS, Spencer SK, Karagas MR. Tea consumption and basal cell and squamous cell skin cancer: Results of a case-control study. *J Am Acad Dermatol.* 2007;56:781–785.

- Sil H, Sen T, Moulik S, Chatterjee A. Black tea polyphenol (theaflavin) downregulates MMP-2 in human melanoma cell line A375 by involving multiple regulatory molecules. *J Environ Pathol Toxicol Oncol.* 2010;29:55–68.
- Zykova TA, Zhang Y, Zhu F, Bode AM, Dong Z. The signal transduction networks required for phosphorylation of STAT1 at Ser727 in mouse epidermal JB6 cells in the UVB response and inhibitory mechanisms of tea polyphenols. *Carcinogenesis.* 2005;26:331–342.

THEARUBIGINS*

Description

Thearubigins are a class of one of the largest polyphenol components of black tea—the other being theaflavins. Black and green teas both come from the plant *Camellia sinesis*; however, they differ in their production techniques. While green teas are rich in catechins, these molecules become oxidized during production (fermentation) resulting in theaflavins, thearubigins, and other polyphenol compounds, which are found in black tea. Like theaflavins, thearubigins have many positive health benefits.

General interest articles

- Haslam E. Thoughts on thearubigins. *Phytochem.* 2003;64:61–73.
- Kuhnert N. Unraveling the structure of the black tea thearubigins. *Arch Biochem Biophys.* 2010;501:37–51.

THIOGLYCOLIC ACID

- *Empirical formula*: $C_2H_4O_2S$
- *MW*: 92.12
- *Synonyms*: Alpha-mercaptoacetic acid; 2-thioglycolic acid; mercaptoacetic acid
- *CAS*: 68-11-1
- *EC Number*: 200-677-4
- *SMILES*: SCC(O)=O

Description

The most common use of thioglycolic acid in cosmetics is in permanent wave formulations, often in a salt form (e.g., ammonium thioglycolate). Application consists of shaping hair into a desired set, followed first by treatment with the reducing agent (it reduces/breaks cystine disulfide bonds in hair), then further treatment with an oxidant, such as H_2O_2, which reforms the disulfide bonds.

Chemical/physical properties

- *Melting point*[50]: −16.5°C
- *Boiling point*[50]: 120°C (20 mm Hg)
- *Color/form*[15]: clear, colorless liquid[8]; water-white liquid
- *Solubilities*[8,37]: Miscible with water, alcohol, ether, chloroform, benzene, and many other organic solvents; miscible with mono- and polyalcohols, ethers, ketones, esters, chlorinated hydrocarbons, and aromatic hydrocarbons, but not with aliphatic hydrocarbons
- *Dissociation constants*[8]: pKa1 = 3.82 ± 0.1; pKa2 = 9.30 ± 0.1 (in $NaClO_4$ solution at 20°C)
- *LogP (exp)*[51]: 0.09
- *ALOGPs*[6]: 0.09
- *Index of refraction*[50]: 1.5080 at 20°C/D
- *Max absorption (water, pH 10)*[52]: 240 nm (log ε = 3.26)

Stability/shelf life

Readily oxidizes upon exposure to air.[37]

Analytical studies

- Cavrini V, Andrisano V, Gatti R, Scapini G. HPLC determination of thioglycolic acid and other aliphatic thiols in cosmetic formulations using ethacrynic acid as precolumn derivatization reagent. *Int J Cosmet Sci.* 1990;12:141–150.
- Rooselaar J, Liem DH. High pressure liquid chromatographic determination of thioglycolic acid in cold wave fluids and depilating creams. *Int J Cosmet Sci.* 1981;3:37–47.
- Zen JM, Yang HH, Chiu MH, Chen YJ, Shih Y. Determination of thioglycolic acid in hair-waving products by disposable electrochemical sensor coupled with high-performance liquid chromatography. *J AOAC Int.* 2009;92:574–579.

General interest articles

- Burnett CL, Bergfeld WF, Belsito DV, Klaassen CD, Marks JGJ, Shank RC et al. Final amended report on the safety assessment of ammonium thioglycolate, butyl thioglycolate, calcium thioglycolate, ethanolamine thioglycolate, ethyl thioglycolate, glyceryl thioglycolate, isooctyl thioglycolate, isopropyl thioglycolate,

---

* For related studies see section on Theaflavin.

magnesium thioglycolate, methyl thioglycolate, potassium thioglycolate, sodium thioglycolate, and thioglycolic acid. *Int J Toxicol.* 2009;28(4 Suppl):68–133.

Skin studies

- Brown MB, Khengar RH, Turner RB, Forbes B, Traynor MJ, Evans CR et al. Overcoming the nail barrier: A systematic investigation of ungual chemical penetration enhancement. *Int J Pharm.* 2009;370:61–67.
- Erra P, Solans C, Azemar N, Parra JL, Touraud D, Clausse M. Reactivity of hair cystine in microemulsion media. *Int J Cosmet Sci.* 1990;12:71–80.
- Gan HF, Meng XS, Song CH, Li BX. A survey on health effects in a human population exposed to permanent-waving solution containing thioglycolic acid. *J Occup Health.* 2003;45:400–404.
- Solans C, Parra JL, Erra P, Azemar N, Clausse M, Touraud D. Influence of microemulsion structure on cystine reactivity with keratin fibres. *Int J Cosmet Sci.* 1987;9:215–222.
- Valks R, Conde-Salazar L, Malfeito J, Ledo S. Contact dermatitis in hairdressers, 10 years later: Patch-test results in 300 hairdressers (1994 to 2003) and comparison with previous study. *Dermatitis.* 2005;16:28–31.

TOCOPHEROLS

Alpha-tocopherol (alpha-Toc) when R_1=CH$_3$, R_2=CH$_3$, and R_3=CH$_3$

Gamma-tocopherol (gamma-Toc) when R_1=H, R_2=CH$_3$, and R_3=CH$_3$

Delta-tocopherol (delta-Toc) when R_1=H, R_2=H, and R_3=CH$_3$

- *Empirical formula*: (alpha-Toc) $C_{29}H_{50}O_2$; (gamma-Toc) $C_{28}H_{48}O_2$; (delta-Toc) $C_{27}H_{46}O_2$
- *MW*: (alpha-Toc) 430.71; (gamma-Toc) 416.68; (delta-Toc) 402.65
- *Synonyms*: (alpha-Toc) 2,5,7,8-tetramethyl-2-(4′,8′,12′-trimethyltridecyl)-6-chromanol; 5,7,8-trimethyltocol; D-alpha-tocopherol; vitamin E; (gamma-Toc) (R,R,R)-gamma-tocopherol; 7,8-dimethyltocol; (delta-Toc) N/A
- *CAS*: (alpha-Toc) 59-02-9; (gamma-Toc) 54-28-4; (delta-Toc) 119-13-1
- *EC Number*: (alpha-Toc) 200-412-2; (gamma-Toc) 200-201-5; (delta-Toc) 204-299-0
- *SMILES*:
(alpha-Toc) c12c(CCC(O2)(CCCC(C)CCCC(C)CCCC(C)C)C)c(C)c(O)c(C)c1C;
(gamma-Toc) c12c(C)c(C)c(O) cc2CCC(CCCC(C)CCCC(C)CCCC(C)C)(C)O1;
(delta-Toc) c12c(CCC(CCCC(C)CCCC(C)CCCC(C)C)(C)O1)cc(O)cc2C

Description

The tocopherols, one of the forms of vitamin E, are an extremely important group of antioxidants. Much of the pioneering work in antioxidant research was conducted on alpha-Toc, due to its importance as one of the principle lipid phase antioxidants in the body. Of the isomer forms shown earlier, alpha-Toc is the most commonly found in tissues. Tocopherols are characterized by their long phytyl tail, which embeds the molecule in lipid membranes, and the chromanol ring structure—present at the lipid membrane-aqueous phase interface. Antioxidant activity by this molecule is rendered by the proton-donating abilities of the hydroxyl group on the chromanol ring. In addition to its commercial availability, vitamin E is obtained in the diet and is found in many plant oils, nuts, and seeds.

Chemical/physical properties

- *Melting point*[27]: 3°C*
- *Boiling point*[27]: 210°C at 0.1 mm Hg*
- *Solubilities*[27]: Insoluble in water; soluble in alcohol, ether, acetone, and chloroform*
- *Color/form*[27]: Pale, yellow viscous oil*
- Decomposes at 350°C[53]
- Slightly viscous, pale yellow oil; not affected by acid up to 100°C; slowly oxidized by atmospheric oxygen; rapidly oxidized by ferric and silver salts; gradually darkens on exposure to light; not precipitated by digitonin (dl-alpha-Toc)[13]
- *ALOGPs*[6]: (alpha-Toc) 8.84; (gamma-Toc) 8.81; (delta-Toc) 8.76
- *Henry's law constant*[7]: (alpha-Toc) 3.60×10^{-6} atm · m^3/mol
- *Hydroxyl radical reaction rate constant*[7]: (alpha-Toc) 2.30×10^{-10} cm^3/molec · s
- *Max absorption (methanol)*[53]: 292 nm (log ε = 3.54)*
- *Specific optical rotation*[13]: +0.65° at 25°C/D (EtOH)*

Stability/shelf life

Unstable to UV light, alkalies, and oxidation; in the absence of oxygen tocopherols are stable to heat, strong acids, and visible light.[54]

Analytical studies

- Fayet B, Fino L, Tisse C, Guerere M. Characterization and quantitative determination of tocopherols and gallates in essential oils. *Sciences des aliments.* 1996;16:89–93.
- Fuchs J, Weber S, Podda M, Groth N, Herrling T, Packer L et al. HPLC analysis of vitamin E isoforms in human epidermis: Correlation with minimal erythema dose and free radical scavenging activity. *Free Rad Biol Med.* 2003;34:170–176.

---

* These data are for vitamin E (CAS 59-02-9), which presumably refers to alpha-Toc.

- Guaratinia T, Gianetia M, Campos P. Stability of cosmetic formulations containing esters of vitamins E and A: Chemical and physical aspects. *Int J Pharm.* 2006;327:12–16.
- Podda M, Weber C, Traber MG, Packer L. Simultaneous determination of tissue tocopherols, tocotrienols, ubiquinols, and ubiquinones. *J Lipid Res.* 1996;37:893–901.

ESR studies

- Kagan V, Witt E, Goldman R, Scita G, Packer L. Ultraviolet light-induced generation of vitamin E radicals and their recycling. A possible photosensitizing effect of vitamin E in skin. *Free Rad Res.* 1992;16:51–64.

General interest articles

- Atkinson J, Epand RF, Epand RM. Tocopherols and tocotrienols in membranes: A critical review. *Free Rad Biol Med.* 2008;44:739–764.
- Azzi A. Molecular mechanism of alpha-tocopherol action. *Free Rad Biol Med.* 2007;43:16–21.
- Bell SJ, Grochoski GT. How safe is vitamin E supplementation? *Crit Rev Food Sci Nutr.* 2008;48:760–764.
- Galli F, Azzi A. Present trends in vitamin E research. *Biofactors.* 2010;36:33–42.
- Ju J, Picinich SC, Yang Z, Zhao Y, Suh N, Kong AN et al. Cancer-preventive activities of tocopherols and tocotrienols. *Carcinogenesis.* 2010;31:533–542.
- Zingg JM. Vitamin E: An overview of major research directions. *Mol Aspects Med.* 2007;28:400–422.

Skin studies

- Azzi A, Meydani S, Meydani M, Zingg J. The rise, the fall and the renaissance of vitamin E. *Arch Biochem Biophys.* 2016;595:100–108.
- Baumann LS, Spencer J. The effects of topical vitamin E on the cosmetic appearance of scars. *Dermatol Surg.* 1999;25:311–315.
- Buettner GR. The pecking order of free radicals and antioxidants: Lipid peroxidation, alpha-tocopherol, and ascorbate. *Arch Biochem Biophys.* 1993;300:535–543.
- Burke KE. Interaction of vitamins C and E as better cosmeceuticals. *Dermatol Ther.* 2007;20:314–321.
- Ekanayake-Mudiyanselage S, Thiele J. [Sebaceous glands as transporters of vitamin E]. *Hautarzt.* 2006;57:291–296.
- Murray JC, Burch JA, Streilein RD, Iannacchione MA, Hall RP, Pinnell SR. A topical antioxidant solution containing vitamins C and E stabilized by ferulic acid provides protection for human skin against damage caused by ultraviolet irradiation. *J Am Acad Dermatol.* 2008;59:418–425.
- Kosari P, Alikhan A, Sockolov M, Feldman SR. Vitamin E and allergic contact dermatitis. *Dermatitis.* 2010;21:148–153.
- Krol ES, Kramer-Stickland KA, Liebler DC. Photoprotective actions of topically applied vitamin E. *Drug Metab Rev.* 2000;32:413–420.
- Lopez-Torres M, Thiele JJ, Shindo Y, Han D, Packer L. Topical application of alpha-tocopherol modulates the antioxidant network and diminishes ultraviolet-induced oxidative damage in murine skin. *Br J Dermatol.* 1998;138:207–215.
- Podhaisky HP, Wohlrab W. Is the photoprotective effect of vitamin E based on its antioxidative capacity? *J Dermatol Sci.* 2002;28:84–86.
- Thiele JJ, Ekanayake-Mudiyanselage S. Vitamin E in human skin: Organ-specific physiology and considerations for its use in dermatology. *Mol Aspects Med.* 2007;28:646–667.
- Thiele JJ, Traber MG, Podda M, Tsang K, Cross CE, Packer L. Ozone depletes tocopherols and tocotrienols topically applied to murine skin. *FEBS Lett.* 1997;401:167–170.
- Traber MG, Rallis M, Podda M, Weber C, Maibach HI, Packer L. Penetration and distribution of alpha-tocopherol, alpha- or gamma-tocotrienols applied individually onto murine skin. *Lipids.* 1998;33:87–91.
- Weber C, Podda M, Rallis M, Thiele JJ, Traber MG, Packer L. Efficacy of topically applied tocopherols and tocotrienols in protection of murine skin from oxidative damage induced by UV-irradiation. *Free Rad Biol Med.* 1997;22:761–769.

TOCOTRIENOLS

Alpha-tocotrienol (alpha-Toc) when $R_1=CH_3$, $R_2=CH_3$, and $R_3=CH_3$

Gamma-tocotrienol (gamma-Toc) when $R_1=H$, $R_2=CH_3$, and $R_3=CH_3$

Delta-tocotrienol (delta-Toc) when $R_1=H$, $R_2=H$, and $R_3=CH_3$

- *Empirical formula*: (alpha-Toc) $C_{29}H_{44}O_2$; (gamma-Toc) $C_{28}H_{42}O_2$; (delta-Toc) $C_{27}H_{40}O$
- *MW*: (alpha-Toc) 424.66; (gamma-Toc) 410.63; (delta-Toc) 380.61
- *Synonyms*: (alpha-Toc) (R)-alpha-tocotrienol; (R-[E, E])-3,4-dihydro-2,5,7,8-tetramethyl-2-(4,8,12-trimethyl-3,7,11-tridecatrienyl)-2H-1-benzopyran-6-ol; (gamma-Toc) (R)-gamma-tocotrienol; (R-[E, E])-3,4-dihydro-2,7,8-trimethyl-2-(4,8,12-trimethyl-3,7,11-tridecatrienyl)-2H-1-benzopyran-6-ol; (delta-Toc) (R-[E, E])-3,4-dihydro-2,8-dimethyl-2-(4,8,12-trimethyl-3,7,11-tridecatrienyl)-2H-1-benzopyran-6-ol
- *CAS*: (alpha-Toc) 58864-81-6; (gamma-Toc) 14101-61-2; (delta-Toc) 25612-59-3

Description

Tocotrienols represent a group of vitamin E isomers, which structurally differ from tocopherols in their long aliphatic tail, which associates with lipid membrane structures. Unlike the tocopherols, the tocotrienol tail contains three isoprenoid units in the tail, which have double-bond character. Otherwise, the chromanol ring portion of the molecule, with the three different isomers (alpha, gamma, and delta), is the same. Historically, the tocopherols were the recipients of most of the attention in the scientific literature. However, in the last several years more research has been conducted on the tocotrienols as they are now deemed to also play a very important role in physiology.

Analytical studies

- Fuchs J, Weber S, Podda M, Groth N, Herrling T, Packer L et al. HPLC analysis of vitamin E isoforms in human epidermis: Correlation with minimal erythema dose and free radical scavenging activity. *Free Rad Biol Med.* 2003;34:170–176.
- Podda M, Weber C, Traber MG, Packer L. Simultaneous determination of tissue tocopherols, tocotrienols, ubiquinols, and ubiquinones. *J Lipid Res.* 1996;37:893–901.

General interest articles

- Aggarwal BB, Sundaram C, Prasad S, Kannappan R. Tocotrienols, the vitamin E of the 21st century: Its potential against cancer and other chronic diseases. *Biochem Pharmacol.* 2010;80:1613–1631.
- Atkinson J, Epand RF, Epand RM. Tocopherols and tocotrienols in membranes: A critical review. *Free Rad Biol Med.* 2008;44:739–764.
- Galli F, Azzi A. Present trends in vitamin E research. *Biofactors.* 2010;36:33–42.
- Ju J, Picinich SC, Yang Z, Zhao Y, Suh N, Kong AN et al. Cancer-preventive activities of tocopherols and tocotrienols. *Carcinogenesis.* 2010;31:533–542.
- Sen CK, Khanna S, Rink C, Roy S. Tocotrienols: The emerging face of natural vitamin E. *Vitam Horm.* 2007;76:203–261.
- Sen CK, Khanna S, Roy S. Tocotrienols: Vitamin E beyond tocopherols. *Life Sci.* 2006;78:2088–2098.
- Sylvester PW, Kaddoumi A, Nazzal S, El Sayed KA. The value of tocotrienols in the prevention and treatment of cancer. *J Am Coll Nutr.* 2010;29 (3 Suppl):324S–333S.
- Weber C, Podda M, Rallis M, Thiele JJ, Traber MG, Packer L. Efficacy of topically applied tocopherols and tocotrienols in protection of murine skin from oxidative damage induced by UV-irradiation. *Free Rad Biol Med.* 1997;22:761–769.

Skin studies

- Packer L, Weber SU, Rimbach G. Molecular aspects of alpha-tocotrienol antioxidant action and cell signalling. *J Nutr.* 2001;131:369S–373S.
- Thiele JJ, Traber MG, Podda M, Tsang K, Cross CE, Packer L. Ozone depletes tocopherols and tocotrienols topically applied to murine skin. *FEBS Lett.* 1997;401:167–170.
- Traber MG, Rallis M, Podda M, Weber C, Maibach HI, Packer L. Penetration and distribution of alpha-tocopherol, alpha- or gamma-tocotrienols applied individually onto murine skin. *Lipids.* 1998;33:87–91.
- Weber SU, Thiele JJ, Han N, Luu C, Valacchi G, Weber S et al. Topical alpha-tocotrienol supplementation inhibits lipid peroxidation but fails to mitigate increased transepidermal water loss after benzoyl peroxide treatment of human skin. *Free Rad Biol Med.* 2003;34:170–176.
- Yamada Y, Obayashi M, Ishikawa T, Kiso Y, Ono Y, Yamashita K. Dietary tocotrienol reduces UVB-induced skin damage and sesamin enhances tocotrienol effects in hairless mice. *J Nutr Sci Vitaminol (Tokyo).* 2008;54:117–123.

TROLOX

- *Empirical formula*: $C_{14}H_{18}O_4$
- *MW*: 250.29
- *Synonyms*: (±)-6-hydroxy-2,5,7,8-tetramethylchromane-2-carboxylic acid
- *CAS*: 53188-07-1
- *EC Number*: 258-422-8
- *SMILES*: c12c(CCC(C(O)=O)(C)O1)c(C)c(O)c(C)c2C

Description

Trolox is a trade name (Hoffman-LaRoche) for 6-hydroxy-2,5,7,8-tetramethylchroman-2-carboxylic acid—a water-soluble vitamin E derivative. Unlike vitamin E isomers, trolox contains a carboxyl group in place of the long phytyl chain. Trolox, an ingredient in cosmetic products, also is used in one of the antioxidant assays discussed in Chapter 6. The Trolox Equivalent Antioxidant Assay, uses Trolox as a reference of antioxidant efficacy to which investigated antioxidants are measured.

Stability/shelf life

- Carlotti ME, Sapino S, Vione D, Pelizzetti E, Trotta M. Photostability of Trolox in water/ethanol, water, and Oramix CG 110 in the absence and in the presence of TiO_2. *J Dispersion Sci Technol.* 2004;25:193–207.
- Cort WM, Scott JW, Araujo M, Mergens WJ, Cannalonga MA, Osadca M et al. Antioxidant activity and stability of 6-hydroxy-2,5,7,8-tetramethylchroman-2-carboxylic acid. *J Am Oil Chem Soc.* 1975;52:174–178.

Analytical studies

- Huang S-W, Frankel EN, Schwarz K, German JB. Effect of pH on antioxidant activity of α-tocopherol and

Trolox in oil-in-water emulsions. *J Agr Food Chem.* 1996;44:2496–2502.
- Oehlkea K, Heinsa A, Stöckmanna H, Sönnichsenb F, Schwarza K. New insights into the antioxidant activity of Trolox in o/w emulsions. *Food Chem.* 2011;124:781–787.

ESR studies
- Davies MJ, Forni LG, Willson RL. Vitamin E analogue Trolox C. *Biochem J.* 1988;255:513–522.
- Guo Q, Packer L. ESR studies of ascorbic acid-dependent recycling of the vitamin E homologue Trolox by coenzyme Q_0 in murine skin homogenates. *Redox Rep.* 1999;4:105–111.

General interest articles
- Ohara K, Kikuchi K, Origuchi T, Nagaoka S. Singlet oxygen quenching by Trolox C in aqueous micelle solutions. *J Photochem Photobiol B: Biol.* 2009;97:132–137.
- Poljsak B, Raspor P. The antioxidant and pro-oxidant activity of vitamin C and Trolox in vitro: A comparative study. *J Appl Toxicol.* 2008;28:183–188.
- Sivonová M, Zitnanová I, Horáková L, Strosová M, Muchová J, Balgavý P et al. The combined effect of pycnogenol with ascorbic acid and Trolox on the oxidation of lipids and proteins. *Gen Physiol Biophys.* 2006;25:379–396.

Skin studies
- Guo Q, Packer L. Ascorbate-dependent recycling of the vitamin E homologue Trolox by dihydrolipoate and glutathione in murine skin homogenates. *Free Rad Biol Med.* 2000;29:368–374.
- Kitazawa M, Podda M, Thiele J, Traber MG, Iwasaki K, Sakamoto K et al. Interactions between vitamin E homologues and ascorbate free radicals in murine skin homogenates irradiated with ultraviolet light. *Photochem Photobiol.* 1997;65:355–365.

UBIQUINONE-10

- *Empirical formula*: $C_{59}H_{90}O_4$
- *MW*: 863.34
- *Synonyms*: coenzyme Q_{10}, coenzyme Q
- *CAS*: 303-98-0
- *EC number*: 206-147-9
- *Beilstein registry number*: 1900141
- *SMILES*: C(C1=C(C(C(OC)=C(OC)C1=O)=O)C)C=C(C)CCC=C(C)CCC=C(C)CCC=C(C)CCC=C(C)CCC=C(C)CCC=C(C)CCC=C(C)CCC=C(C)C

Description
Ubiquinone-10, also referred to as coenzyme Q, is a lipid-soluble antioxidant that is naturally found in the body and is also available from commercial sources. In vivo it is found in lipid membranes, most prominently in the inner membrane of the mitochondrion where it carries out the function of electron transport carrier. This process, known as oxidative phosphorylation, is the principal energy producing (in the form of ATP) event in the cell. Structurally, ubiquinone-10 consists of 10 isoprenoid units that provide it with a long aliphatic tail to anchor into lipid membranes. The quinone portion of the molecule contributes to its antioxidant properties. The structural form shown earlier is fully oxidized—with two ketone groups. There is also a semiquinone (ubisemiquinone) and fully reduced structure (ubiquinol), in which there are one or two hydroxy groups, respectively, at the location of the ketone groups. Coenzyme Q's unique behavior—electron transfer agent and antioxidant—is a result of these molecular forms, in which case the quinone structure is involved with electron transport and ubiquinol with antioxidation.

Chemical/physical properties
- $ALOGPs^6$: 9.94

Stability/shelf life
- Bulea MV, Singhala RS, Kennedy JF. Microencapsulation of ubiquinone-10 in carbohydrate matrices for improved stability. *Carbohyd Polym.* 2010;82:1290–1296.

Analytical studies
- Lunetta S, Roman M. Determination of coenzyme Q10 content in raw materials and dietary supplements by high-performance liquid chromatography-UV: Collaborative study. *J AOAC Int.* 2008;91:702–708.
- Podda M, Weber C, Traber MG, Packer L. Simultaneous determination of tissue tocopherols, tocotrienols, ubiquinols, and ubiquinones. *J Lipid Res.* 1996;37:893–901.
- Rodríguez-Acuña R, Brenne E, Lacoste F. Determination of coenzyme Q10 and Q9 in vegetable oils. *J Agr Food Chem.* 2008;56:6241–6245.

ESR studies
- Stoyanovsky DA, Osipov AN, Quinn PJ, Kagan VE. Ubiquinone-dependent recycling of vitamin E radicals by superoxide. *Arch Biochem Biophys.* 1995;323:343–351.

General interest articles
- Choi JH, Ryu YW, Seo JH. Biotechnological production and applications of coenzyme Q10. *Appl Microbiol Biotechnol.* 2005;68:9–15.
- Cluis CP, Burja AM, Martin VJ. Current prospects for the production of coenzyme Q10 in microbes. *Trends Biotechnol.* 2007;25:514–521.
- Crane FL. Biochemical functions of coenzyme Q10. *J Am Coll Nutr.* 2001;20:591–598.
- Ernster L, Dallner G. Biochemical, physiological and medical aspects of ubiquinone function. *Biochim Biophys Acta.* 1995;24:195–204.
- Ernster L, Forsmark-Andrée P. Ubiquinol: An endogenous antioxidant in aerobic organisms. *Clin Investig.* 1993;71(8 Suppl):S60–S65.

- Hidaka T, Fujii K, Funahashi I, Fukutomi N, Hosoe K. Safety assessment of coenzyme Q10 (CoQ10). *Biofactors.* 2008;32:199–208.
- Littarru GP, Tiano L. Bioenergetic and antioxidant properties of coenzyme Q10: Recent developments. *Mol Biotechnol.* 2007;37:31–37.
- Nohl H, Gille L, Staniek K. The biochemical, pathophysiological, and medical aspects of ubiquinone function. *Ann New York Acad Sci.* 1998;854:394–409.
- Nohl H, Staniek K, Kozlov AV, Gille L. The biomolecule ubiquinone exerts a variety of biological functions. *Biofactors.* 2003;18:23–31.

Skin studies

- Fuller B, Smith D, Howerton A, Kern D. Anti-inflammatory effects of CoQ10 and colorless carotenoids. *J Cosmet Dermatol.* 2006;5:30–38.
- Hojerová J. Coenzyme Q10—Its importance, properties and use in nutrition and cosmetics. *Ceska Slov Farm.* 2000;49:119–123.
- Hoppe U, Bergemann J, Diembeck W, Ennen J, Gohla S, Harris I et al. Coenzyme Q10, a cutaneous antioxidant and energizer. *Biofactors.* 1999;9:371–378.
- Inui M, Ooe M, Fujii K, Matsunaka H, Yoshida M, Ichihashi M. Mechanisms of inhibitory effects of CoQ10 on UVB-induced wrinkle formation in vitro and in vivo. *Biofactors.* 2008;32:237–243.
- Vinson J, Anamandla S. Comparative topical absorption and antioxidant effectiveness of two forms of coenzyme Q10 after a single dose and after long-term supplementation in the skin of young and middle-aged subjects. *IFSCC Mag.* 2005;8(4):1–6.
- Yue Y, Zhou H, Liu G, Li Y, Yan Z, Duan M. The advantages of a novel CoQ10 delivery system in skin photoprotection. *Int J Pharm.* 2010;392:57–63.

REFERENCES

1. Zafarullah M et al. *Cell Mol Life Sci.* 2003;60:6–20.
2. Lide D. *Handbook of Chemistry and Physics*, 88th ed. Boca Raton, FL: CRC Press; 2008.
3. Sigma-Aldrich Online Catalog, www.sigmaaldrich.com, 2018.
4. Osol A et al. *Remington's Pharmaceutical Sciences.* Easton, PA: Mack Publishing; 1980.
5. Serjeant EP, Dempsey B (Eds.). *Ionisation Constants of Organic Acids in Aqueous Solution.* International Union of Pure and Applied Chemistry (IUPAC). New York: Pergamon Press; 1979.
6. Tetko IV et al. *J Comput Aid Mol Des.* 2005;19:453–463; VCCLAB, Virtual Computational Chemistry Laboratory, http://www.vcclab.org, 2005.
7. USEPA. United States Environmental Protection Agency, Estimation Programs Interface (EPI) Suite, Vers. 4.0, http://www.epa.gov/oppt/exposure/pubs/episuitedl.htm, 2008.
8. Gerhartz W (Ed.). *Ullmann's Encyclopedia of Industrial Chemistry*, 6th ed. Deerfield Beach, FL: VCH Publishers; 1985–1996.
9. Osol A, Hoover JE (Eds.). *Remington's Pharmaceutical Sciences*, 14th ed. Easton, PA: Mack Publishing; 1970.
10. Perrisoud D, Testa B. *Arzneim-Forsch.* 1986;36:1249–1253.
11. Cayman Chemical. Apigenin (item no. 10010275) product information, www.caymanchem.com, 2010.
12. Poretz RD, Goldstein IJ. *Arch Biochem Biophys.* 1968;125:1034–1036.
13. O'Neil MJ (Ed.). *The Merck Index*, 13th ed. Rahway, NJ: Merck; 2001.
14. PentaPharm. Alpha-arbutin product information, www.pentapharm.com, 2011.
15. Seidel A (Ed.). *Kirk-Othmer Encyclopedia of Chemical Technology.* Hoboken, NJ: John Wiley & Sons; 2007.
16. Takacs-Novak K, Avdeef A. *J Pharm Biomed Anal.* 1996;14:1405–1413.
17. Lide DR, Milne GWA (Eds.). *Handbook of Data on Organic Compounds*, 3rd ed. Boca Raton, FL: CRC Press; 1994.
18. Windholz M, Budavari S, Stroumtsos LY, Fertig MN (Eds.). *The Merck Index*, 9th ed. Rahway, NJ: Merck; 1976.
19. Furia TE (Ed.). *CRC Handbook of Food Additives*, 2nd ed. Boca Raton, FL: CRC Press; 1972.
20. Budavari S (Ed.). *The Merck Index*, 11th ed. Rahway, NJ: Merck; 1989.
21. O'Brien RD. *Fats and Oils: Formulating and Processing for Applications*, 2nd ed. Boca Raton, FL: CRC Press; 2004.
22. Weast RC, Astle MJ (Eds.). *CRC Handbook of Data on Organic Compounds.* Boca Raton, FL: CRC Press; 1985.
23. Hites RA (Ed.). *Handbook of Mass Spectra of Environmental Contaminants.* Boca Raton, FL: CRC Press; 1985.
24. Hanai T, Hubert J. *J Chromatogr.* 1982;239:527–536.
25. Bors W, et al. *Oxygen Radicals in Chemistry and Biology.* Berlin, Germany: de Gruyter & Co.; 1984.
26. Weast RC (Ed.). *CRC Handbook of Chemistry and Physics*, 60th ed. Boca Raton, FL: CRC Press; 1979.
27. Lide DR (Ed.). *Handbook of Chemistry and Physics*, 86th ed. Boca Raton, FL: CRC Press; 2006.
28. FDA. *187 Fake Cancer 'Cures' Consumers Should Avoid.* Silver Spring, MD: U.S Food and Drug Administration, U.S. Department of Health and Human Services, www.fda.gov; 2018.
29. O'Neil M. *The Merck Index*, 15th ed. Cambridge, UK: The Royal Society of Chemistry; 2013.
30. Taylor CK, et al. *Nutr Rev.* 2009;67:398–415.
31. Lewis RJ (Ed.). *Hawley's Condensed Chemical Dictionary*, 15th ed. Hoboken, NJ: John Wiley & Sons; 2007.
32. Kontoghiorghes GJ. *Inorg Chim Acta.* 1988;151:101–106.
33. Su EG. Formulating with Skin Lighteners. Sino Lion (USA), Ltd.; 2011.

34. Csomós G, Leuschner U. Gallbladder and Liver Therapy. In: Bohnet, M (Ed.). *Ullmann's Encyclopedia of Industrial Chemistry*, 7th ed. Hoboken, NJ: John Wiley & Sons; 2002.
35. Volpi A, Toffoli F. *Boll Chim Farm*. 1979;118:594–609.
36. Hata TR et al. *J Invest Dermatol*. 2000;115:441–448.
37. Budavari S (Ed.). *The Merck Index*, 12th ed. Rahway, NJ: Merck; 1996.
38. Trevithick-Sutton CC et al. *Molecul Vis*. 2006;12:1127–1135.
39. Human Metabolome Database (HMDB), www.hmdb.ca/metabolites/HMDB0030703.
40. Lide DR (Ed.). *Handbook of Chemistry and Physics*, 75th ed. Boca Raton, FL: CRC Press; 1995.
41. Boyd I, Beveridge EG. *Microbios*. 1979;24:173–184.
42. Herrmann K. *Int J Food Sci Tech*. 1976;11:433–448.
43. Rothwell, J et al. *J Agric Food Chem*. 2005;53:4355–4360.
44. Brown J, et al. *Biochem J*. 1998;330:1173–1178.
45. Meylan W *J Pharm Sci*. 1995;84:83–92.
46. Baumann LS. *Cosmetic Dermatology: Principles and Practice*, 2nd ed. New York: McGraw-Hill; 2009.
47. Hansch C, Clayton JM. *J Pharm Sci*. 1973;62:1–21.
48. Windholz M (Ed.). *The Merck Index*, 10th ed. Rahway, NJ: Merck; 1983.
49. Jhoo JW et al. *J Agr Food Chem*. 2005;53:6146–6150.
50. Lide DR (Ed.). *Handbook of Chemistry and Physics*, 79th ed. Boca Raton, FL: CRC Press; 1999.
51. Hansch C, Leo A. *The Log p Database*. Claremont, CA: Pomona College; 1987.
52. McCurdy PP (Ed.). *Chemical Week Buyer's Guide 87*. New York: McGraw-Hill; 1987.
53. Weast RC (Ed.). *CRC Handbook of Chemistry and Physics*, 57th ed. Boca Raton, FL: CRC Press; 1976.
54. Lewis RJ (Ed.). *Hawley's Condensed Chemical Dictionary*, 14th ed. Hoboken, NJ: John Wiley & Sons; 2001.

Appendix 1: Glossary of terms

antibody: large Y-shaped proteins produced by immune cells (B cells). The antibody has two active sites that identify and bind with antigens from viruses and bacteria. The binding site of the antibody has a section known as a paratope that binds with an epitope on the antigen. By binding to the antigen, the antibody tags the bacterium or virus, thereby rendering it inactive or allowing other immune cells to attack and destroy. The immunoglobins constitute the protein family of antibodies.

antigen: by definition, an antigen is any foreign substance introduced into the body that results in the production of an antibody, hence a specific immune response. In most cases, antigens are proteins or polysaccharides from a pathogen that bind at the active site of an antibody. The binding portion of the antigen is known as an epitope. Antigens are presented by antigen-presenting cells to T cells of the immune system.

apoptosis: a form of programmed cell death. Complex biochemical mechanisms result in the destruction of cellular components, especially the nucleus and its contents. Apoptosis is a normal process in the body, and defective apoptosis could lead to the over-proliferation of cells and, possibly, carcinogenesis.

atrophy: the wasting away of tissue due to genetic mutations, lack of blood flow, or biochemical dysfunction.

axilla: the armpit or underarm area of the body.

chemotaxis: a process in which chemical signals (e.g., peptides) are secreted by a source leading other cells to migrate to the origin of the signals. The process of migration is chemotaxis. This is very common in the immune system when cells that are damaged by foreign pathogens release chemical signals that attract white blood cells (neutrophils) from the blood. The neutrophils migrate to the tissue and destroy the pathogens.

coenzyme: an organic molecule that aids an enzyme in carrying out its function. Often the term coenzyme is used interchangeably with cofactor. Two examples of coenzymes are NADH and $FADH_2$, which are involved in many important electron transfer reactions.

cofactor: typically, cofactors are metal ions that assist an enzyme in its catalytic activity. Biochemically important cofactors consist of Mn^{2+}, Zn^{2+}, Fe^{2+}, and Mg^{2+}. Often, the term cofactor is used interchangeably with coenzyme.

cytoplasm: the aqueous compartment of the cell. Most eukaryotic cells are surrounded by a cell membrane that encloses an aqueous interior (interior ~70% water) that contains the cell's organelles.

cytotoxicity: when a substance is toxic to cells. Endogenous chemical agents can be cytotoxic to resident cells while immune cells can be cytotoxic to foreign pathogens and cells.

dismutation: a redox reaction in which a reactive oxygen species is simultaneously reduced and oxidized, resulting in the formation of two distinct products. Such a process occurs with the enzyme superoxide dismutase, discussed in Chapter 3.

dorsal: relating to or situated near or on the back, especially of an animal or of one of its parts. In many studies involving skin biology the dorsal region of mice is studied.

endogenous: from within the organism. For example, endogenous antioxidants refer to those that are synthesized by the body or come from the diet and are incorporated into the skin structure, but not those that are exogenously introduced by topical treatment.

endoplasmic reticulum: an organelle in eukaryotic cells composed of membranous tubules and sacs called cisternae. The rough endoplasmic reticulum is directly adjacent to the nucleus and studded with ribosomes. Protein synthesis (translation) takes place on the ribosomes where mRNA is translated to polypeptide. Lipid synthesis and drug metabolism take place in the smooth endoplasmic reticulum (does not contain ribosomes).

enzyme: a protein that catalyzes a specific biochemical reaction by lowering the barrier of activation energy. Enzymes contain active sites and often work together with coenzymes or cofactors. Much of our own endogenous antioxidant system is composed of enzymes that neutralize reactive oxygen species by electron transfer reactions.

exogenous: derived or developed from outside of the body. Throughout the text we refer to exogenous antioxidants. For example, topical treatment is achieved with exogenous antioxidants.

genotoxic: an agent that is damaging to DNA. Genetic mutations caused by genotoxic substances could eventually result in carcinomas.

Golgi apparatus: an organelle in eukaryotic cells, which receives proteins from the endoplasmic reticulum then packages them in transport vesicles before they are delivered to other locations.

homeostasis: the ability of a cell to maintain a steady state or internal equilibrium by carefully controlling its physiological processes.

intraperitoneal: existing within or administered by entering the peritoneum (body cavity). In some studies of animal models, antioxidant treatments are administered by intraperitoneal injection.

isozyme: enzymes that have different amino acid sequences but carry out the same function.

keratohyalin granules: granular structures found in the stratum granulosum of the epidermis that contain profilaggrin (precursor of filaggrin), keratin intermediate filaments, and loricrin (a protein of the cornified envelope).

lamellar bodies: membrane-bound organelles that originate in the Golgi apparatus that contain lipids and enzymes. Their primary site of activity is at the stratum granulosum in the epidermis where they deliver precursors of stratum corneum lipids to intercellular space. As a result, lamellae are formed at the stratum granulosum-stratum corneum interface.

lysosome: cellular organelles that contain digestive enzymes that process old organelles, food particles, viruses, and bacteria.

mammary areola: areola refers to an anatomical region of the body that contains a different color tissue than that of the surrounding area. The mammary areola is the red tissue of the breast including the nipple.

melanogenesis: the synthesis of melanin (eumelanin or pheomelanin) by melanocytes, resulting in the production of melanin granules that are packaged in organelles called melanosomes.

MED: minimal erythemal dose (MED) refers to the amount of UVB light that produces redness 24 hours after exposure.

mitochondrion: cellular organelle found in eukaryotic cells that is responsible for energy production. Many important metabolic pathways take place in the mitochondrion, including oxidative phosphorylation, beta-oxidation, citric acid cycle, and amino acid oxidation pathways. As an important energy source for the cell, it is most well known for oxidative phosphorylation (final stage of cellular respiration) in which adenosine triphosphate is synthesized due to the activity of the electron transport chain.

necrosis: the death of body tissue resulting from lack of blood flow due to injury, radiation, or chemicals.

nucleus: the cell nucleus is a membrane-bound organelle in eukaryotic cells that contain chromosomes—thread-like structures that contain the cell's DNA. Important biological processes, such as DNA replication and transcription (DNA is transcribed to RNA), take place in the nucleus.

oxidation: the reaction of a substance with oxygen. It is a reaction in which the atoms of a molecule or an ion lose electrons (or protons). As a result, the valence state of the species increases.

perineal region: anatomically, the perineal region is the area of the trunk below the pelvic diaphragm. In general, it refers to the regions between the anal and female vaginal or male genital regions.

peritoneum: the smooth transparent serous membrane that lines the cavity of the abdomen of a mammal and is folded inward over the abdominal and pelvic viscera.

peroxisome: cellular organelle in eukaryotes that contains enzymes that rid the cell of toxic peroxides. Beta-oxidation also takes places in this organelle, although the mitochondrion is the major site of beta-oxidation.

phagocytosis: common in macrophages of the immune system, phagocytosis is a process in which a cell engulfs a particle and packages it in a membrane-bound sac, which is presented to lysosomes that contain hydrolytic enzymes capable of degrading its contents.

photosensitizer: a chromophore that absorbs light then enters an excited state, eventually leading to the formation of reactive oxygen species.

ping-pong mechanism: this describes the mechanism of an enzymatic reaction when one substrate is bound to the enzyme then released followed by the subsequent binding and releasing of a second substrate.

reduction: a type of redox reaction in which a species gains electrons (or protons). As a result, the valence state of the molecule or ion increases.

replication: a biochemical process in which an identical copy is made of DNA. A DNA double helix produces a copy of itself in which each strand of the parent DNA is unwound and used as a template for the two new strands. An important part of mitosis and occurring in the nucleus, DNA replication is the biological basis of heredity.

ribosome: a large molecular complex consisting of two subunits and composed of RNA and proteins. They are bound to the rough endoplasmic reticulum and are responsible for the translation (protein synthesis) of mRNA to polypeptides.

senescence: the normal process of chronological aging in the cell due to endogenous factors, ultimately leading to cell death.

tautomerism: interconversion between two isomers. One common example in biochemistry is keto-enol tautomerism, which is an equilibrium state between a keto (a ketone or aldehyde) and enol (an alcohol) form of a molecule.

telangiectasia: an epithelial condition in which small, dilated blood vessels are found near the surface of skin or mucous membranes.

transcription: the synthesis of RNA from a DNA template by the enzyme RNA polymerase. Essentially, the enzyme opens the DNA double helix and chains together RNA nucleotides corresponding to base-pairs with one of the DNA strands. Transcription occurs in the nucleus of the cell.

transcription factor: proteins that facilitate the activity (binding) of RNA polymerase and initiate transcription.

translation: a biochemical process that takes place in ribosomes resulting in the synthesis of proteins. Produced by transcription, mRNA is decoded by tRNA, which contains an amino acid corresponding to the sequence of three nucleotide bases in mRNA (codon). At the ribosome, tRNA corresponding to each codon carry amino acids to the ribosome where they are linked together as a polypeptide (see Appendix 2).

Appendix 2: Biologically important molecules and mechanisms

AMINO ACIDS

There are 20 common alpha-amino acids that link together by peptide bonds to form the building blocks of the proteins found in the body. The naturally occurring amino acids are L stereoisomers and are optically active (they rotate the plane of linear polarized light). They contain an amine group, carboxylic acid group, and alpha-carbon to which a pendant functional group (usually referred to as an R group) is bound and makes each amino acid distinct. The primary structure of proteins is the sequence of amino acids along the polypeptide backbone. The nature of each amino acid's R group governs the secondary structure of the protein, which can be alpha helix, beta sheet, or beta turn. The tertiary structure of the protein is the actual three-dimensional arrangement of atoms in space and ultimately depends on the chemistry of the amino acids as well as the primary and secondary structure. The amino acids are typically classified by the nature of the R group (Figure A2.1). The most common categorization breaks them down into the following groups: aliphatic (nonpolar or hydrophobic), uncharged polar, basic, acidic, and aromatic side chains. The structures of the amino acids are shown as they exist in free form (not part of a protein) at pH 7.0. Please keep in mind that the surface pH of skin is approximately 5.4 and this may affect the protonation state of some of the amino acids close to the surface.

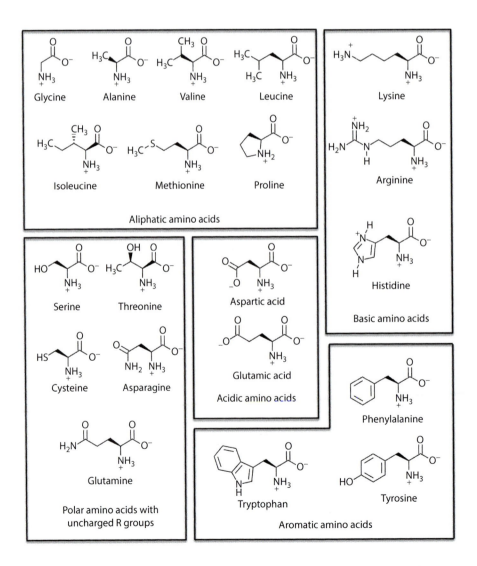

Figure A2.1 The 20 standard amino acids found in proteins, categorized into their respective classification according to R group.

NUCLEIC ACIDS

The genetic diversity of organisms is due to the hereditary information that is encoded in the deoxyribonucleic acid (DNA), which is stored in chromosomes in the nuclei of all living cells. Nucleotides (monomer units) are the building blocks of DNA and their specific sequence determines genetic code. As shown in Figure A2.2, DNA nucleotides contain a deoxyribose ring, phosphate group, and nitrogen-containing base. DNA is formed by linkages between the phosphate group and the pendant hydroxyl group on the adjacent carbon (3 position) on the deoxyribose ring. The nitrogen-containing bases are adenine, guanine, cytosine, and thymine. When two strands of DNA form an alpha helix, complementary bases adjacent to each other help to stabilize the helical structure. For example, adenosine and thymine form one pair while guanosine and cytosine form another. Ribonucleic acid (RNA) is also comprised of the same nucleotides as DNA with the exception of thymine, which is replaced by uracil. Unlike DNA, RNA contains a ribose ring with a hydroxyl group at the 2 position of the ring (DNA has a deoxyribose ring without a hydroxyl group at the 2 position). Based on their molecular structure the nucleotide bases of DNA and RNA are classified as purines or pyrimidines. The purines are adenine and guanine, while pyrimidines are cytosine, thymine, and uracil (Figure A2.3).

Transcription, Translation, and Replication

From the storage of genetic information to the expression of proteins, there are core processes at work in the cell, which facilitate transcription, translation, and replication.[1] Transcription and translation are two biochemical processes that convert information stored in the genetic code (DNA) to a functional protein with the help of RNA.

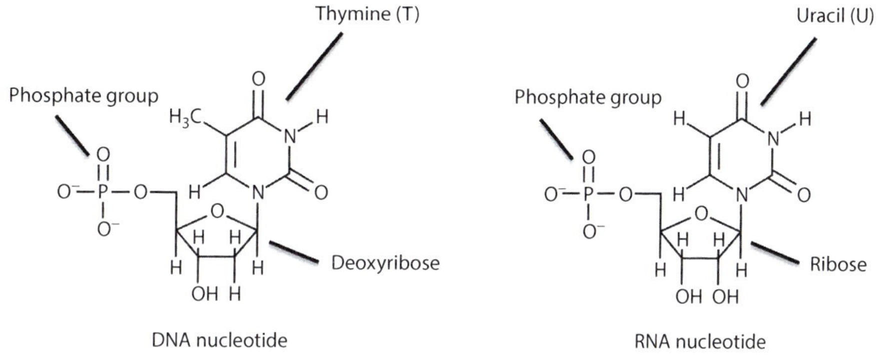

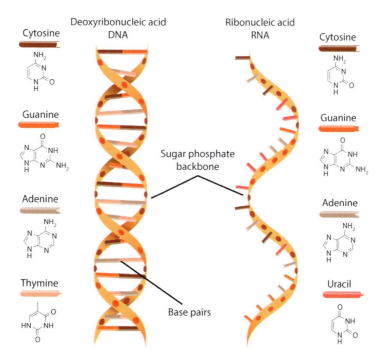

Figure A2.2 Example of a DNA and RNA nucleotide based on the thymine and uracil bases.

Figure A2.3 Illustration of the double-stranded DNA (left) structure and a single-stranded RNA (right) molecule along with the nitrogenous bases that distinguish the five different nucleotides.

In the process of transcription, one of the strands of DNA from a double helix is transcribed into a single strand of mRNA by the action of the enzyme RNA polymerase. The new RNA strand contains complementary bases to the DNA template (Figure A2.3). For example, guanine replaces cytosine, cytosine replaces guanine, adenine replaces thymine, and uracil replaces adenine.

Each series of three consecutive nucleotides in mRNA forms a codon, which corresponds to a particular amino acid that will form part of a newly synthesized protein by the process known as translation. Before protein synthesis can occur, mRNA must be decoded by tRNA. As illustrated in Figure A2.4, there is a specific tRNA molecule for each amino acid.[2] It contains an anticodon, which binds to

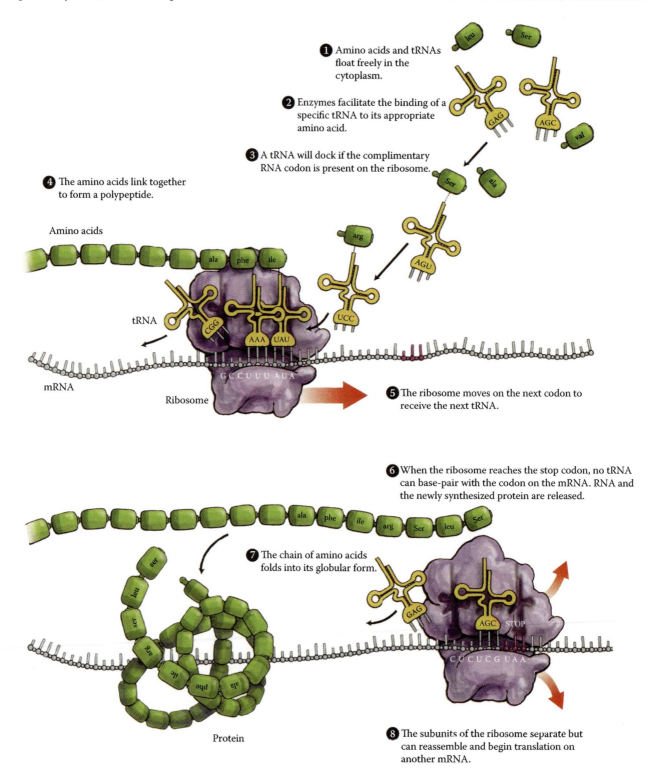

Figure A2.4 Illustration of translation (protein synthesis) that occurs on ribosomes of the rough endoplasmic reticulum. (From Elk, C. and Maier, V.B., *Human Biology*, 1st ed., Copyright 2009. Reprinted by permission of Pearson Education, Inc., New York.)

the corresponding codon site of mRNA. This mechanism occurs in ribosomes, and as each tRNA carries an amino acid to the active site, a polypeptide chain is formed with an amino acid sequence corresponding to the order of the codons of the mRNA. Finally, a tRNA molecule containing a stop anticodon matches up with the stop codon of mRNA and protein synthesis ceases, at which time the protein folds into its three-dimensional structure and is released to the cytoplasm of the cell. Throughout this book, there are many circumstances where we mention transcription factors and their activation. Transcription factors are proteins that bind to DNA and control the transfer of genetic information from DNA to mRNA, eventually leading to the upregulation of proteins by translation.

DNA integrity is preserved when cells divide (mitosis) by a process known as DNA replication. The double helix unwinds and each polynucleotide strand (parental strands) serves as a template for the synthesis of a complementary DNA strand (daughter strands). Normally, DNA synthesis proceeds by a conservative or semi-conservative mechanism. In the conservative mechanism the two daughter strands form a new double helix. In contrast, following the semi-conservative mechanism each parent strand forms a new double helix with one of the daughter strands. There are many other phenomena associated with DNA, especially repair mechanisms, which play an integral role in cellular homeostasis.

Oxidation and Reduction of Cystine

In many proteins, the amino acid cysteine forms disulfide crosslinks in which two cysteine amino acid residues produce one cystine unit. This form of crosslinking in proteins may be found in globular proteins, but more often than not they are responsible for tightly binding structural fibrous proteins together. This is especially true for many of the structural proteins that constitute the various morphological components of human hair and nail. As shown in Figure A2.5, the disulfide bond in cystine can undergo reduction (gain of electrons or protons) or oxidation (loss of electrons or protons), resulting in the formation of two cysteine residues or two cysteic acid residues. Reduction occurs when hair undergoes certain chemical procedures such as permanent waving. First, hair is treated with a reducing agent to break the cystine bonds (resulting in sulfhydryl groups), then it is set into its desired hair style and oxidized with H_2O_2 to reform the cystine bonds in the new hair set. Likewise, oxidation of hair occurs during chemical treatments as well as upon exposure to UV light, which may result in the formation of cysteic acid residues.

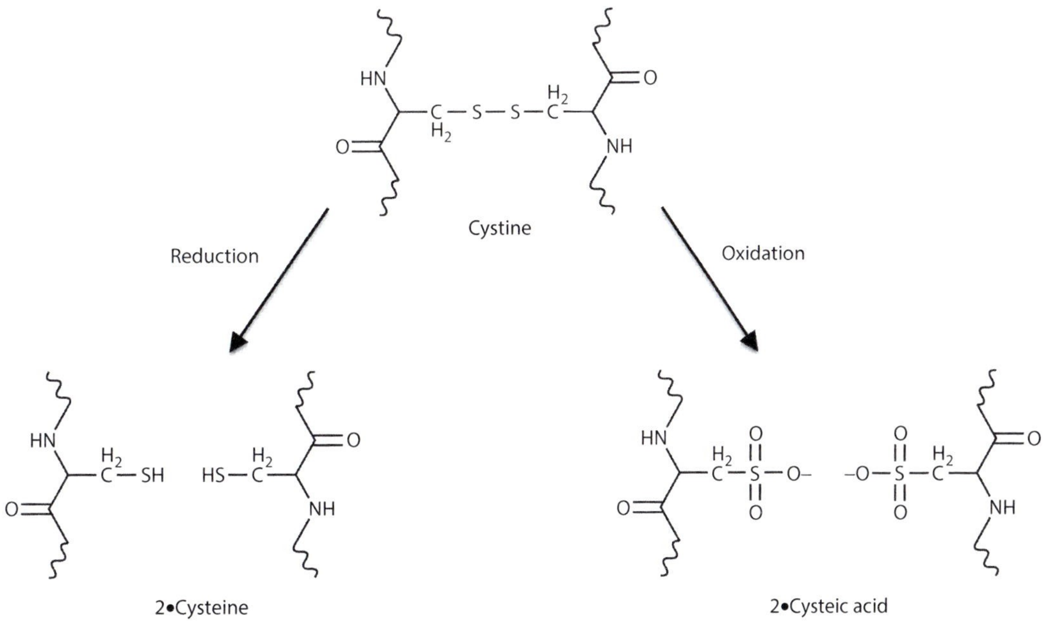

Figure A2.5 Reduction and oxidation of cystine, resulting in the formation of cysteine and cysteic acid.

Important Enzyme Cofactors and Coenzymes

Discussed mostly in Chapter 3 in regard to antioxidant enzymes, cofactors/coenzymes are an essential component for enzyme activity, usually binding to the enzyme active site to aid in catalysis. Cofactors are typically metal ions (e.g., Mn^{2+}, Zn^{2+}, Fe^{2+}, and Mg^{2+}) while coenzymes are more complex organic molecules that may contain an inorganic ion. The reader should bear in mind that the terms cofactor and coenzyme are often used interchangeably. Regardless, in most cases their function includes the transfer of electrons, atoms, or functional groups.

Two important cofactors, based on the nucleic acid base adenine, are nicotinamide adenine dinucleotide (NAD^+) and flavin adenine dinucleotide (FAD). The structure of NAD^+ (reduced form) and its oxidized counterpart (NADH) are shown in Figure A2.6. In both NAD^+ and NADH, one of the nucleotides contains the adenine base while the other contains nicotinamide. The nucleotides are joined together by two phosphate groups. NAD^+/NADH is mostly involved in electron transfer reactions, where NADH acts as a reducing agent and donates electrons to other substrates. The electron transfer reactions take place at the nicotinamide portion of the molecule. A variant of NAD^+/NADH is $NADP^+$/NADPH, which includes an additional phosphate group at the 2 position on the ribose ring. The structure of FAD and $FADH_2$ is provided in Figure A2.7. FAD/$FADH_2$ contains a riboflavin (vitamin B2) group attached to the adenosine portion of the molecule. Like NAD^+/NADH, FAD/$FADH_2$ is an electron transfer agent. FAD is reduced to $FADH_2$ by the transfer of two electrons.

Adenosine triphosphate (ATP) is another important cofactor and chief energy source for the cell (Figure A2.8). Structurally, it is composed of an adenosine group (adenine base and ribose) and a moiety containing three phosphate groups. It is produced by cellular respiration (mitochondrial electron transport chain) and is later utilized in reactions requiring the input of energy, which is provided by the cleavage of one of its phosphate groups. This biochemical reaction results in the conversion of ATP to adenosine diphosphate (ADP), which as indicated by its name contains one less phosphate group than ATP.

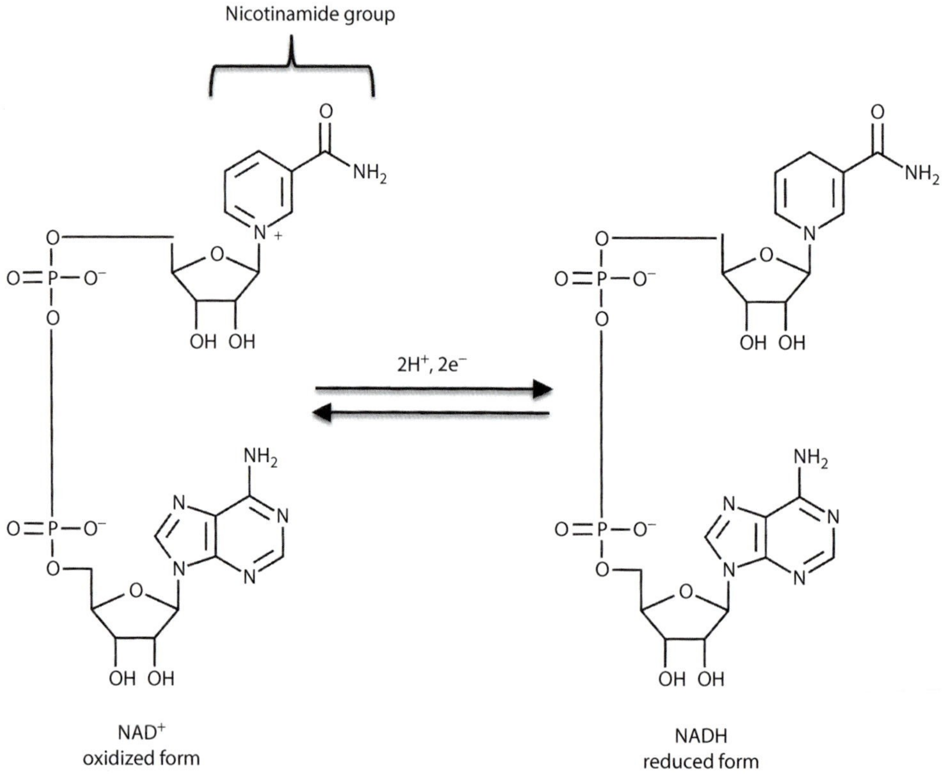

Figure A2.6 Redox interconversion of NAD^+ and NADH.

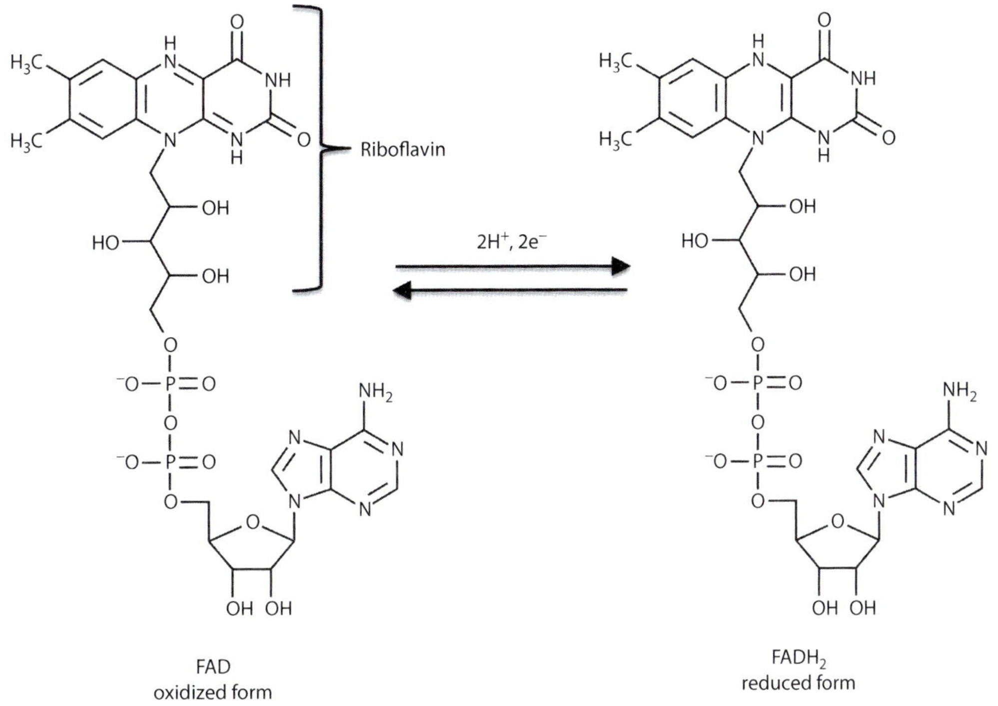

Figure A2.7 Redox interconversion of FAD and FADH$_2$.

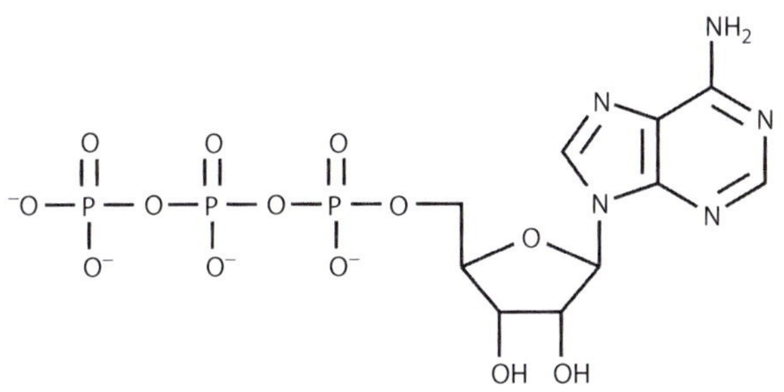

Figure A2.8 Molecular structure of ATP.

Furthermore, ADP is also involved in many biochemical reactions and may undergo conversion to adenosine monophosphate (AMP) with the liberation of another phosphate group.

Synthesis of Melanin

In Chapter 3, we briefly discussed the structure of melanin, a pigmentation molecule responsible for conferring protection to hair and skin from UV radiation. In hair, melanin granules are found in the cortex region and protect the alpha-keratin proteins of the inner core. In skin, melanin surrounds the nuclei of basal cell keratinocytes in order to protect the UV-sensitive DNA. There are two types of melanin, the brown/black pigment eumelanin and the yellow/red pigment pheomelanin. The biosynthetic pathway for both types of melanin follows a mechanism that depends on the action of the enzyme tyrosinase on the amino acid tyrosine. As illustrated in Figure A2.9, tyrosine is first converted to 3,4-dihydroxyphenylalanine (DOPA) and then to dopaquinone. At that point, one of two pathways may be followed. The eumelanin pathway results in the generation of oligomers of 5,6-dihydroxyindole and its derivatives. Alternatively, dopaquinone can follow the pheomelanin route by reacting with cysteine, resulting in the production of oligomers containing benzothiazine and benzothiazole units.

MOLECULES THAT CONSTITUTE THE NATURAL MOISTURIZING FACTOR IN STRATUM CORNEUM

Profilaggrin is a large protein precursor (350 kDa) composed of smaller subunits of filaggrin (26–45 kDa). Profilaggrin is present in keratohyalin granules in the epidermis and is released prior to undergoing proteolysis at the border of the stratum granulosum and stratum corneum to form filaggrin. There are two principle roles carried out by filaggrin in skin. The first is to align/aggregate keratin intermediate filaments in keratinocytes so that the formed corneocyte contains a very planar structure. Second, once filaggrin is finished arranging keratin intermediate filaments, it breaks down into the natural moisturizing factor (NMF), which is a group of compounds responsible for maintaining a hydrated stratum corneum. These consist of amino acids, organic acids, inorganic ions, urea, pyrrolidone carboxylic acid, sodium lactate, and *trans*-urocanic acid (Figure A2.10).

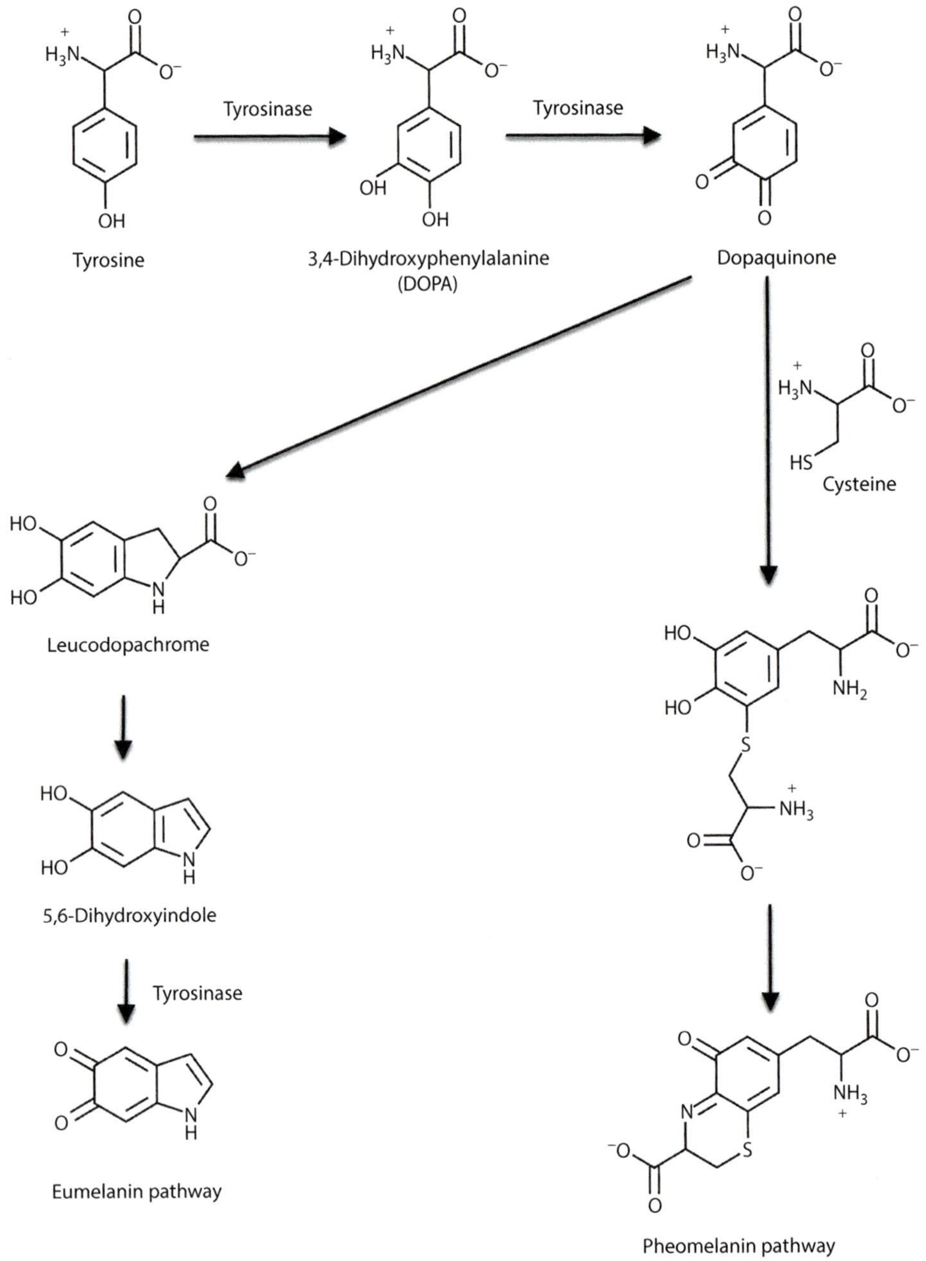

Figure A2.9 Schematic of eumelanin and pheomelanin synthesis catalyzed by tyrosinase.

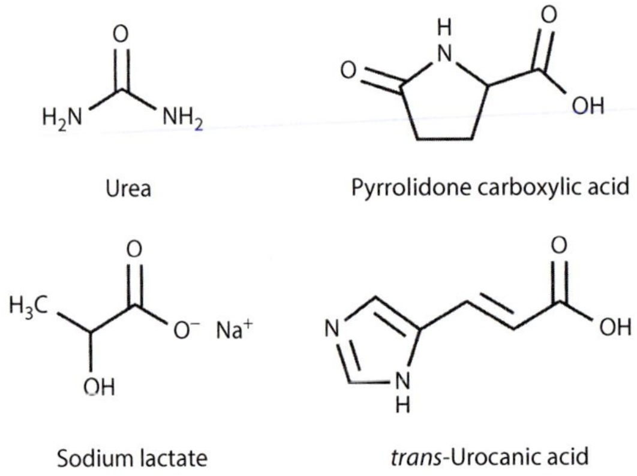

Figure A2.10 Molecular structure of key components of the NMF found in stratum corneum.

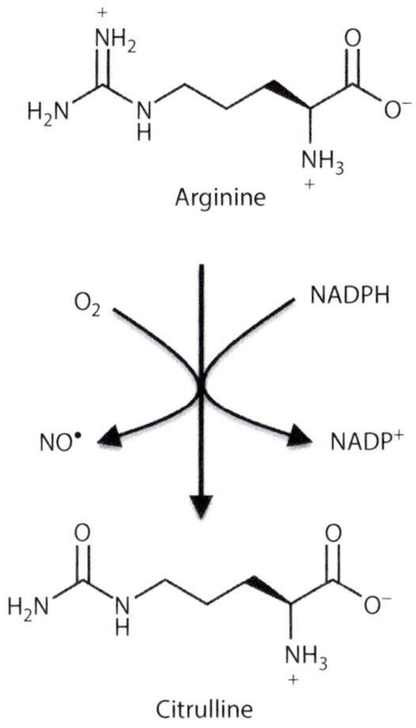

Appendix 2 191

CONVERSION OF ARGININE TO CITRULLINE

In Chapter 2 we discussed the synthesis of nitric oxide (NO·) that results from the conversion of arginine to citrulline. The reaction proceeds according to the scheme shown in Figure A2.11. L-arginine in combination with NADPH and O_2 produces citrulline, NO·, and the oxidized cofactor, NADP$^+$. This reaction is carried out by enzymes belonging to the NO· synthase family. A similar reaction takes place in proteins and is called citrullination; however, it is a distinct process from the one described herein.

HORMONES AND NEUROTRANSMITTERS

Throughout the text, reference is made to the activity of several hormones and neurotransmitters. Compounds classified as catecholamines (Chapter 2) can undergo autoxidation in the presence of O_2, resulting in the formation of superoxide anion ($O_2^{·-}$). Examples of these molecules are L-3,4-dihydroxyphenylalanine (L-DOPA), dopamine, adrenalin (epinephrine), and noradrenalin (norepinephrine). Their structures are shown in Figure A2.12.

Figure A2.11 Conversion of arginine to citrulline.

REFERENCES

1. Urry L, Cain M, Wasserman S, Minorsky P, Reece J. *Campbell Biology*. New York: Pearson; 2017.
2. Elk C, Maier VB. *Human Biology*, 1st ed. New York: Pearson Education; 2009.

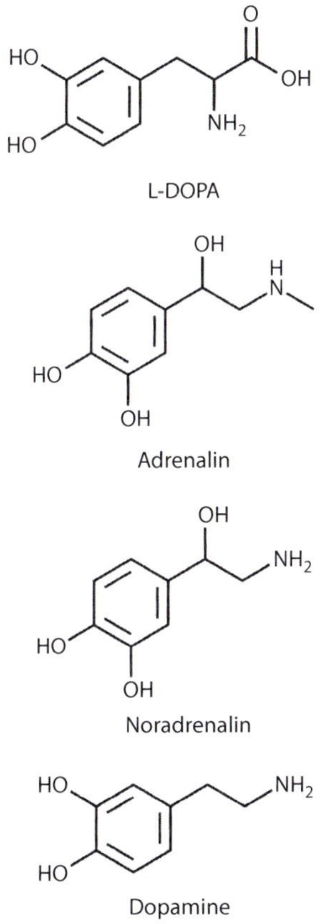

Figure A2.12 Molecular structures of several catecholamines.

Appendix 3: Cellular signaling in skin

An important aspect of the molecular biology of skin is the ability of cells to communicate with each other by extracellular means such as cell signaling. The importance of cell signaling stems from its role in the regulation of cell proliferation, differentiation, growth, and death.[1] For example, one cell (in distress) can send signals to other cells instructing them to manufacture a particular protein, which may help all cells to act in unison during times of necessity. Cellular signaling usually occurs by a process in which a molecule is secreted by one cell and the molecule, typically a protein or peptide, can travel in extracellular space until it reaches its destination cell where it finds a receptor on the plasma membrane of that cell. As a result of binding, the receptor (membrane-bound protein) undergoes some change (e.g., conformational changes) and this is followed by a series of steps within the cell (e.g., phosphorylation), ultimately leading to a cellular response, which is usually the activation or deactivation of a transcription factor (a molecule responsible for the transcription of DNA to RNA, ultimately leading to the expression of the corresponding protein). For demonstration, this mechanism is illustrated in Figure A3.1. A signal molecule binds to the membrane-bound surface receptor, which is followed by a series of events inside the cell, known as a signal transduction pathway. The pathway shown in the figure is a phosphorylation cascade in which a protein kinase is activated as a result of a conformation change in the membrane-bound receptor molecule. This leads to subsequent phosphorylations, eventually phosphorylating the inactive form of the transcription factor. This scheme is only provided as an example of the possibilities for the relay of the signal from the receptor to the nucleus of the cell. If activated, the transcription factor triggers the synthesis of mRNA by RNA polymerase, the

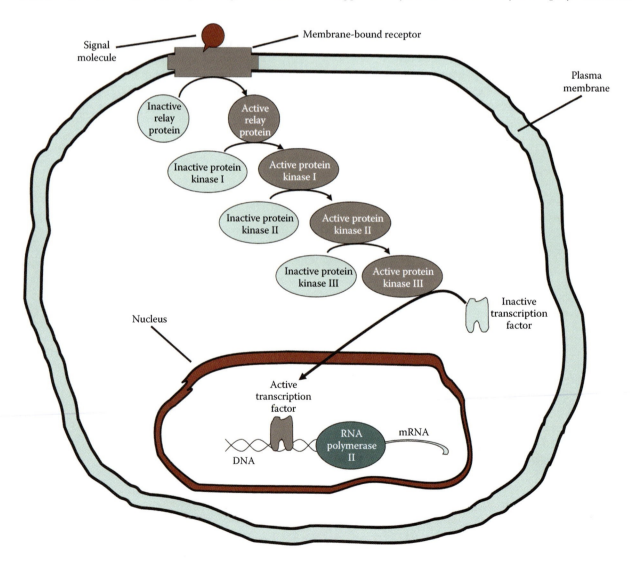

Figure A3.1 Signal transduction pathway leading to transcription.

process known as transcription. In the paragraphs that follow a brief description is provided of some of the most common classes of receptors, signal transduction pathways, and signal molecules in skin.

RECEPTORS

Receptors can either be membrane-bound or nuclear receptors. Table A3.1 includes a list of membrane-bound receptors. Structurally, membrane-bound receptors typically contain three domains, the extracellular, transmembrane, and intracellular domains.[1] Nuclear receptors, on the other hand, typically bind to lipid soluble hormones such as steroid, thyroid, and vitamin D_3 hormones as well as to vitamin A. In this case, the lipid-soluble hormones are able to freely cross the plasma membrane and travel through the cytoplasm until they meet their receptor in the nucleus. There are also membrane-bound receptors that are linked to G proteins. The G protein is inactive when guanosine diphosphate (GDP) is bound to the protein; however, it becomes active after phosphorylation in which the protein contains bound gaunosine triphosphate (GTP). There is also the cytokine family of membrane-bound receptors.

SIGNAL TRANSDUCTION PATHWAYS

As stated earlier, signal transduction is the process by which a conformation change in the receptor results in a subsequent series of molecular events, allowing a signal to reach the nucleus of the cell. Listed in Table A3.2 are three of the most well-known signal transduction pathways. The mitogen activated protein (MAP) kinase cascade, as its name implies, utilizes protein kinases to relay the transduction signal via phosphorylation. There are three subcategories within the MAP kinase cascade: ERK cascade, SAPK/JNK cascade, and the p38 kinase system. A description of the three different pathways is provided in Figure A3.2.[2] ERK and SAPK/JNK represent extracellular-related protein kinases and stress-activated protein kinases, respectively. The ERK cascade is probably the most well-studied in skin and is initiated by binding of the epidermal growth factor (EGF) to the receptor.[3]

Table A3.1 Classes of membrane-bound receptors.

- Receptor tyrosine kinases
- Serine/threonine kinase receptors
- Cytokine receptor family
- G protein-coupled receptors

Table A3.2 Signal transduction pathways.

- MAP kinase cascade
- JAK/STAT pathway
- Adenylate cyclase/cAMP system

The SAPK/JNK cascade can be induced by UV irradiation, heat shock, inflammatory cytokines, and osmotic imbalance, and involves the protein, Jun N-terminal kinase (JNK).[1] The MAP kinase cascade has received considerable attention in the literature as it represents one of the most common signal transduction cascades.

The JAK/STAT pathway involves janus kinases as well as signal transducers and activators of transcription, respectively. In comparison to the MAP kinase cascade, which follows an indirect route, the JAK/STAT pathway is much more direct in its signaling from the cytokine receptor to the nucleus, where the activated transcription factor (which happens to be a STAT protein) can perform its function. Upon activation of the cytokine receptor, inactive STAT proteins come to the receptor where they encounter a protein from the JAK family, which is associated with the receptor. The STAT proteins are then phosphorylated at tyrosine residues by the JAK protein. This results in dimerization of two STAT proteins, thereby producing an active transcription factor, which is able to enter the nucleus.

The last pathway listed in Table A3.2, the adenylate cyclase/cyclic adenosine monophosphate (cAMP) system, involves the membrane-bound enzyme (adenylate cyclase) which is responsible for the conversion of adenosine triphosphate (ATP) to cAMP.[1] As shown in Figure A3.3, the membrane-bound receptor in this system is associated with G protein, which contains three subunits (alpha, beta, and gamma). After ligand binding to the receptor, the alpha-subunit of the G protein becomes active and breaks away from the other two subunits. The alpha-subunit renders the enzyme adenylate cyclase active, thereby allowing conversion of ATP to cAMP. The production of cAMP results in the activation of protein kinase, which serves as the catalyst for a transcription factor. In the example shown in the figure, the cAMP response element binding protein (CREB) transcription factor is then activated followed by subsequent gene expression. It is also noteworthy to add that in addition to the complex signal transduction pathways already described, cellular signaling is also achieved by phospholipids as well as Ca^{2+}.

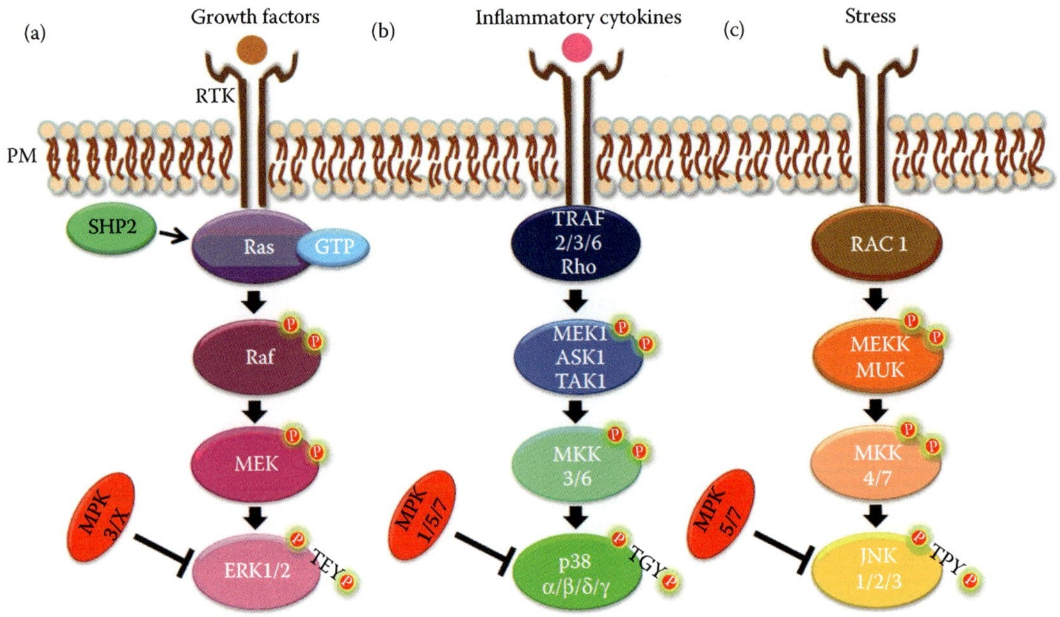

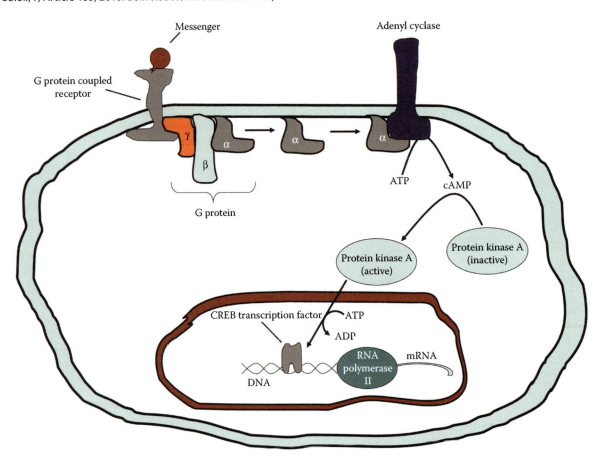

Figure A3.2 MAP kinase pathways in mammalian cells. The function or full name of all of the different kinases is not provided, only their acronyms. They are shown to illustrate the complexity of the different pathways. It is sufficient to define the activity of the kinases, which are enzymes that transfer energy in the form of ATP to specific substrates by phosphorylation reactions. The three MAP kinase pathways shown are ERK cascade, SAPK/JNK cascade, and p38 kinase system. (From Soares-Silva, M. et al., *Front. Microbiol.*, 7, Article 183, 2016. doi:10.3389/fmicb.2016.00183.)

Figure A3.3 Activation of a G protein-coupled receptor by an intracellular messenger leading to the migration of the G protein alpha subunit, which catalyzes the conversion of ATP to cAMP. Protein kinase A is then made active by cAMP, leading to the eventual activation of the CREB transcription factor.

CELL SIGNALING MOLECULES

Another key component of the cellular signaling system is the molecules that serve as the intercellular messengers, which are typically cytokines, growth factors, or hormones (Table A3.3). The most well-known and largest family of molecules to serve as these signaling agents is a structurally and functionally diverse group of proteins called cytokines. As such, this family of proteins serves as the communication between cells of the immune system as well as the immune cells and the cells of other tissues. Typically, the secretion of cytokines results in proliferation or differentiation of specific cells as well as the induction of the secretion of other cytokines. In addition to cytokines, various growth factors and hormones also serve as messengers in the scheme of cellular communication.

The field of cytokine research has evolved over the last few decades, with the first molecules of this group being discovered in the sixties. There have been numerous cytokines that have been identified and structurally characterized. The most well-studied of these are interleukin-1 (IL-1), interleukin-6 (IL-6), and tumor necrosis factor-alpha (TNF-alpha). In relation to skin, these three molecules represent the cytokines with the most diverse set of functions. They are typically secreted by cells in order to mediate and regulate the immune response. For example, TNF-alpha, which is a proinflammatory cytokine, can be secreted by a number of cells including monocytes, macrophages, eosinophils, natural killer cells, B cells, T cells, keratinocytes, fibroblasts, and mast cells.[4] Several examples of the activity of TNF-alpha are included in Table A3.4. Like TNF-alpha, many cytokines are said to be pleiotropic, that is they have many functions, while others behave in a more specific capacity and may only have one or two functions. Furthermore, the keratinocyte serves as a crucial component of the cutaneous immune system. In response to invasion by foreign pathogens, UV

Table A3.3 Activity of TNF-alpha.

Interleukins	**Interferons**
• Interleukin-1alpha (IL-1alpha)	• Interferon-alpha (IFN-alpha)
• Interleukin-1beta (IL-1beta)	• Interferon-beta (IFN-beta)
• Interleukin-2 (IL-2)	• Interferon-gamma (IFN-gamma)
• Interleukin-4 (IL-4)	**Colony-Stimulating Factors (CSF)**
• Interleukin-5 (IL-5)	• Granulocyte-CSF (G-CSF)
• Interleukin-6 (IL-6)	• Macrophage-CSF (M-CSF)
• Interleukin-10 (IL-10)	• Granulocyte/Macrophage-CSF (GM-CSF)
• Interleukin-12 (IL-12)	**Epidermal Growth Factor Family**
• Interleukin-13 (IL-13)	• EGF Amphiregulin (AR)
• Interleukin-15 (IL-15)	• Transforming Growth Factor-alpha (TGF-alpha)
• Interleukin-18 (IL-18)	
Lymphokines	**Platelet-Derived Growth Factor (PDGF) Family**
• Tumor necrosis factor-alpha (TNF-alpha)	• Platelet-derived growth factor (PDGF)
• Tumor necrosis factor-beta (TNF-beta)	• Vascular endothelial growth factor (VEGF)
Fibroblast Growth Factor (FGF) Family	
• Acidic FGF (aFGF)	**Chemokines**
• Basic FGF (bFGF)	**Transforming Growth Factor-Beta Family**
• Keratinocyte Growth Factor (KGF)	**Nerve Growth Factor**

Table A3.4 Activity of TNF-alpha.

- T cell and B cell proliferation
- Enhances expression of MHC class I and MHC class II molecules
- Activation of vascular endothelial cells[a]
- Induction of fever
- Stimulates the secretion of IL-1 and IL-6
- Angiogenesis

Source: Burbach, G. et al., Cytokines in skin, in *The Biology of the Skin*, Freinkel, R. and Woodley, D. (Eds.), Parthenon, New York, 2001.

[a] This results in the expression of intercellular adhesion molecules on the plasma membrane of vascular endothelial cells, such as intercellular adhesion molecules (ICAM-1) and vascular cell adhesion molecules (VCAM-1).

irradiation, trauma, and so on, keratinocytes are able to secrete numerous cytokines, which quickly mobilize cells of the immune system such as leukocytes as well as activate T cells and B cells (see Chapter 4).

TRANSCRIPTION FACTORS

The last component of the cellular signaling system is constituted by the transcription factors, which become activated as a result of the original signal. Typically, transcription factors reside in the cytoplasm as their inactive form and upon activation are able to cross the nuclear membrane where they can bind to the explicit DNA they are associated with. As a result, transcription results in mRNA synthesis and is followed by translation of a particular protein. Relevant transcription factors in skin cells are included in Table A3.5 with a brief description of their activity.

Table A3.5 Transcription factors and their functions.

AP-1	Regulates cell proliferation. Assembled from subunits of Jun, Fos, or ATF.
NF-kappa beta	Involved in inflammatory responses.
p53	Controls the cell cycle by acting as a tumor suppressor.
ATFs	Regulation of cell proliferation and apoptosis. Bind to CREB proteins.
c-Myc	Promoter of cell proliferation.

REFERENCES

1. Petrazzuoli M, Goldsmith L. Molecular mechanisms of cell signaling. In: Freedberg I, Eisen A, Wolff K, Austen K, Goldsmith L, Katz S et al. (Eds.). *Fitzpatrick's Dermatology in General Medicine*, 5th ed. New York: McGraw-Hill; 1999, pp. 114–131.
2. Soares-Silva M et al. *Front Microbiol.* 2016;7. doi:10.3389/fmicb.2016.00183.
3. Rittié L, Fisher G. *Ageing Res Rev.* 2002;1:705–720.
4. Burbach G, Ansel J, Armstrong C. Cytokines in skin. In: Freinkel R, Woodley D (Eds.). *The Biology of the Skin*. New York: Parthenon; 2001.

Appendix 4: Thermodynamic and kinetic factors that contribute to antioxidant behavior

The reactions between antioxidants and free radicals are governed by thermodynamics and kinetics. Thermodynamics allows us to ask if a particular reaction will be feasible, and if so, kinetics determines the speed at which the process occurs. Oftentimes, a reaction may appear to be thermodynamically possible; however, the rate constant of the reaction may be extremely low and the reaction may not even proceed. Using standard electrode reduction potentials, we can predict with some certainty the degree at which an oxidation/reduction should occur. Another thermodynamic parameter, bond dissociation energy, helps us to examine the O–H bond in phenol-based antioxidants and understand what type of structure provides the weakest bond—therefore, the best antioxidant. In addition, we examine how kinetic measurements can help us to identify whether or not a reaction will proceed and how efficacious a particular antioxidant will be toward various reactive oxygen species.

OXIDATION AND REDUCTION

At the most basic level, redox reactions describe a situation in which the oxidation state of atoms in a molecule change as a result of oxidation or reduction. Oxidation refers to the case when an electron (or proton) is lost by a reductant whereas reduction describes the gain of an electron (or proton) by an oxidant. As already touched upon in other chapters, skin and other biological systems are subjected to free radical reactions, which result in a change of oxidation state of a particular molecule. Likewise, such processes may also occur in formulation or in complex carrier systems. By knowing the propensity of a moiety to be an oxidant or reductant, we can better understand how multiple species (i.e., antioxidants and free radicals) interact with each other endogenously, or what types of systems can best be formulated together (e.g., a mixture of antioxidants) to exert a synergistic effect that relies on their redox properties. In the following paragraphs, we discuss the use of a measured thermodynamic quantity, standard electrode potential, to determine how oxidative or reductive a particular species may be.

Standard electrode potentials in voltaic cells

The energy released in an oxidation or reduction process can be measured using a voltaic cell containing an electrode and anode. Oxidation occurs at the anode and reduction occurs at the cathode; that is, anions flow to the anode and cations migrate to the cathode.

In voltaic cells, the overall cell potential (electromotive force) is the sum of the standard oxidation and reduction potentials.

$$E^{\circ}_{cell} = E^{\circ}_{ox} + E^{\circ}_{red} \quad (A4.1)$$

To provide a reference value, the standard reduction potential of the half-reaction involving the reduction of H^+ to H_2 is measured and set to zero ($E^{\circ}_{cell} = 0$ V).

$$2H^+ + 2e^- \rightarrow H_2 \quad (A4.2)$$

An electrode designed to produce this reaction is known as a standard hydrogen electrode. In a common voltaic cell, we can use the standard hydrogen electrode as the anode and a cathode fabricated from Zn. In this system, oxidation of Zn occurs in the anode while reduction of H^+ takes place in the cathode. The ensuing reaction for this process is:

$$Zn + 2H^+ \rightarrow Zn^{2+} + H_2 \quad (A4.3)$$

The cell potential for this reaction is 0.76 V. Utilizing Equation A4.1—with $E^{\circ}_{cell} = 0.76$ V and $E^{\circ}_{red} = 0$—the standard oxidation potential (E°_{ox}) is 0.76. The corresponding half-reaction corresponding to the oxidation process is:

$$Zn \rightarrow Zn^{2+} + 2e^- \quad (A4.4)$$

By convention, half-cell potentials are usually referenced as standard reduction potentials.

$$E^{\circ}_{red} = E^{\circ}_{ox} \quad (A4.5)$$

Therefore, in the case of the zinc cathode, hydrogen anode voltaic cell, $E^{\circ}_{red} = -0.76$ and the corresponding half-reaction is:

$$Zn^{2+} + 2e^- \rightarrow Zn \quad (A4.6)$$

In general, the half-cell potential (E°_{red}) provides us with information related to the tendency for a reaction to proceed. *A negative reduction potential indicates that something is more difficult to reduce, which means that it will be more easily oxidized.* In contrast, a half reaction defined by a positive reduction potential will more easily be reduced and less easily be oxidized. In electrochemistry, half-reactions and standard reduction potentials are known for many inorganic species. These same concepts apply to free radical processes in biological systems.

Standard electrode potentials of free radicals and antioxidants

Most radical reactions follow first- and second-order kinetics, making their outcome rather predictable. In terms of thermodynamics, reduction potential is an important quantity that allows us to predict how easily a molecular species will undergo oxidation or reduction. Instead of using voltaic cells, photolysis and pulse radiolysis measurements provide standard reduction potentials for many organic species. Table A4.1 provides a list of standard one-electron reduction potentials for many relevant species of interest in free radical chemistry. Table A4.1 is arranged from the most oxidizing species (at the top) to the most reducing species (at the bottom). Therefore, one should expect that a more oxidizing species is able to abstract an electron (or a proton) from anything that is below it on the scale. For example, the hydroxyl radical (HO·) is the most reactive radical species and is at the top of the list. In addition, standard reduction potentials help explain how endogenous antioxidants work in synergy. For example, we know that once alpha-tocopherol neutralizes a free radical species, the alpha-tocopheroxyl radical can react with the more reductive ascorbate⁻, thus regenerating alpha-tocopherol. Likewise, highly reductive glutathione disulfide regenerates ascorbate⁻ by neutralizing the ascorbyl radical (ascorbate·⁻). For comparison, epicatechins and theaflavins—polyphenols from tea extracts—provide values between 0.43 and 0.57 V.[1] While the thermodynamic parameters presented in Table A4.1 may explain many phenomena, there are times when kinetics favors a reaction type other than electron transfer. In those cases, standard electrode potential cannot be used as an indicator of oxidation or reduction.

BOND DISSOCIATION ENERGIES OF O–H BONDS IN ANTIOXIDANTS

Bond dissociation energy is the enthalpy required to break a specified bond. In antioxidants we commonly encounter the O–H bond, which is often responsible for the antioxidant activity of the molecule in question. By donating a proton from the hydroxyl group to a free radical, the antioxidant in effect neutralizes the radical, which could otherwise react with other biological molecules and result in damage. The stronger this O–H bond, the less likely the antioxidant will give up the proton to a free radical. The optimum strength of this bond is reached at a threshold that depends on the molecule's structure. In the case of phenolic antioxidants, the nature and arrangement of substituent groups around the aromatic rings ultimately determines the bond dissociation energy of the O–H bond.

Using instrumental techniques, such as photoacoustic calorimetry or electron spin resonance, one may determine the bond dissociation energy of an O–H bond by reacting an antioxidant with an in situ-generated free radical.[2,3] It may also be calculated from kinetic rate constants determined by other experimental means. The strength of an O–H bond—that is, how readily a proton may be donated to a free radical species—helps us to determine the anticipated efficacy of an antioxidant. Figure A4.1 contains a diagram of the bond dissociation enthalpies for a series of substituted phenolic antioxidants. The most basic molecule, phenol, with the lowest degree of substitution on the aromatic ring, has the highest bond dissociation enthalpy (hence the strongest O–H bond), which indicates that it is the least likely (of the molecules shown) to act as an antioxidant. As we increase the complexity of the substituent groups, the O–H bond dissociation energy decreases, indicating that the bond will be more labile and more easily donate a proton to a free radical. The nature of the constituent groups will greatly affect the energy of the O–H bond. They destabilize the O–H bond by funneling electron density into the ring either through induction (e.g., through carbon-carbon sigma bonds) or by resonance (through pi bonds). The more electron density substituent groups are able to donate to the ring, the more destabilized the O–H bond will be. In addition, steric effects also play an important role. A good example is to compare 2,4,6-tri-*tert*-butylphenol (I) with 2,4,6-trimethylphenol (II). The bond dissociation is lower for 2,4,6-tri-*tert*-butylphenol due to

Table A4.1 Standard reduction potential values for selected systems important in biology at pH 7.

Half reaction	Standard reduction potential (V)
HO·, H⁺/H₂O	2.31
RO·, H⁺/ROH (aliphatic alkoxyl radical)	1.60
HOO·, H⁺/H₂O₂	1.06
ROO·, H⁺/ROOH (alkylperoxyl radical)	1.00
O₂·⁻, H⁺/H₂O₂	0.95
O₂ (¹Δg)/O₂·⁻	0.65
PUFA·, H⁺/PUFA-H (polyunsaturated fatty acid, *bis*-allylic-H)	0.60
Alpha-tocopheroxyl·, H⁺/alpha-tocopherol (TO·, H⁺/TOH)	0.50
Ascorbate·⁻, H⁺/ascorbate⁻ (vitamin C)	0.28
Semiubiquinone, H⁺/ubiquinol (CoQ·⁻, 2H⁺/CoQH₂)	0.20
Ubiquinone, H⁺/semiubiquinone (CoQ, H⁺/CoQ·⁻)	−0.36
Dehydroascorbate/ascorbate·⁻	−0.17
O₂/O₂·⁻	−0.33
O₂, H⁺/HO₂·	−0.46
RSSR/RSSR·⁻ (cystine or glutathione disulfide, GSSG)	−1.50

Source: Reprinted from *Arch. Biochem. Biophys.*, 300, Buettner, G.R., The pecking order of free radicals and antioxidants: Lipid peroxidation, alpha-tocopherol, and ascorbate, 535–543, Copyright 1993, with permission from Elsevier.

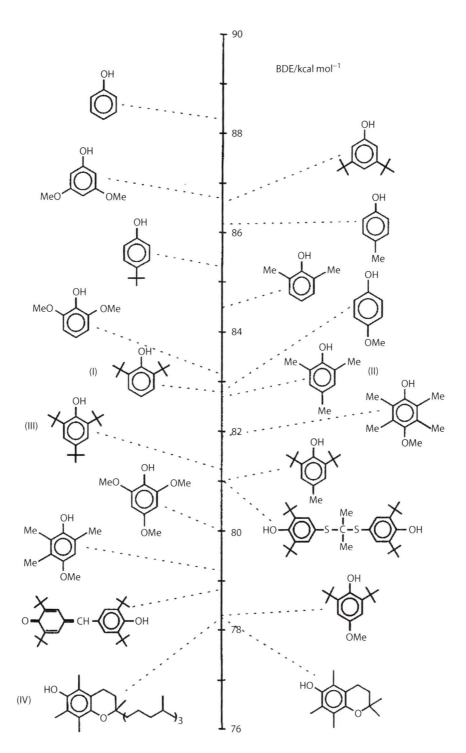

Figure A4.1 Bond dissociation energy values for substituted phenols. (Reprinted with permission from Lucarini, M. et al., *J. Org. Chem.*, 61, 9259–9263, 1999. Copyright 1999 American Chemical Society.)

both induction and steric destabilization. The influence of resonance destabilization is clearly illustrated by comparing 2,4,6-tri-methoxyphenol (III) with either of the two examples just mentioned. In this case, resonance destabilization through pi bonds occurs via the oxygen atom of the methoxy groups. As illustrated in Figure A4.1, there are a number of structure-property relationships that can be resolved to help us understand which types of substituent groups are the most important for providing the best antioxidant. Alpha tocopherol (IV), shown at the bottom left of the chart, has the lowest bond dissociation energy due to the uniqueness of the chromanol ring in combination with the other substituents (methyl groups) on the aromatic ring.

Table A4.2 Bond dissociation energy values for O–H bonds in natural polyphenols.

Antioxidant	D_{O-H} (Kcal/mol)
Alpha-tocopherol	78.82
Tannic acid	80.75
Caffeic acid	81.16
Delta-tocopherol	81.57
Quercetin	81.92
(–)-Epicatechol	81.97
Rutin	82.09
Coenzyme Q	82.47
Nordihydroguaiaretic acid	83.91

Source: Denisova, T. and Denisov, E., *Russ. Chem. Bull. Int. Ed.*, 57, 1858–1866, 2008.

Table A4.3 $^1O_2$ quenching constants ($k_q + k$) of several antioxidants obtained from Stern–Volmer plots.

Antioxidant	$k_q + k_r$ ($10^6\,M^{-1}\,s^{-1}$)
Lycopene	31,000
Gamma-carotene	25,000
Beta-carotene	14,000
Lutein	8000
Bilirubin	3200
Alpha-tocopherol	280
Delta-tocopherol	160
Lipoic acid	130
Glutathione	59

Source: Di Mascio, P. et al., *Biochem. Soc. Trans.*, 18, 1054–1056, 1990.

Over the years, a great deal of work was completed to fully characterize simple substituted phenols like the ones shown in Figure A4.1 and other antioxidants.[4] More recently, efforts have been made to better understand the bond dissociation energies of polyphenols from botanical sources.[5] In an attempt to provide a broad survey of common natural antioxidants, such as coenzyme Q, catechins, vitamin E forms, and various flavonoids, a comprehensive tabulation of bond dissociation enthalpies was constructed from kinetic data (reaction rates for antioxidants and peroxy radicals). Table A4.2 contains a summary of some of these values. Overall, alpha-tocopherol is taken as the standard and provides the lowest bond dissociation energy values for the O–H bond of the hydroxyl group. Even delta-tocopherol, which only differs from alpha-tocopherol by two substituents on the aromatic ring, has a significantly stronger O–H bond, making it a less effective antioxidant. Relative to the other polyphenols, caffeic and tannic acids have bond dissociation enthalpies significantly lower than the other polyphenols shown. This most certainly has to do with a unique feature of their molecular structure. While bond dissociation energies provide a nice guide for the likelihood of an antioxidant to react with a free radical, other factors must also be considered, such as molecular environment and bioavailability.

REACTION RATES AND SCAVENGING ACTIVITY OF ANTIOXIDANTS

The thermodynamic parameters discussed in the preceding sections demonstrate the tendency for free radical reactions to take place with antioxidants. Once that has been established, reaction kinetics will ultimately govern the rate at which reactions will take place. While a reaction may be thermodynamically feasible, if the reaction rate is too slow it may not even occur. Kinetics involving antioxidants may be broken down into two parts. In the first case, we could refer to the rate of the reaction between a free radical (reactive oxygen species) and various in vivo substrates such as lipids, proteins, or DNA. Alternatively, we may be more interested in the rate of the reaction between an antioxidant and reactive oxygen species such as HO·, peroxyl radical species (ROO·), superoxide anion ($O_2^{\cdot-}$), singlet oxygen ($^1O_2$), and hydrogen peroxide (H_2O_2). Many of the assays in Chapter 6 are designed to measure the kinetics between antioxidants and free radical probes. In this section, we will limit our discussion to the interactions between antioxidants and reactive oxygen species.

All antioxidants are not equal. One antioxidant may be more effective at quenching $^1O_2$ while another might be more suited to neutralize HO· or $O_2^{\cdot-}$. As an example, Table A4.3 contains rate constants for the quenching of $^1O_2$ by carotenoids and several other notable antioxidants.[6] As discussed in Chapter 3, carotenoids are known for their ability to quench $^1O_2$, which explains their high $^1O_2$ quenching constants as compared to other small molecule antioxidants, such as alpha-tocopherol, glutathione, and lipoic acid. Equally intriguing is the scavenging activity of antioxidants towards various reactive oxygen species. One way to generate such data is to use spin traps in combination with electron spin resonance.

Table A4.4 summarizes the scavenging activity of a selection of botanical extracts and two key antioxidants towards $O_2^{\cdot-}$ and HO·.[7] In the case of both reactive oxygen species, alpha-tocopherol is by far the greatest free radical scavenger. Ascorbic acid follows suit in the presence of $O_2^{\cdot-}$, but performs rather poorly compared to the botanical extracts in the presence of HO·. Although comparisons were made on a dry material weight basis, it is likely that pure antioxidants will have a much greater advantage over plant extracts, which are a mixture of phytoantioxidants and other biological molecules. Curiously, the plant extracts are more efficacious at quenching $^1O_2$ than ascorbic acid. Such activity might be explained by the complex conjugated structure of polyphenols present in the extracts.

Table A4.4 Scavenging activity of botanical extracts and antioxidants against $O_2^{\cdot-}$, $HO^{\cdot}$, and $^1O_2$. Reported as IC_{50} μg (dry material)/mL.

Plant	$O_2^{\cdot-}$	$HO^{\cdot}$	$^1O_2$
Aesculus hippocastanum L.	0.24 ± 0.01	7.79 ± 0.26	72.98 ± 6.20
Hamamelis virginiana L.	0.17 ± 0.01	7.79 ± 0.49	44.08 ± 3.39
Polygonum cuspidatum SIEB.	2.38 ± 0.25	30.73 ± 0.60	—
Quercus robur L.	1.00 ± 0.07	14.07 ± 0.27	16.13 ± 1.00
Rosemarinus officinalis L.	1.47 ± 0.11	50.64 ± 5.77	—
Salvia officinalis L.	2.14 ± 0.20	30.63 ± 3.91	—
Sanguisorba officinalis L.	0.75 ± 0.03	12.70 ± 0.46	99.79 ± 1.49
L-Ascorbic acid	4.10 ± 0.39	3.30 ± 0.03	21.18 ± 0.39
Alpha-tocopherol	576.20 ± 38.70	253.70 ± 38.70	—

Source: Masaki, H. et al., *Biol. Pharm. Bull.*, 18, 162–166, 1995.

REFERENCES

1. Buettner G. *Arch Biochem Biophys*. 1993;300:535–543.
2. Lucarini M et al. *J Org Chem*. 1996;61:9259–9263.
3. Wayner D *J Org Chem*. 1996;61:6430–6433.
4. Denisov E. *Handbook of Antioxidants: Bond Dissociation Energies, Rate Constants, Activation Energies, and Enthalpies of Reactions*. Boca Raton, FL: CRC Press; 2000.
5. Denisova T, Denisov E. *Russ Chem Bull, Int Ed*. 2008;57:1858–1866.
6. DiMascio P et al. *Biochem Soc Trans*. 1990;18:1054–1056.
7. Masaki H et al. *Biol Pharm Bull*. 1995;18:162–166.

Index

Note: Page numbers followed by f and t refer to figures and tables respectively.

2,2′-Azino-*bis*(3-ethylbenzothiazoline-6-sulfonic acid) (ABTS) assay
  absorbance spectra of, 95f, 96f
  experimental approaches, 94–95
  generating systems for, 94t
  radical cationic form conversion, 94f
  TEAC, 93
2,2-Diphenyl-1-picrylhydrazyl (DPPH) assay, 92f, 92–93, 93f, 94f
2,4,6-Tripyridyl-*s*-triazine (TPTZ), 97, 97f
2,4-Dinitrophenylhydrazine (DNPH), 82, 86
3,4-Dihydroxyphenylalanine (DOPA), 45, 189
4-Hydroxy-2-trans-nonenal (HNE), 73, 82
7-Dehydrocholesterol, 53, 54f
8-Hydroxy-2′-deoxyguanosine (8-OHdG), 56
8-Iso-prostaglandin F2alpha (8-iso-PGF2alpha), 82f

A

Absorption spectra of chromophores, 51f, 52f
Accelerated stability tests
  AOM, 87
  OSI, 87
  Schaal Oven Test, 87
  Weight Gain, 86–87
N-acetyl cysteine, 145–146
Acini, 14, 14f
Acne vulgaris, 67
Action spectrum for UV-induced cancer, 63f
Active Oxygen Method (AOM), 87
Adaptive immune system, 16–17, 17f
Adenosine diphosphate (ADP), 188
Adenosine monophosphate (AMP), 39, 189
Adenosine triphosphate (ATP), 26, 188, 193
Adherens junctions, 5
ADP (adenosine diphosphate), 188
Age spots, 57
Aging skin, histological features of, 57t
Air pollution effects on skin, 63–64
  O_3, 64
  oxides, 64
  PAHs, 65–66
  PM, 64–65
  protection strategies, 66–67
  tobacco smoke, 66
  VOCs, 66
Alkoxyl and peroxyl radicals, 23
ALOGPS, 145
Alpha-lipoic acid, 46, 163–164
Alpha-tocopherol, 112–113, 113t
  regeneration, 41f
Alpha-tocopherylquinone reduction, 36
American Oil Chemists' Society (AOCS), 79, 84
Amide-linked fatty acid, 74
AMP (adenosine monophosphate), 39, 189
Androgens, 14
p-anisidine value (AV) test, 85–86, 85f
Antibody, 181
Antigen, 181
  APCs, 16
  infected cell, 17
  isoprostane, 83
  tracer, 83
Antigen-presenting cells (APCs), 3, 16
Antimicrobial proteins, 16
Antioxidant assays
  ABTS, 93–95, 93f, 93t, 95f, 96f
  deoxyribose, 99–100
  DPPH, 92–93, 93f, 94f
  FRAP, 97–98, 97f
  ORAC, 98, 98f, 99f
  review and benchmarking studies, 101t
  TRAP, 95–97, 96f
Antioxidant properties and application
  N-acetyl cysteine, 145–146
  apigenin, 146–147
  arbutin, 147–148
  L-ascorbic acid, 148–149
  BHA, 150–151
  BHT, 151–152
  caffeic acid, 152–153
  beta-caroten, 153–154
  curcumin, 154–155
  ellagic acid, 155–156
  (-)-epicatechin, 156–157
  (-)-epicatechin gallate, 157
  (-)-epigallocatechin, 157
  (-)-epigallocatechin gallate, 157–158
  equol, 158–159
  ferulic acid, 159–160
  genistein, 160–161
  glutathione, 161–162
  kojic acid, 162–163
  alpha-lipoic acid, 163–164
  lycopene, 164–165
  nordihydroguaiaretic acid, 165–166
  pogostone, 166–167
  propyl gallate, 167–168
  quercetin, 168–169
  resorcinol, 169
  resveratrol, 169–171
  rosmarinic acid, 171–172
  silibinin, 172
  TBHQ, 149–150
  theaflavin, 173–174
  thearubigins, 174. *See also* Theaflavin
  thioglycolic acid, 174–175
  tocopherols, 175–176
  tocotrienols, 176–177
  trolox, 177–178
  ubiquinone-10, 178–179
Antioxidants combinations, 135–137
Antiquated organ, apocrine gland, 10
AOCS (American Oil Chemists' Society), 79, 84
AOM (Active Oxygen Method), 87
Apigenin, 146–147
Apocrine sweat gland, 7, 9–10
Apoeccrine sweat gland, 10
Apoptosis, 58, 62, 181
Arachidonic acid, 73, 82
Arbutin, 147–148
Arctostaphylos uva-ursi, 147
Arginine to citrulline conversion, 191, 191f
$AscH_2$ (L-ascorbic acid). *See* L-ascorbic acid ($AscH_2$)
Ascorbate ($AscH^-$), 38
  regeneration, 41f
Ascorbate free radical ($Asc^{•-}$), 107
L-ascorbic acid ($AscH_2$), 38–39, 114
  antioxidant properties/ application information, 148–149
  with DPPH, 94
  molecular structure, 115f
  reaction kinetics for FRAP experiment, 97f
  stability of, 115
  structure of, 38f
  as terminal reductant, 107
Atom abstraction, 25
ATP (adenosine triphosphate), 26, 188, 193
Atrophy, 181
Axilla, 181

B

Basal cell carcinoma, 61–62
Basal lamina/basement membrane zone. *See* Dermal-epidermal junction
Basolateral membrane, 9
B cells, 16–17
BHA (butylated hydroxyanisole), 150–151
BHT (butylated hydroxytoluene), 84, 151–152
Bilirubin, 44, 50
Black tea, 122, 122f, 173
Blois, M., 93
Blue light effects on skin, 67
Bond dissociation energies of O–H bonds, 198–200, 199f, 200t
Botanical extracts
  Ginkgo biloba, 129–130
  grape seed, 130
  Prunis persica flower, 130
Brown/black pigment eumelanin, 189
Buckminster Fullerenes/ Buckyballs, 131
Bulb, hair, 11
Burke, K., 136
Butylated hydroxyanisole (BHA), 150–151
Butylated hydroxytoluene (BHT), 84, 151–152

C

Cadherins, 5
Caffeic acid, 121, 121f, 152–153
Camellia sinensis (green tea), 122, 156–158
CAMP (cyclic adenosine monophosphate), 193
CAMP response element binding protein (CREB), 193
Canities, 12
Carbonyls with 2,4-dinitrophenyl-hydrazine, 86f
Carcinogenesis in skin, 62f
Carcinomas, 61
L-carnitine, 46
Beta-caroten/carotene, 116–117, 153–154
Carotenoids, 43, 43f, 116
CAS (chemical abstract service), 145
Catalase, 31, 32f
Catechins, 157
Cell
  envelope, 1
  -mediated immune response, 16–17
  membrane complex of cortex, 13
  potential, 197
  signaling molecules, 195–196
Cellular signaling during inflammatory response, 18f
Cellular signaling in skin, 192–193
  molecules, 195–196
  receptors, 193
  signal transduction pathways, 193–194
  transcription factors, 196
Ceramides
  lipids, 74
  molecular structures of, 4f
Chapman cycle, 64
Chemical abstract service (CAS), 145
Chemotaxis, 181
Cholesterol esters, 74
Chromophores in skin
  absorption spectra of, 51f, 52f
  amino acids, 50
  bilirubin, 50
  coenzymes (cofactors), 50
  7-dehydrocholesterol, 53, 54f
  elastin, 51
  enzyme cofactors, 50
  flavins, 50
  lipofuscin granules, 50
  nucleotides, 50
  quinones, 50
  spectrum absorbers, 50
  trans-urocanic acid, 53
CHS (contact hypersensitivity response), 124
Citrullination, 191
Citrus fruits, vitamin C source, 114f, 119, 120f
Coenzyme. *See* Cofactor
Coenzyme Q (coQ), 42–43
  oxidization by NADP:quinone reductase, 36f

in personal care products, 118
radical form, 42f
reduced/oxidized forms, 42f
Cofactor, 181, 188
AscH⁻, 38
ATP, 188
enzyme, 50
FAD, 34, 188
GSH, 39
NAD⁺, 188
oxidized form of, 50
vitamin C, 114
Condensed tannins, 126
Conjugated diene, 78, 79f
Contact hypersensitivity response (CHS), 124
Corneodesmosomes, 5
Cosmetic
essential oils, 107
formulations, lipid peroxidation in, 75–76
fullerenes in, 130–131
lipid ingredients in, 76
oleic acid, 76
Covalent bond, 21
COX (cyclooxygenase), 82
CREB (cAMP response element binding protein), 193
Creosote bush (*Larrea tridentata*), 165
Criegee ozonation of unsaturated molecules, 24, 24f
Cuboidal/columnar-shaped secretory cells, 10
Curcuma longa (turmeric), 124, 124f, 154
Curcumin, 124–125, 125f, 154–155
Curcumoids, 124
Cutaneous appendages, 7
apocrine sweat gland, 7, 9–10
apoeccrine sweat gland, 10
eccrine glands, 7–9
nail unit, 15
pilosebaceous unit, 7, 10–15
Cuticle
eponychium, nail, 15, 15f
layer, 11
morphological components, 13f
Swift description on, 13
Cyclic adenosine monophosphate (cAMP), 193
Cyclooxygenase (COX), 82
Cystine, oxidation/reduction of, 187, 187f
Cytokines, 59, 195
Cytoplasm, 3–4, 10, 181
Cytotoxicity, 181

D
Dark (mucoid) cells, 8
Decolorization assay, 95
Defense systems of oxidative damage, 31f
Dehydroascorbate (DHA), 38
Deoxyribonucleic acid (DNA), 48, 185, 185f, 187
Deoxyribose assay, 99–100
Dermal-epidermal junction, 2, 5–6, 6f
Dermis, 1
cell types, 7t
collagen types, 7
connective tissue proteins, 6
elastic fibers, 7
fibrillar bundles, 6
glycoproteins, 7
glycosaminoglycans, 7
ground substance, 7
papillary, 6, 7f

primary cell types, 6
residence for vascular network, 6
reticular, 6, 7f
Desmosomes, 5
Detoxication enzymes, 30
DHA (dehydroascorbate), 38
Dietary intake effects on skin, 131–134
Differentiation process, hair, 10
Dimeric form enzyme, 30
Dipalmitoylphosphatidylcholine (DPPC), 83
Dismutation, 181
DNPH (2,4-dinitrophenyl-hydrazine), 82, 86
Domain mosaic model, stratum corneum lipids, 4–5
DOPA (3,4-dihydroxyphenylalanine), 45, 189
Dorsal, 181
DPPC (dipalmitoylphosphatidylcholine), 83
DT-diaphorase, 34

E
Eccrine sweat glands
basolateral membrane, 9
component structure, 9f
duct of, 9
intradermal duct, 8
intraepidermal duct, 8
ion recuperation, 9
Na⁺/K⁺-ATPase function, 9
secretory coil, 8
transmembrane proteins, 8
ultrafiltrate of plasma, 7
ECM. *See* Extracellular matrix (ECM)
EC (European commission) number, 145
EDTA (ethylenediaminetetraacetic acid), 76
EGF (epidermal growth factor), 193
EIA (enzyme immunoassay), 83
Elastic fibers, 7
Elastotic material, 58
Electrode potentials
free radicals/antioxidants, 198
in voltaic cells, 197
Electromagnetic spectrum, 48, 49f
Electron paramagnetic resonance (EPR), 103
Electron spin resonance (ESR), 92, 103
for exogenous antioxidant efficacy measure, 107–109
free radicals detection by, 107
imaging, 109–110
spectra of DPPH, 93f
spectrometer, 106f
spectrum characteristics, 105–106
theory, 103f, 103–106
Electron transfer, 26
Electron transport chain, 22
coQ functioning, 117–118
and H₂O₂, 23
mitochondrial, 27, 27f
Electrostatic interactions, 77
Ellagic acid, 155–156
Emblica antioxidant, 127
Emulsifiers, 76
Endogenous, 181
Endogenous antioxidant network
alpha-lipoic acid, 46
enzymatic, 30–38
ferritin, 46
L-carnitine, 46

levels and distribution in skin, 46
melanins, 44–46
metallothioneins, 46
small-molecule antioxidants, 38–44
Endogenous enzymatic antioxidants, 30
catalase, 31, 32f
GSH peroxidase, 32, 32f, 33f
NAD(P)H:quinone reductase, 32–34, 35f
SODs, 30–31, 31f, 31t
Trx system, 35–38, 37f
Endogenous sources of free radical, 26–27
endoplasmic reticulum, 28
enzymatic sources, 28
heme proteins, 28
mitochondrial electron transport chain, 27
peroxisomes, 27–28
phagocytic cells, 27
transition metals, 28
Endoplasmic reticulum, 28, 181
Enzymatic sources, 28
Enzyme, 181
Enzyme cofactors and coenzymes, 188–189
Enzyme immunoassay (EIA), 83
(−)-epicatechin, 156–157
(−)-epicatechin gallate, 157
Epidermal-dermal junction in skin, 6f
Epidermal growth factor (EGF), 193
Epidermis, 1–5, 2f
keratinocyte adhesion/cell junctions, 5
stratum basale, 2–3
stratum corneum, 1, 4–5
stratum granulosum, 3–4
stratum spinosum, 3
(−)-epigallocatechin, 157
Epigallocatechin-3-gallate, 122
(−)-epigallocatechin gallate, 157–158
Epithelial tissue, 15
EPR (electron paramagnetic resonance), 103
Epsilon-(gamma-glutamyl) lysine isopeptide cross-links, 4
Equol, 158–159
ERK (extracellular signal related kinase) cascade, 58, 193
Erythema, 56–57
ESR. *See* Electron spin resonance (ESR)
Essential fatty acids, 73
Esterbauer, H., 82
Esterification, 113
Estrogens, 14
Ethylenediaminetetraacetic acid (EDTA), 76
Eumelanin, 45–46, 45f
synthesis, 190f
European commission (EC) number, 145
Exogenous, 181
Extracellular matrix (ECM), 51
MMPs in, 58t
pyridinium compounds in, 52
UV damage symptoms, 57
Extracellular signal related kinase (ERK) cascade, 58, 193
Extrinsic skin aging, 57, 64

F
FAD (flavin adenine dinucleotide), 22, 34, 50, 188

Fats/oils oxidation tests
AV test, 85f, 85–86
2,4-dinitrophenylhydrazine, 86
Kreis test, 85
PV determination by iodometric titration, 84–85
TOTOX value, 86
Fenton reaction, 22
Ferric reducing ability of plasma (FRAP) assay, 97f, 97–98
Ferritin, 46
Ferrous oxidation in xylenol orange (FOX) assay, 77, 80–81
Ferulic acid, 121, 121f, 159–160
Fever, 16
Fibroblasts, 6
Filaggrin, 189
Filaggrin/filament aggregating protein, 3
Fisher, M., 59
Flavanols, 122
Flavin adenine dinucleotide (FAD), 22, 34, 50, 188
Flavin mononucleotide (FMN), 50
Fluorescein reaction, 99f
Follicle, hair, 10–12
FOX (ferrous oxidation in xylenol orange) assay, 77, 80–81
FRAP (ferric reducing ability of plasma) assay, 97f, 97–98
Free electron
magnetic field effects on, 103f
magnetic moment of, 104
Free radical, 21
atom abstraction, 25
in biology, 21–28
cellular sources of, 26f
detection by ESR, 107
electron transfer, 26
endogenous sources of, 26–28
radical addition, 26
reactions, 25–26
sink, 46
terminology, 21
trapping by beta-carotene, 44f
French Paradox, 127, 170
Fullerenes in cosmetics, 130–131
Fullerenols, 131

G
Gallic acid, 121, 121f
Gap junctions, 5
Gas chromatography–mass spectrometry (GC-MS), 82
Gaunosine triphosphate (GTP), 193
GDP (guanosine diphosphate), 193
Genistein, 160–161
Genotoxic, 181
Ginkgo biloba extract, 129–130
Glutathione (GSH), 161–162
alpha-tocopherol/ascorbate regeneration by, 41f
peroxidase, 32, 32f, 33f
selenium-dependent, 34t
water-soluble antioxidants, 39–41
Glycine max (soy beans), 160
Glycoproteins, dermis, 7
Glycosaminoglycans, 7
GMP (guanosine monophosphate), 39
Golgi apparatus, 181
Gout, 39

Grape seeds (*Vitis vinifera*), 130
Green tea (*Camellia sinensis*), 122, 156–158
Ground substance, dermis, 7
GSH. See Glutathione (GSH)
GTP (gaunosine triphosphate), 193
Guanosine diphosphate (GDP), 193
Guanosine monophosphate (GMP), 39

H
Haber–Weiss reactions, 22, 26, 72, 76
Hair
  alpha-keratin, 12
  bulb, 11
  dead tissue, 10
  follicle, 10–12, 11f
  graying/whitening, 12
  lanugo, 10
  shaft, 12–14, 12f
  terminal, 10
  vellus, 10
Half-cell potential, 197
Hardening process, hair, 10
Hard keratins, nail, 15
Heme group, 31
Heme proteins, 28
Heme to bilirubin degradation, 45f
Henle layer, 11
Henry's law constant, 145
High-performance liquid chromatography (HPLC), 78, 80
Histidine derivatives, chemical structures of, 53f
HNE (4-hydroxy-2-transnonenal), 73
HOCl (hypochlorous acid), 23, 39
Homeostasis, 181
Homolytic scission reaction, 22
Hormones and neurotransmitters, 191
Humoral immune response, 16
Huxley layer, 11
Hydrogen peroxide (H_2O_2), 23
Hydrolyzable tannins, 126
Hydroxyl radical (HO·), 22, 55
Hypercarotenodermia, 116
Hypochlorous acid (HOCl), 23, 39
Hypodermis, 1

I
IARC (International Agency for Research on Cancer), 132
Immediate pigment darkening, 57
Immune suppression, UV-induced, 48
Induction Period, 87
Inflammatory response, 16
Infrared light effects on skin, 63
Inhibition assay, 95
Innate immune system, 15–16, 17f
Inner root sheath, 11
Integrins, 3
International Agency for Research on Cancer (IARC), 132
International Union of Pure and Applied Chemistry (IUPAC), 87
Intraperitoneal, 181
Intrinsic skin aging, 57
In vitro lipid peroxidation assays
  accelerated stability tests, 86–87
  fats/oils oxidation tests, 84–86
In vitro test, DPPH assay, 92
In vivo, lipid peroxidation, 72–74
Involucrin, 3–4
Iodometric titration technique, 84–85
Iron in lipid peroxidation, 72, 76
Isoflavones, 122–123
Isoprostane antigen, 83
Isozyme, 182
IUPAC (International Union of Pure and Applied Chemistry), 87

J
JAK/STAT pathway, 193
Japanese knotweed (*Polygonum cuspidatum*), 127
Jun N-terminal kinase (JNK), 58, 193

K
Keratin intermediate filaments (KIFs), 1, 15
Keratinization, 10
Keratinocyte
  adhesion/cell junctions, 5
  cells, 1–2
Keratohyalin granules, 3, 182, 189
KIFs (keratin intermediate filaments), 1, 15
Klystron tubes, 106
Kojic acid, 162–163
Kreis, H., 85
Kreis test, 85
Kripke, M., 59

L
L-3,4-dihydroxyphenylalanine (L-DOPA), 191
Lag time measurement assay, 95
Lamellar bodies, 74, 182
Lamellar granules, 3–4
Lamina lucida, 5
Laminins, 5–6
Landé factor, 104
Langerhans cells, 3
Lanugo hair, 10
Larrea tridentata (creosote bush), 165
Lateral nail fold, 15
LC-MS (liquid chromatography–mass spectrometry), 83
Lentigines, 57
Light effects on skin, UV photosensitization reactions from UVA radiation, 54–55
  UVA-induced DNA damage, 55–56
  UVB-induced DNA damage, 54
Light interaction with skin, 48–49, 48f
Linoleic acid, 73, 76
Lipid, 71
  Bo Forslind on, 4–5
  hydroperoxide formation, 79
  oxidation/antioxidants, 76–77
  peroxidation in vivo, 72–74
  phases, 5
Lipid hydroperoxide (ROOH), 23
Lipid peroxidation, 60
  in cosmetic formulations, 75–76
  iron, 72
  measurement techniques, 77–84
  mechanism of, 71–72
  products formed during, 78f
  with reference to skin, 74–75
  in vitro. See In vitro lipid peroxidation assays
  in vivo, 72–74
Lipid peroxidation measurement techniques, 77–78
  cytotoxic aldehydes—HNE measurement, 82
  diene conjugation, 78
  F_2-isoprostanes quantification, 82–83
  FOX assay, 80–81
  model lipid systems, 83
  TBARS assay, 78–80
  in vivo/ex vivo/in vitro samples analysis, 83–84
Lipid peroxyl radical ($L_1OO·$), 71
Lipid-soluble antioxidants, 30, 38
Lipofuscin granules, 50
Liquid chromatography–mass spectrometry (LC-MS), 83
Liver spots, 50
Lorentzian curve, 103, 103f
Loricrin, 3
Lumen, 8
Lunula, 15
Lycopene, 164–165
Lymphocytes, 3, 16
Lysosome, 182

M
Macrofibrils, 13
Macrophages, 18
Malignant melanoma, 61–62
Malondialdehyde (MDA)/malonaldehyde, 73, 78
  formation by DR degradation products, 99–100
  formation from PUFAs, 80f
  quercetin and, 126
Mammary areola, 182
MAP (mitogen activated protein), 193
MAP kinase pathways, 193, 194f
MAPKs (mitogen-activated protein kinases), 58, 123
Matrix metalloproteinases (MMPs), 58, 58t, 113
Matrix, nail unit, 15
Mature sebaceous cells, 14
MDA. See Malondialdehyde (MDA)/malonaldehyde
MED (minimal erythemal dose), 117, 137, 182
Melanin, 189
Melanocytes, 3, 11, 44
Melanogenesis process, 12, 182
Melanosomes, 3, 45
Melatonin, 44, 45f
Membrane-bound receptors, 193, 193t
Membrane lipid peroxidation, 72f
Merkel cell/disc, 3
Mesenchymal, hair follicle illustration, 11f
Metallothioneins, 46
Methods in Enzymology series (book), 100
Microencapsulation, 135
Microfibril, 13
Microvilli, 10
Milk thistle plant (*Silybum marianum*), 123, 172
Minimal erythemal dose (MED), 117, 137, 182
Mitochondrial electron transport chain, 27
Mitochondrion, 27, 182
Mitogen activated protein (MAP), 193
Mitogen-activated protein kinases (MAPKs), 58, 123
MM (molecular mass), 30
MMPs (matrix metalloproteinases), 58, 58t
Model lipid systems, 78, 83, 84t
Molecular mass (MM), 30
Molecular structures
  ascorbic acid derivatives, 115f
  ATP, 189f
  C_{60} fullerene, 130f
  catecholamines, 191f
  ceramides, 4f
  coQ, 118f
  epigallocatechin-3-gallate, 122f
  flavonoid class, 121f
  genistein, 123f
  hesperidin, 120f
  hydroxydecyl ubiquinone, 118f
  8-iso-PGF2alpha, 82f
  NMF in stratum corneum, 190f
  phenolic acids, 121f
  polycyclic aromatic hydrocarbons, 66f
  redox couple, 119f
  resveratrol, 128f
  retinoids, 116, 116f
  rutin, 125f
  L-selenocysteine, 117f
  silibinin, 123f
  tannic acid, 126f
  tea polyphenol, 122f
  thiol-containing compounds, 119f
  tocopheryl acetate/phosphate, 113f
  tocoquinone, 118f
Montagna, W., 10

N
NADH (nicotinamide adenine dinucleotide), 26, 34, 50
NADPH (nicotinamide adenine dinucleotide phosphate), 22, 31, 50
NAD(P)H:quinone reductase, 32–34, 35f
Nail unit, 15, 15f
Natural killer cells, 16
Natural moisturizing factor (NMF), 189
Necrosis, 182
Negative reduction potential, 197
Nicotinamide adenine dinucleotide (NADH), 26, 34, 50
Nicotinamide adenine dinucleotide phosphate (NADPH), 22, 31, 50
Nitric oxide (NO·), 24
NMF (natural moisturizing factor), 189
NMR (nuclear magnetic resonance), 103
Nordihydroguaiaretic acid, 165–166
Nuclear magnetic resonance (NMR), 103
Nuclear receptors, 193
Nucleic acids, 185
Nucleotides, 50
Nucleus, 182

O

Oil-in-water (o/w) emulsion, 76–77
Oil Stability Index (OSI), 87
Oleic acid, 76
ORAC (oxygen radical absorbance capacity) assay, 98, 98f, 99f, 139
OSI (Oil Stability Index), 87
Outer root sheath, hair follicle, 11
O/w (oil-in-water) emulsion, 76–77
Oxidation, 21, 182, 197
Oxidation/reduction of cystine, 187, 187f
Oxidative phosphorylation, 178
Oxides, air pollution effects on skin, 64
Oxidized coenzyme Q reduction, 36
Oxygen radical absorbance capacity (ORAC) assay, 98, 98f, 99f, 139
Ozone (O$_3$), 24, 48, 64

P

P53 gene, 63–64
PAF (platelet activating factor), 60
PAHs (polycyclic aromatic hydrocarbons), 65–66, 66f
Pannexins, 5
Papillary dermis, 6, 7f
Particulate matter (PM), 48, 64–65
Patched gene, 63
Perineal region, 10, 182
Peritoneum, 182
Peroxide value (PV), 84–85
Peroxisomes, 27–28, 182
Peroxyl and alkoxyl radicals, 23
Persistent pigment darkening, 57
Phagocytes, 16, 16t, 27
Phagocytosis, 182
Phenolic acids, 121–122
Pheomelanin, 45, 45f
  synthesis, 190f
Phosphatidylinositol 3-kinase/AKT, 58
Phospholipids, 74
Photoaging of skin, 48, 57–58
Photocarcinogenesis, 61–63
Photodamaged skin
  biochemical alterations in, 57–58
  clinical/histological characteristics of, 57
Photoimmunology, 59
Photoimmunosuppression, 48, 59–61
Photosensitization
  of chromophore, 56f
  reactions from UVA radiation, 54–55
Photosensitizer, 23, 67, 182
Phyllanthus emblica, 127
Phytochemicals, 120
Pilosebaceous unit, 7, 10–15
  sebaceous gland, 14–15
  with sudoriferous glands, 8f
Ping-pong mechanism, 182
Plakins, 5
Platelet activating factor (PAF), 60
PM (particulate matter), 48, 64–65
Pogostemon cablin, 166
Pogostone, 166–167
Polar paradox, 76
Polycyclic aromatic hydrocarbons (PAHs), 65–66, 66f
Polygonum cuspidatum (Japanese knotweed), 127

Polyphenols, 120
  curcumin, 124–125, 125f
  description of, 120–121
  phenolic acids, 121–122
  quercetin, 125–126
  resveratrol, 127–128
  silymarin, 123–124
  soy isoflavones, 122–123
  tannins, 126–127
  tea polyphenols, 122
Polyunsaturated fatty acids (PUFAs), 71, 73f
Porphyridium cruentum, 98
Postmitotic cells, 2
Potential skin care evaluation, 100
Preventive antioxidants, 30
Primary dermis cell types, 6
Primary terminal fibers, 10
Principal dermal cell types, 7t
Profilaggrin, 3, 189
Propagation/chain reaction, 71
Propionibacterium acnes, 14, 67
Propyl gallate, 167–168
Proteoglycan structure, 8f
Proximal nail fold, 15
Prunis persica flower extract, 130
PUFAs (polyunsaturated fatty acids), 71, 73f
Purine nucleotide metabolism, 40f
Purpura, 57
Pyridine nucleotide oxidoreductases, 35
Pyridinium compounds in ECM, 52f

Q

Quercetin, 125–126, 168–169
Quinones, 32, 32f

R

Radical, 21
  addition, 26
Ras gene, 62
Reaction rates of antioxidants, 200, 201t
Reactive nitrogen species (RNS), 21, 21t, 24–25, 25f
Reactive oxygen species (ROS), 21, 21t, 30, 48
  $^1O_2$, 22–23
  generation by PM, 65f
  H_2O_2, 23
  HO•, 22
  HOCl, 23
  $O_2^{•-}$, 22
  O_3, 24
  RO•/RO$_2$•/HO$_2$•, 23
Receptors, 193
Redox interconversion
  FAD and FADH$_2$, 189
  NAD$^+$ and NADH, 188f
Redox reactions, 197
Reduction, 21, 182, 197
Reflection, 48
Replication, 182
Resorcinol, 169
Resveratrol, 127–128, 169–171
Reticular dermis, 6, 7f
Retinoids, 116, 116f
Retinyl derivatives on skin, 116
Riboflavin, 50
Ribonucleic acid (RNA), 185, 185f
Ribosome, 182
Rickets, 53
RNA (ribonucleic acid), 185, 185f
RNS (reactive nitrogen species), 21, 21t, 24–25, 25f
ROS. See Reactive oxygen species (ROS)
Rosmarinic acid, 171–172

S

Saccharide-containing antioxidants, 119f, 119–120
Sandwich model, stratum corneum lipids, 5
SAP (Skin Antioxidative Protection), 139
SAPK/JNK cascade, 193
Saturated ceramides, 76
Scavenging activity of antioxidants, 200, 201t
Schaal Oven Test, 87
Scurvy, 114
SDS (sodium dodecyl sulfate), 107
Sebaceous gland, 14f
  anatomical distribution, 14
  context of antioxidants, 14–15
  morphological structure, 14
  in terminal/vellus hair, 14
Sebum, 14
Secondary terminal fibers, 10
Secretory cells in apocrine glands, 10
Secretory coil, eccrine glands, 8
Secretory segment, apocrine gland, 10
Selenium, 32, 117
L-selenomethionine, 117
Semidehydroascorbate, 38
Senescence, 182
Sensation, 1
Shaft, hair, 12–14
Signaling cascades, UV-induced, 58–59
Signal transduction pathway, 192f, 192–194, 193t
Silibinin, 172
Silybum marianum (milk thistle plant), 123, 172
Silymarin, 122–124
Simplified molecular-input line-entry system (SMILES) formula, 145
Singlet oxygen ($^1O_2$), 22–23
Sink, free radical, 46
Skin
  air pollution and, 63–67
  blue light and, 67
  cancer, 62–63
  damage, UV-induced, 56–58
  dietary intake and, 131–134
  structure, 1f
  UV light and, 54–56
Skin Antioxidative Protection (SAP), 139
Skin immune system, 15
  adaptive immune system, 16–17
  important features, 17–18
  innate immune system, 15–16
  physical barrier to invaders, 15
Skin treatment with antioxidants
  botanical extracts, 129–130
  combinations, 135–137
  dietary intake effect, 131–134
  formulation challenges, 134–135
  fullerenes in cosmetics, 130–131
  polyphenols, 120–128
  rating systems, 137–139
  saccharide-containing, 119–120
  selenium, 117
  in sunscreen formulations, 137–139, 138t
  thiol-based, 118–119

topical application, 134
ubiquinone derivatives, 117–118
vitamin A, 116–117
vitamin C, 114–115
vitamin E, 112–114
Small-molecule antioxidants, 38–44
  AscH$_2$, 38–39, 39f
  bilirubin, 44
  carotenoids, 43f
  coenzyme Q, 42–43
  GSH, 39–41
  melatonin, 44
  uric acid, 39, 39f
  vitamin E, 41–42
SMILES (simplified molecular-input line-entry system) formula, 145
Sodium dodecyl sulfate (SDS), 107
SODs (superoxide dismutases), 30–31, 31f, 31t
Soft keratins, nail, 15
Solar radiation penetration into skin, 48–49, 49f
Soy beans (Glycine max), 160
Soy isoflavones, 122–123
Spin trapping, 106, 107f
Squalene photooxidation, 74–75
Squamous cell carcinoma, 61–62
Standard hydrogen electrode, 197
STAT proteins, 193
Stereoisomers of alpha-tocopherol, 41
Sterol esters, 74
Strata of epidermis, 2
Stratum basale, 2–3
Stratum corneum, 1
  bricks and mortar structure, 4, 4f
  ceramides, 74
  conversion to cis-urocanic acid, 60, 60f
  domain mosaic model, 4–5
  lipid conformation, 107
  lipid hydroperoxides in, 139
  lipids components, 74
  natural moisturizing factor in, 189
  NMF molecular structures in, 190f
  sandwich model, 5
  trans-urocanic acid in, 53, 59
Stratum germinativum, 2–3
Stratum granulosum, 3–4
Stratum lucidum, 2
Stratum spinosum, 3
Subcutaneous layer, 1
Sudoriferous glands, 7
Sunflower seeds, vitamin E source, 112f
Sunscreen formulations, antioxidants in, 137–139, 138t
Superoxide anion ($O_2^{•-}$), 22
Superoxide dismutases (SODs), 30–31, 31f, 31t
Support structure, nail, 15
Sweat gland
  apocrine, 7, 9–10
  apoeccrine, 10
  eccrine. See Eccrine sweat glands
Sweating, 1
Swift, JA, 13

T

Tannins, 126–127
Tautomerism, 182

TBARS assay. *See* Thiobarbituric acid reactive substances (TBARS) assay
TBHQ (*tert*-butylhydroquinone), 149–150
T cells, 16–17
TEAC (Trolox equivalent antioxidant assay), 93–94
Tea polyphenols, 122
Telangiectasia, 57, 182
Terminal hair, 10
Tert-butylhydroquinone (TBHQ), 149–150
Testosterone, 14
Tetrameric form enzyme, 30
TEWL (transepidermal water loss), 1, 76
TGF-beta (transforming growth factor-beta), 58
Theaflavin, 173–174
Thearubigins, 174. *See also* Theaflavin
Thermodynamics, 197
Thin-layer chromatography (TLC), 82
Thiobarbituric acid reactive substances (TBARS) assay, 77
  caveats of, 79
  in detection of MDA, 78–79
  MDA-TBARS complex, 81f
  methods to improve, 88
  in skin utilizing various substrates, 81t
Thioglycolic acid, 174–175
Thiol-based antioxidants, 118–119
Thioredoxin (Trx) system, 35–38, 37f
Thiyl radicals (RS·), 25

Tight junctions, 5
TLC (thin-layer chromatography), 82
TNF-alpha (tumor necrosis factor-alpha), 15, 195, 195t
Tobacco smoke, air pollution effects on skin, 66
Tocopherols, 175–176
Tocotrienols, 176–177
Tonofilaments, 3
Topical application of antioxidants, 134
TOTal OXidation value (TOTOX) value, 86
Total (peroxyl) radical trapping parameter (TRAP) assay, 95–97, 96f
TOTOX (TOTal OXidation value) value, 86
TPTZ (2,4,6-tripyridyl-*s*-triazine), 97, 97f
Tracer antigen, 83
Transcription
  factor, 182, 187, 192, 196, 196t
  process, 54, 185–186
Transepidermal water loss (TEWL), 1, 76
Transforming growth factor-beta (TGF-beta), 58
Transglutaminases, 4
Transient amplifying cells, 2
Transition metals, 28
Translation process, 183, 185–186
Trans-urocanic acid chemical structure, 53, 53f
TRAP (total (peroxyl) radical trapping parameter) assay, 95–97, 96f
T regulatory cells, 61
Triplet sensitizer (^{3}S·), 54–55

Trolox, 177–178
Trolox equivalent antioxidant assay (TEAC), 93–94
Trx (thioredoxin) system, 35–38, 37f
TSGs (tumor suppressor genes), 62f
Tumor development in tissues, 61f
Tumor necrosis factor-alpha (TNF-alpha), 15, 195, 195t
Tumor suppressor genes (TSGs), 62f
Turmeric (*Curcuma longa*), 124, 124f
Two-step reaction, catalase, 31

U
Ubiquinol, 42
Ubiquinone-10, 178–179
Ubiquinone derivatives, 117–118
Ultraviolet (UV), 21, 48
  cancer in hairless mouse, 63
  epidermal free radicals, 73f
  immune suppression, 48
  immunosuppression, 60f
  signaling cascades, 58–59, 59t
  skin damage, 56–58
Undifferentiated sebaceous cells, 14
Universal antioxidant, alpha-lipoic acid, 118, 163
Unsaturated molecules, Criegee ozonation of, 24f
Urate, 39
Uric acid, 39, 39f
UVA-induced DNA damage, 55–56
UVB-induced DNA damage, 54, 55f

V
Vasoconstriction, 1
Vasodilation, 1, 16
Vellus hair, 10
Visible light effects on skin, 63
Vitamin A, 116–117
Vitamin C, 38, 114–115. *See also* L-ascorbic acid (AscH$_2$)
Vitamin E, 41–42
  alpha-tocopherol, 112–113
  esterification, 113
  example studies, 114t
  in mammalian tissues, 113
  MMP expression, 113
  pro-oxidant, 114
  sunflower seeds, 112f
  tocopherol derivatives, 113t
  topical treatment problems, 113
Vitis vinifera (grape seeds), 130
Volatile organic compounds (VOCs), 66
von Allwörden, K., 13

W
Water-in-oil (w/o) emulsion, 76
Wax esters, 74
Weak photon emission, 118
Weight Gain Test, 86–87
W/o (water-in-oil) emulsion, 76
Wolff, S.P., 80

X
Xenobiotics, 34

Y
Yellow/red pigment pheomelanin, 189